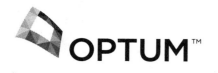 OPTUM™

MW00758185

SAVE UP TO 25%

when you renew your coding essentials.

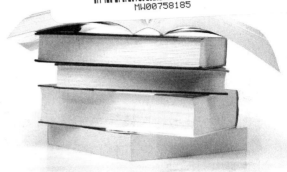

>> Buy 1–2 items, save 15%
Buy 3–5 items, save 20%
Buy 6+ items, save 25%

ITEM #	TITLE INDICATE THE ITEMS YOU WISH TO PURCHASE	QUANTITY	PRICE PER PRODUCT	TOTAL
		Subtotal		
	(AK, DE, HI, MT, NH & OR are exempt)	Sales Tax		
	1 item $10.95 • 2–4 items $12.95 • 5+ CALL	Shipping & Handling		
		TOTAL AMOUNT ENCLOSED		

Save up to 25% when you renew.

 Visit **www.optumcoding.com** and enter your promo code.

 Call **1.800.464.3649, option 1,** and mention the promo code.

 Fax this order form with purchase order to **801.982.4033.** *Optum no longer accepts credit cards by fax.*

PROMO CODE
FOBA13C

Mail this order form with payment and/or purchase order to:
OptumInsight, PO Box 88050, Chicago, IL 60680-9920.

Name _____

Address _____

_____

Customer Number _____ Contact Number _____

○ CHECK ENCLOSED (PAYABLE TO OPTUMINSIGHT)

CHARGE MY: ○ MCard ○ Visa ○ AMEX ○ Discover

Card Number _____ Exp. mm / yr _____

Signature _____

○ BILL ME ○ P.O.# _____

( ) _____
Telephone
( ) _____
Fax
_____ @ _____
E-mail

Optum respects your right to privacy. We will not sell or rent your email address or fax number to anyone outside Optum and its business partners. If you would like to remove your name from Optum promotions, please call 1.800.464.3649, option 1.

INGENIX®

Ingenix is now Optum
—a leading health services business.

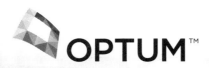
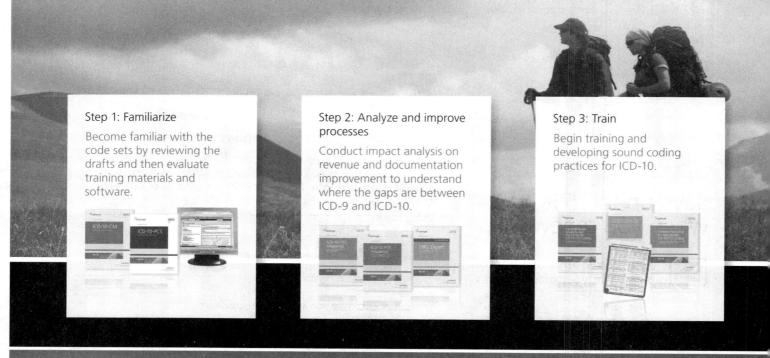
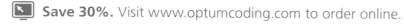

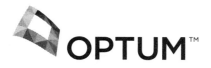
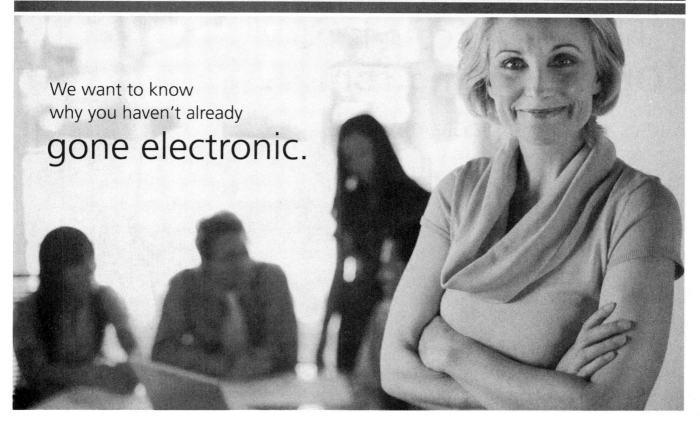

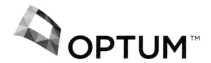

ShopIngenix.com is now
OptumCoding.com

NEW ADDRESS. SAME GREAT WEBSITE.

- Find the products you need quickly and easily with our powerful search engine

- View all available formats and edition years on the same page with consolidated product pages

- Browse our eCatalog online

- Chat live with a customer service representative; ask questions about the site or the checkout process

- Visit Coding Central for expert resources including articles, *Inside Track to ICD-10,* and coding scenarios to test your knowledge

Register on OptumCoding.com for a customized website experience:

- **View special website promotions/ discounts**

- **Get product recommendations based on your order history**

- **Research your order history**

- **Check on shipment status and tracking**

- **View invoices and payment history**

- **Pay outstanding invoices online**

- **Manage your address book**

- **Ship orders to multiple locations**

- **Renew your order with a single click**

- **Compile a wish list of the products you want and purchase when you're ready**

- **Receive a $50 coupon for every $500 you spend on OptumCoding.com (for customers who are not a part of our Medallion or Reseller programs). When logged in, the eRewards meter keeps track of purchases toward your next reward**

Don't have an OptumCoding.com account yet?

It's easy to create one:

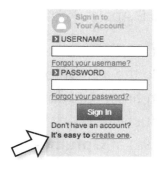

>> **REGISTER TO SAVE 15% ON YOUR NEXT ONLINE ORDER.**

Call toll-free 1.800.464.3649, option 1

FOBA13D

INGENIX.

Ingenix is now Optum
—a leading health services business.

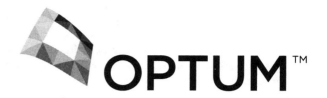

Optum Learning: Detailed Instruction for Appropriate ICD-10-CM Coding

An educational guide to the structure, conventions, and guidelines of ICD-10-CM coding

2013

Optum Notice

Our Commitment to Accuracy

Optum is committed to producing accurate and reliable materials.

To report corrections, please visit www.optumcoding.com/accuracy or email accuracy@optum.com. You can also reach customer service by calling 1.800.464.3649, option 1.

Copyright

Acknowledgments

Julie Orton Van, CPC, CPC-P, *Product Manager*
Karen Schmidt, BSN, *Technical Director*
Stacy Perry, *Manager, Desktop Publishing*
Lisa Singley, *Project Manager*
Beth Ford, RHIT, CCS, *Clinical/Technical Editor*
Brigid T. Caffrey, BA, BS, CCS, *Clinical/Technical Editor*
Tracy Betzler, *Senior Desktop Publishing Specialist*
Hope M. Dunn, *Senior Desktop Publishing Specialist*
Katie Russell, *Desktop Publishing Specialist*
Regina Heppes, *Editor*

Technical Editors

Beth Ford, RHIT, CCS

Ms. Ford is a clinical/technical editor for OptumInsight. She has more than 25 years experience in both physician and facility ICD-9-CM and CPT/HCPCS coding and compliance. Ms. Ford has extensive experience in a variety of health care settings including acute and post-acute facilities, occupational health and ambulatory care. She has provided coding education and consulting services to hospitals and physician practices, and has developed curriculum for medical terminology and ICD-9-CM and CPT coding education for a large healthcare system and multi-specialty physician groups. Formerly, she served as a coding specialist, coding manager, coding trainer/educator, coding consultant, and a health information management director. Her areas of specialization include coding auditing and training for DRG, inpatient, outpatient and physician coding. She is credentialed by the American Health Information Management Association (AHIMA) as a registered health information technologist (RHIT) and a certified coding specialist (CCS). She is an active member of the AHIMA and is an AHIMA-approved ICD-10-CM/PCS trainer.

Brigid T. Caffrey, BA, BS, CCS

Ms. Caffrey has expertise in hospital inpatient and outpatient coding and compliance and ICD-9-CM and CPT/HCPCS coding. Her experience includes conducting coding audits, providing staff education inclusive of physician education, and creating internal coding guidelines. She has a background in professional component coding, with expertise in radiology procedure coding. Most recently Ms. Caffrey was responsible for coding audits and compliance of a health information management services company. She is an active member of the American Health Information Management Association (AHIMA).

Contents

Chapter 1: Introduction

It is a reality in today's modern medical science that the codes within ICD-9-CM fall woefully short of our ever-changing medical reporting needs. The ninth revision of the International Classification of Diseases (ICD) was released more than 30 years ago as a modern and expansive system that was then only partially filled. Thousands of codes have been added to ICD-9-CM to classify new procedures and diseases over the years, and today the remaining space in ICD-9-CM procedure and diagnosis coding systems cannot accommodate our new technologies or our new understanding of diseases. An overhaul of our coding systems is needed.

New coding systems have been developed. Through the World Health Organization (WHO), ICD-10 was created and adopted in 1994. This is the system upon which the 10th revision of ICD that is used as the U.S. diagnosis coding system (ICD-10-CM) is based. Concurrent to the clinical modification of ICD-10 by the National Center for Health Statistics (NCHS), the Centers for Medicare and Medicaid Services (CMS) commissioned 3M Health Information Management to develop a new procedure coding system to replace volume 3 of ICD-9-CM, used for inpatient procedure coding.

Now that the coding systems have been drafted and modified, they need only to be implemented; but progress is slow. The government has been moving cautiously toward implementation, partly because: (1) the medical reimbursement industry has been adjusting to the impact of the Health Insurance Portability and Accountability Act (HIPAA) of 1996; (2) the scope of change is massive and will have a profound effect upon all care providers, payers, and government agencies; and (3) the change is big enough and costly enough to carry considerable political impact.

Two important events occurred late in 2002 that affected ICD-10-CM and ICD-10-PCS and their implementation. First, a subcommittee on coding for the National Committee on Vital and Health Statistics (NCVHS) forwarded a recommendation to the full committee that ICD-10-CM and ICD-10-PCS be adopted by the secretary of Health and Human Services (HHS). ICD-10-CM and ICD-10-PCS took one step closer to national rule making, which opened up a formal public comment period. The second event was the posting of a near-final draft of ICD-10-CM on the CMS website. While an earlier draft included only the tabular section of ICD-10-CM, the 2002 draft included the index as well.

In June 2003, NCHS posted a pre-release draft of ICD-10-CM on the NCHS website. That pre-release draft contained both index and tabular sections and a table of drugs and chemicals, which could be downloaded from the NCHS website. Since that time, Ingenix has published updated versions of the complete text.

On August 22, 2008, HHS published a notice of proposed rule making (NPRM) to adopt the ICD-10 coding systems (ICD-10-CM and ICD-10-PCS) to replace ICD-9-CM in transactions under HIPAA.

Proposed rule NPRM CMS-0013-P called for updated versions of HIPAA electronic transaction standards. Specifically, the rule urged adoption of version

 DEFINITIONS

CMS. Centers for Medicare and Medicaid Services. Federal agency that administers the public health programs.

NCHS. National Center for Health Statistics. Division of the Centers for Disease Control and Prevention that compiles statistical information used to guide actions and policies to improve the public health of U.S. citizens. The NCHS maintains the ICD-9-CM coding system.

WHO. World Health Organization. International agency comprising UN members to promote the physical, mental, and emotional health of the people of the world and to track morbidity and mortality statistics worldwide. WHO maintains the International Classification of Diseases (ICD) medical code set.

5010 to facilitate electronic health care transactions to accommodate the ICD-10 code sets. This NPRM also proposed implementing ICD-10-CM for diagnosis coding and ICD-10-PCS for inpatient hospital procedure coding, effective October 1, 2011. The comment period for this proposed rule was closed on October 21, 2008.

On January 16, 2009, HHS published a final rule in the *Federal Register*, 45 CFR, part 162, "HIPAA Administrative Simplification: Modifications to Medical Data Code Set Standards to Adopt ICD-10-CM and ICD-10-PCS." This rule may be downloaded at http://edocket.access.gpo.gov/2009/pdf/E9-743.pdf.

This final rule adopts modifications to standard medical data code sets for coding diagnoses and inpatient hospital procedures by adopting ICD-10-CM for diagnosis coding, including the Official ICD-10-CM Guidelines for Coding and Reporting, and ICD-10-PCS for inpatient hospital procedure coding, effective October 1, 2013. On April 17, 2012, a one-year delay was proposed to 45 CFR Part 162; 77 FR 22949) to postpone ICD-10-CM implementation until October 1, 2014. This proposal was adopted as a final rule and published in the September 5, 2012 *Federal Register*. Although the last regular, annual update to both ICD-9-CM and ICD-10 occurred on October 1, 2011, the ICD-9-CM Coordination and Maintenance Committee established a partial code freeze to both code sets. The limited updates allowed to ICD-10 are intended only to capture new technologies and diseases as required by section 503(a) of Pub. L. 108-173. This limited code set freeze remains in effect throughout the remainder of the transition period. The most current 2013 draft update release is available for public viewing, and additional updates are expected prior to implementation. At this time, ICD-10-CM codes are not valid for any purpose or use other than for reporting mortality data for death certificates.

A successful transition from ICD-9-CM to the ICD-10-CM coding system will require focused training for individuals and organizations. The first step in transitioning to the new coding system is to develop a firm foundation in understanding the coding conventions and guidelines in ICD-10-CM to prepare the medical office, practice, department or facility for the significant changes that the new coding system will bring. *Optum Learning: Detailed Instruction for Appropriate ICD-10-CM Coding* provides a new resource to create a solid foundation for all levels of ICD-10-CM coding. The knowledge gleaned from this book will prepare facilities or offices for the impact of the new coding system. Nearly everyone will be affected: human resources staff, accountants, information systems staff, physicians—just to name a few. ICD-10-CM provides tremendous opportunities for disease tracking, but also creates enormous challenges. Computer hardware and software, medical documentation, and the revenue cycle are just three elements of medical reimbursement that will require adjustment when implementation occurs.

This book is suitable for all specialties, facilitating a firm foundation of ICD-10-CM knowledge to ease the transition of the implementation process and reduce the margin for error and delay. The following features assist in providing a heightened awareness of the issues unique to ICD-10-CM:

- An easy-to-follow guide to ICD-10-CM that explains the content, structure, and key features of each chapter of the ICD-10-CM coding system.

 KEY POINT

Two federal agencies, NCHS and CMS, are responsible for the development of the ICD-9-CM replacement (i.e., ICD-10-CM and ICD-10-PCS).

- The official draft ICD-10-CM coding and reporting guidelines released by NCHS that provide essential insight into coding concepts and classification changes.

- Coding examples that illustrate key contrasts and similarities between systems.

- Knowledge assessments to help quantify understanding of the ICD-10-CM system. Answers, with decision logic, are provided for all test questions.

HISTORY OF MODIFICATIONS TO ICD

The original intent of the World Health Organization for ICD was as a statistical tool for the international exchange of mortality data. A subsequent revision was expanded to accommodate data collection for morbidity statistics. An eventual seventh revision, published by WHO in 1955, was clinically modified for use in the United States based upon a joint study on the efficiency of hospital diseases indexing by the American Hospital Association (AHA) and the American Association of Medical Record Librarians (AAMRL). Results of that study led to the 1959 publication of the *International Classification of Diseases, Adapted for Indexing Hospital Records (ICDA)*, by the federal Public Health Service. The ICDA uniformly modified ICD-7, and it gave the United States a way to classify operations and treatments.

Hospitals were initially slow in their acceptance of ICDA, though momentum picked up. An eighth edition of ICD, published by WHO in 1965, eventually lacked the depth of clinical data required for America's emerging health care system. In 1968, two widely accepted modifications were published in the United States: the Eighth Revision International Classification of Diseases Adapted for Use in the United States (ICDA-8) and the Hospital Adaptation of ICDA (H-ICDA). Hospitals used either of these two systems through the latter years of the next decade.

ICD-9 and ICD-9-CM

The ninth revision by WHO in 1975 prompted the typical American response: clinical modification. This time, the impetus flowed from a process initiated in 1977 by NCHS to modify ICD-9 for hospital indexing and retrieving case data for clinical studies. The NCHS and the newly created Council on Clinical Classifications modified ICD-9 according to U.S. clinical standard, and developed a companion procedural classification. This classification, published as volume 3 of ICD-9-CM, revised a portion of WHO's International Classification of Procedure Modification (ICPM). In 1978, the three-volume set was published in the United States for use one year later. There were no further changes in the direction to ICD-9-CM until the October 1983 implementation of diagnosis related groups (DRG), which gave ICD-9-CM a new significance. After more than 30 years since ICD's arrival in the United States, the classification system proves indispensable to hospitals interested in payment schedules for health care services.

ICD-10-CM

The evolution of ICD took another turn in 1994 when WHO published ICD-10. Again, the NCHS wanted to modify the latest revision, but with an emphasis on problems that had been identified in the current ICD-9-CM and resolved by the improvements to ICD-10 for classifying mortality and morbidity data. The Center for Health Policy Studies (CHPS) was awarded the NCHS

 KEY POINT

NCHS is responsible for developing the diagnostic portion of the ICD-10 coding system, ICD-10-CM. CMS is responsible for developing the procedure portion of the ICD-10 coding system, ICD-10-PCS.

 DEFINITIONS

morbidity. Diseased condition or state.

mortality. Condition of being mortal (subject to death).

 QUICK TIP

The Centers for Disease Control in Atlanta publishes a weekly epidemiologic report on the incidence of communicable diseases and deaths (morbidity and mortality) in selected urban areas of the United States.

KEY POINT

WHO's seventh edition of ICD was the first edition modified by the United States. Two versions of a modified ICD-8 were published in 1968. A procedure classification was created by the U.S. government and accompanied the clinical modification of ICD-9, which was published in 1978.

contract to analyze ICD-10 and to develop the appropriate clinical modifications.

Phase I provided the analysis for clinical modification. According to CHPS, ICD-10 must be modified to do the following:

- Return the level of specificity found in ICD-9-CM
- Facilitate an alphabetic index to assign codes
- Provide code titles and language that complement accepted clinical practice
- Remove codes unique to mortality coding

Phase II followed protocol. CHPS developed modifications based on the analysis, including the following:

- Increasing the five-character structure to six characters
- Incorporating common fourth- and fifth-digit subclassifications
- Creating laterality
- Combining certain codes
- Adding trimesters to obstetric codes
- Creating combined diagnosis/symptoms codes
- Deactivating procedure codes

In the second phase, CHPS expanded the codes for alcohol/drug abuse, diabetes mellitus, and injuries.

A draft of ICD-10-CM for public comment was released at the conclusion of phase II. Since that time, the drafts have been revised and updated concurrent with the changes in ICD-9-CM, and to accommodate classification needs as they have been identified. The final version will draw on an analysis of the comments by NCHS and phase III reviewers.

Regulatory Process

This section outlines the regulatory process as defined by HIPAA for adoption of a new standard code set. Legislation has been introduced in both houses of Congress that address national health information issues. Bills that have been introduced include provisions for adopting ICD-10. Both the House and Senate must approve legislation before the bill advances to the president for signature. The inclusion of ICD-10 adoption provisions within current legislation is separate from the process outlined in HIPAA. Bills that pass both the House and Senate require the president's signature, and the regulatory process must still take place.

Background

On Wednesday, November 5, 2003, the National Committee on Vital and Health Statistics (NCVHS) voted to recommend that the secretary of HHS take steps toward national adoption of ICD-10-CM and ICD-10-PCS as replacements under HIPAA standards for the current uses of ICD-9-CM, volumes 1, 2, and 3.

 KEY POINT

The following websites post updated versions of the ICD-10-CM code set, guidelines and mappings:

- The 2013 release of ICD-10-CM is available on the NCHS website at: http://www.cdc.gov/nchs/icd/icd10cm.htm.
- The 2013 release of ICD-10-CM is also available on the CMS website at: http://www.cms.gov/Medicare/Coding/ICD10/2013-ICD-10-CM-and-GEMs.html.

Administrative Simplification

Congress addressed the need for a consistent framework for electronic transactions and other administrative simplification issues in HIPAA, which became part of the Social Security Act titled "Administrative Simplification." Sections 1171 through 1179 require any standard adopted by the secretary of HHS (including the standard code sets):

- To be developed, adopted, or modified by a standard-setting organization
- To adopt code standards applicable to health plans, health care clearinghouses, and health care providers who transmit any health information in electronic form
- To adopt transaction standards and data elements for the electronic exchange of health information for certain health care transactions
- To ensure that procedures exist for the routine maintenance, testing, enhancement, and expansion of code sets
- To set a compliance date not later than 24 months after the date on which an initial standard or implementation specification is adopted for all covered entities except small health plans

The transactions and code sets final rule (2000) adopted a number of standard medical data code sets for use in those transactions, including:

- ICD-9-CM, volumes 1 and 2, for coding and reporting diseases, injuries, impairments, other health problems and their manifestations, and causes of injury, disease, impairment, or other health problems
- ICD-9-CM, volume 3, for the following procedures reported by hospitals: prevention, diagnosis, treatment, and management
- CPT codes for physician services and all other health care services
- HCPCS codes for other substances, equipment, supplies, and other items used in health care

The rule also included adoption of a procedure for maintaining existing standards, adopting modifications to existing standards, and adopting new standards.

Process

The committee formulated a letter of recommendation requesting that the secretary of HHS initiate the regulatory process for the concurrent national adoption of the two classification systems with an implementation period of at least two years following issuance of a final rule.

The NCVHS recommendation was the first step of the regulatory process. The next step was the acceptance of the recommendation by the secretary of Health and Human Services. In the meantime, American Health Information Management Association (AHIMA) had urged the secretary to issue a notice of proposed rule making (NPRM).

On August 22, 2008, the NPRM was published in the *Federal Register* with a proposed implementation date of October 1 of 2011. A two-year implementation period after establishment of the final rule is required under the HIPAA two-year window for compliance.

The comment period for the NPRM closed on October 21, 2008. However, a final rule was not published at that time.

Upon publishing the ICD-10 and version 5010/NCPDP[1] version D.0 (electronic transaction standards) final rules, both CMS and the industry will begin documenting the requirements for both ICD-10 and version 5010 system changes, initiate and/or complete any gap analyses, and then undertake design and system changes. Version 5010 is progressing first, based on the need to have this transaction standard in place prior to ICD-10 implementation to accommodate the increase in the size of the fields for the ICD-10 code sets.

In the United States, the clinical modification of the code set is maintained by the ICD-9-CM Coordination and Maintenance Committee (NCHS, CMS, AHA, and AHIMA). However, the code set standard is approved by legislative process.

The administrative simplification provision of HIPAA encourages the development of health care information systems by establishing standards, including code sets for each data element for health care services. HIPAA requires the secretary of HHS to adopt the code set standards. The secretary then tasked the NCVHS with studying and recommending the standard code sets. These impact studies have been completed, and reports have been made to Congress and HHS.

In summary, the necessary steps to implementation include:

1. Development of recommendations for standards to be adopted by HHS/NCVHS (November 2003)

2. Publication of the proposed rule in the *Federal Register* with a 60-day public comment period (August 2008)

3. Analysis of the public comments and publication of the final rule in the *Federal Register* with the effective date of the rule being 60 days after publication (October 2008)

4. Distribution of standards and coordinated preparation and distribution of implementation guidelines and crosswalks. Implementation is 24 months from the effective date, excluding small health plans (fewer than 50 participants), which have 36 months to comply.

Step 1 of this process ended up lasting until 2008. Cost/benefit analyses were performed. According to the regulatory process, implementation was no sooner than October 1, 2009. However, the NPRM was not released before May 1, 2007, making the 2009 implementation date impossible.

On August 22, 2008, HHS published an NPRM to adopt the ICD-10 coding systems (ICD-10-CM and ICD-10-PCS) to replace ICD-9-CM in HIPAA transactions.

Proposed rule NPRM CMS-0013-P called for updated versions of HIPAA electronic transaction standards. Specifically, the rule urged adoption of version 5010 to facilitate electronic health care transactions to accommodate the ICD-10 code sets. This NPRM also proposed implementing ICD-10-CM for diagnosis coding and ICD-10-PCS for inpatient hospital procedure coding,

1. National Council for Prescription Drug Programs

effective October 1, 2011. The comment period for this proposed rule was closed on October 21, 2008.

On January 16, 2009, HHS published a final rule in the *Federal Register*, 45 CFR, part 162, "HIPAA Administrative Simplification: Modifications to Medical Data Code Set Standards to Adopt ICD-10-CM and ICD-10-PCS." This final rule adopts modifications to standard medical data code sets for coding diagnoses and inpatient hospital procedures by adopting ICD-10-CM for diagnosis coding, including the "ICD-10-CM Draft Official Guidelines for Coding and Reporting," and ICD-10-PCS for inpatient hospital procedure coding, effective October 1, 2013.

On April 17, 2012, a proposed rule was released (45 CFR Part 162; 77 FR 22949) that provides a one-year delay of ICD-10-CM and ICD-10-PCS implementation until October 1, 2014. This proposal was adopted as a final rule and published in the September 5, 2012 *Federal Register*. The intent of this delay was stated by HHS to provide HIPAA-covered entities the additional time needed to synchronize system and business process preparations, and to make necessary changes to accommodate the new code sets. The last regular, annual update to both ICD-9-CM and ICD-10 occurred on October 1, 2011. Effective October 1, 2012, only limited updates are allowed to both the ICD-9-CM and ICD-10 code sets to capture new technologies and diseases as required by section 503(a) of Pub. L. 108-173. This limited code set freeze remains in effect throughout the remainder of the transition period. The proposed rule announced in April is the third in a series of administrative simplification rules in the new health care law. HHS released the first in July of 2011, the second in January of 2012, and the third in September of 2012.

Optum Learning: Implementing ICD-10

Based on the recent passage of legislation, those affected by the version 5010 and ICD-10 transitions (e.g., health care providers, payers, software vendors, clearinghouses, third-party billers) should prepare to meet the following timeline to ensure compliance.

ICD-10 Implementation Timeline

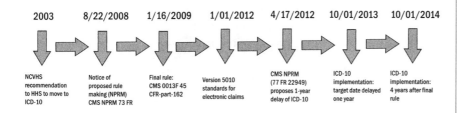

2003	8/22/2008	1/16/2009	1/01/2012	4/17/2012	10/01/2013	10/01/2014
NCVHS recommendation to HHS to move to ICD-10	Notice of proposed rule making (NPRM) CMS NPRM 73 FR	Final rule: CMS 0013F 45 CFR-part-162	Version 5010 standards for electronic claims	CMS NPRM (77 FR 22949) proposes 1-year delay of ICD-10	ICD-10 implementation: target date delayed one year	ICD-10 implementation: 4 years after final rule

DOCUMENTATION

The ICD-10 classification and coding systems are constructed with future reporting needs in mind. Their architecture has been constructed on a grand scale. Therefore, we will focus on the diagnosis coding system (ICD-10-CM), which will affect both hospital and physician providers in the near future. The documentation principles and concepts, however, may apply to documentation considerations created by the impact of both systems.

In creating the clinical modification for ICD-10 in this country, the National Center for Health Statistics has made significant changes. The number of diagnostic codes available for use in the ICD-10-CM coding system is larger than the number available in ICD-9-CM by thousands.

This greater level of detail, called "granularity," is good news for the nosologists and government researchers tracking disease in the United States. Do not underestimate the importance of this work; their statistics help drive health care reform, research, payment systems, and social programs. The granularity of ICD-10-CM does indeed provide benefits for everyone in our society.

DOCUMENTATION NEEDS

ICD-10-CM will pose certain significant challenges to coders in both physician and facility settings.

As additional detail is to be reported with ICD-10-CM, more detail will be required in the medical records from which the data for coding are extracted. For coders who are already facing these challenges on a daily basis, the increased specificity required to report ICD-10-CM may seem daunting. The following examples illustrate some of the documentation gaps that coders should be prepared to address:

Example 1

Term	Coding Component	Codes	
Chalazion	**Specify laterality and anatomic site:** Right upper eyelid Right lower eyelid Right eye, unspecified eyelid Left upper eyelid Left lower eyelid Left eye, unspecified eyelid Unspecified eye, unspecified	H00.11	Chalazion, right upper eyelid
		H00.12	Chalazion right lower eyelid
		H00.13	Chalazion right eye, unspecified eyelid
		H00.14	Chalazion left upper eyelid
		H00.15	Chalazion left lower eyelid
		H00.16	Chalazion left eye, unspecified eyelid
		H00.19	Chalazion unspecified eye, unspecified

In example 1, a single code, 373.2 Chalazion, was used to classify this diagnosis in ICD-9-CM. In ICD-10-CM, an expanded classification was created to facilitate data capture of the specific anatomic site and laterality. Providers should be made aware of the classification specificity within ICD-10-CM so that documentation practices can be adjusted prior to implementation. However, in most cases, specific information about laterality and the anatomic site may be readily available in the patient record.

In this example, the information listed in the coding component column is information that has not been required under the ICD-9-CM coding system, but will be required with ICD-10-CM. One may find that information not essential to choosing the code in ICD-9-CM, but necessary for selecting the code in ICD-10-CM, may already be present in the medical record, such as laterality and specific site.

However, certain issues such as laterality are not documentation issues for ICD-10-CM alone. Physicians must meet the legal and professional standards for documentation that demand a level of granularity in the medical record.

DEFINITIONS

nosologist. Scientist who studies the classification of diseases.

GENERAL INFO

The code examples provided are intended for academic purposes to illustrate the differences between ICD-9-CM and ICD-10-CM. They are not intended to represent direct mappings, except where specifically noted.

Example 2

Term	Coding Component	Codes	
Pregnancy	**With bladder infection, specify trimester:** first second third	O23.10	Infections of bladder in pregnancy, unspecified trimester
		O23.11	Infections of bladder in pregnancy, first trimester
		O23.12	Infections of bladder in pregnancy, second trimester
		O23.13	Infections of bladder in pregnancy, third trimester

In example 2, the new documentation component required for ICD-10-CM code selection is one that should currently exist in the medical record documentation. In ICD-10-CM, code selection in pregnancy includes a trimester component. One would normally expect medical charts to include this information, or that the data could be derived from the patient's due date.

Example 3

Term	Coding Component	Codes	
Sarcoidosis	**Specify anatomic site and/or nature of manifestation**	D86.0	Sarcoidosis of lung
		D86.1	Sarcoidosis of lymph nodes
		D86.2	Sarcoidosis of lung with sarcoidosis of lymph nodes
		D86.3	Sarcoidosis of skin
		D86.8	Sarcoidosis of other sites
		D86.81	Sarcoid meningitis
		D86.82	Multiple cranial nerve palsies in sarcoidosis
		D86.83	Sarcoid iridocyclitis
		D86.84	Sarcoid pyelonephritis
		D86.85	Sarcoid myocarditis
		D86.86	Sarcoid arthropathy
		D86.87	Sarcoid myositis
		D86.89	Sarcoidosis of other sites
		D86.9	Sarcoidosis, unspecified

Example 3 illustrates that additional information is more often necessary to classify conditions in ICD-10-CM than was required in ICD-9-CM. The natures of manifestation, severity, laterality, or specific affected anatomic site, are variables that must be considered in choosing the most appropriate code.

The data granularity of ICD-10-CM in comparison to ICD-9-CM requires education of medical staff members in order to ensure adequate documentation from which to assign appropriately descriptive codes. Documentation improvement audits are useful tools in determining the need for improvement. Focused in-services that address changes in the coding components and documentation requirements for conditions often encountered within certain specialties may prove to be an effective method of ensuring that provider documentation meets the demands of the ICD-10-CM system.

 KEY POINT

One physician, upon hearing a coder from another clinic complain about her doctor's documentation, offered this anecdote:

My daughter came home from school yesterday with a report card and all subjects were marked with the grade "incomplete." I scheduled an appointment with the teacher, since my daughter said she had turned in all of her homework and felt the tests were very easy. At the meeting with the teacher, I asked how a student who does such sterling work could be awarded "incomplete" in every class. The teacher looked me straight in the eye and said, with a bit of a chip on his shoulder, "You know, I didn't get into teaching to do paper work…"

"Doctors," this physician continued, "could learn a lot from that story. Your job isn't done until your paper work is done."

 DEFINITIONS

data granularity. Degree or detail contained in data; the fineness in which data fields are subdivided.

DOCUMENTATION AND THE REIMBURSEMENT PROCESS

Documentation plays an integral role in the reimbursement process. Without it, bottlenecks that delay billing and payment can ensue.

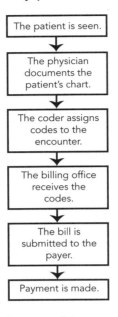

The resulting blockage occurs because of the increased granularity and documentation requirements of ICD-10-CM and is most likely to happen in the early steps of the process. The coder will be the first to recognize that important information is missing. A query is then generated for the doctor in order to gather more information. The doctor must then ensure that the necessary information is included in the medical record before the coding piece of the process can proceed.

It is therefore essential to disseminate information about ICD-10-CM granularity and the accompanying documentation requirements. By studying the differences in coding components and adjusting documentation habits now, future paperwork hurdles can be minimized.

A certain amount of "documentation chasing" is a normal expectation within the course of business; however, billing delays during the implementation phase of ICD-10-CM will not remain a constant. As the learning curve is conquered, the time spent on these steps should return to the usual, pre-implementation operating levels.

Advantages of ICD-10-CM within the Reimbursement Process

There are also some definite advantages to using ICD-10-CM within the reimbursement cycle that occur at the coding stage and beyond. The data granularity of the classification system is likely to reduce time associated with the manual process of choosing the most appropriate codes. Coders are also much more likely to choose the correct code on the first attempt, since there is much less ambiguity in ICD-10-CM. For payers, the clarity afforded by the ICD-10-CM coding system is likely to greatly enhance and assist in supporting medical necessity. With ICD-10-CM, the diagnosis comes significantly closer to being "married" to the procedure; further, it intrinsically gives a more complete description of the condition, thereby leaving less room for denials.

✓ **QUICK TIP**

Medical practices should start by auditing their medical records to assess whether current documentation practices will support the level of detail required to code in the new systems. Provide medical staff with examples of where their current practices fall short, and inform them of the resultant backlogs in the deficiency process and revenue cycles.

INCREASED GRANULARITY

The primary reason for creating a coding system that assigns a number to the diagnosis or condition is simply to record and retrieve information in an efficient way. One of the main purposes we use this for is—and always has been—to gather data for research and statistics.

Nosologists, medical researchers, and epidemiologists are constantly tracking disease in the United States based on the coded data. A coding system for documenting and reporting cases allows the researchers, the statisticians, and the epidemiologists to gather the information upon which many important health care decisions are made. As such, the integrity of statistics and research findings are extremely important. Data drives health care reform, supports decisions regarding most effective and appropriate treatments, determines which clinical research endeavors to pursue, and aids in structuring and funding social programs concerned with health and well-being.

Data affects outcomes. Good data can help change the health care delivery system for the better. Coders are literally building the database that drives our future every time they choose the codes that are used for painting our statistical pictures and conducting research.

The increased granularity, or in other words, the greater level of detail afforded by ICD-10-CM provides the quality data needed to support improved clinical outcomes and more cost-effective disease management.

Improving Treatment Management

ICD-10-CM can improve the management and treatment of disease for the individual. Code classifications for complications of medical and surgical care have been expanded to include the following categories:

Y62	**Failure of sterile precautions during surgical and medical care**
Y63	**Failure in dosage during surgical and medical care**
Y64	**Contaminated medical or biological substances**
Y70–Y82	**Medical devices associated with adverse incidents in diagnostic and therapeutic use**

The increased level of detail in chapter 20, "External Causes of Morbidity (V00–Y99)," provides a means to improve care by putting forth a mechanism for increased efficiency in tracking nosocomial and iatrogenic incidents that were previously either loosely defined by the code categories 996–999 in ICD-9-CM, or missing from the classification altogether.

Establishing Better Clinical Outcomes and Treatment Protocols

ICD-10-CM will not only aid in improving disease management and treatment for all individuals within a certain diagnostic group, but will also assist in achieving better treatment protocols that yield improved clinical outcomes for future cases. The increased data granularity of ICD-10-CM enables researchers to study diseases, together with the current treatments being used, on a more refined level. Statistical patterns are easily identified, linking critical connections necessary to expedite research and develop new treatments.

For example, carcinoma in situ of the breast can be tracked by only one code in ICD-9-CM, 233.0. There are 12 separate codes in the category for carcinoma in situ of the breast (D05) in ICD-10-CM, with axes for lobular, intraductal, other, and unspecified carcinoma. Together with the ICD-10-PCS system for reporting the procedures with greater detail, researchers can track the specific outcomes of the different types of radioactive materials versus surgical procedures used in treating those cases. They may start discovering certain trends that would have been very difficult, if not impossible, to see with less specific data.

Researchers may discover, for instance, that one particular isotope used for treating lobular cancer results in a better response than other isotopes, or that the same treatment does not yield the same outcome on intraductal carcinoma, or surgical intervention proves more effective than radiation in females; these are only a few examples of the kinds of trends and patterns that could be discovered when research is done with better data. Data always affect the outcome. When the procedure data are linked to the diagnosis, the result provides definitive trackable outcomes. This may also significantly decrease the margin for denial based on medical necessity for reimbursement purposes.

Additional advantages may also be identified with the implementation of ICD-10-CM. For example, in ICD-9-CM, there is only one code available for reporting Down syndrome, 758.0. However, ICD-10-CM provides three distinct classification types of Down syndrome: nonmosaicism (meiotic nondisjunction), mosaicism (mitotic nondisjunction), and translocation. The following codes available to choose from are:

Q90.0	**Trisomy 21, nonmosaicism (meiotic nondisjunction)**
Q90.1	**Trisomy 21, mosaicism (mitotic nondisjunction)**
Q90.2	**Trisomy 21, translocation**
Q90.9	**Down syndrome, unspecified**

Once the distinction is made in the clinical coding system, the data gathered are relevant on a much higher level of clinical detail. Researchers may then use this improved quality data to refine genetic testing that broadens the possibilities for advances in medicine. As such, the increased granularity permitted by the ICD-10-CM coding system offers many deep and extensive advantages that are well worth celebrating.

Chapter 2:
Introduction to ICD-10-CM

OVERVIEW OF CHANGES

Before the clinical modifications to ICD-10 are reviewed and understood, one must first become familiar with the changes made by the World Health Organization (WHO) when it moved from ICD-9 to ICD-10. The first clue to the revisions is in the full title: International Statistical Classification of Diseases and Related Health Problems. WHO felt this change would not only clarify the classification's content and purpose, but show how the scope of the classification has moved beyond the classification of disease and injuries to the coding of ambulatory care conditions and risk factors frequently encountered in primary care.

Overall, the 10th revision results in an increase in clinical detail and addresses information about previously classified diseases as well as those diseases discovered since the last revision. Conditions are grouped according to the most appropriate for general epidemiological purposes and the evaluation of health care. Organizational changes are made and new features added. However, for the most part, the format and conventions of the classification remain unchanged.

Other adaptations of the ICD include:

- International Classification of Diseases for Oncology, third edition (ICD-O-3)

- International Classification of External Causes of Injury (ICECI)

- International Classification of Primary Care, second edition (ICPC-2)

- The ICD-10 for Mental and Behavioural Disorders Diagnostic Criteria for Research

- The ICD-10 for Mental and Behavioral Disorders Clinical Descriptions and Diagnostic Guidelines

In the United States, the clinical modification of ICD-10, ICD-10-CM, will replace the clinical modification of ICD-9, ICD-9-CM. The parent classification system, the International Classification of Disease (ICD), is owned and copyrighted by WHO, which publishes the classification. As with ICD-9-CM, WHO authorized the development of an adaptation of ICD-10 for use in the United States. This adaptation, the clinical modification (CM), must conform to WHO conventions for the ICD.

Many of the codes considered new in ICD-10 may seem familiar to users of ICD-9-CM. This is because ICD-10 is a further evolution of the ICD-9 classification, as the ICD-10-CM is a further evolution of the ICD-9-CM. The underlying basic structure, conventions, and philosophy remain the same. The clinical modification in use in the United States (ICD-9-CM) has been maintained and updated annually since 1985. The following example illustrates the evaluation of these systems by showing how angina pectoris classifications

 OBJECTIVES

In this chapter you will learn:

- The purpose of ICD-10-CM
- The motivations for clinically modifying ICD-10
- About the many important uses of ICD-10 and ICD-10-CM beyond reimbursement

 KEY POINT

This publication refers to the 2013 ICD-10-CM update.

 GENERAL INFO

The code examples provided are intended for academic purposes to illustrate the differences between ICD-9-CM and ICD-10-CM. They are not intended to represent direct mappings, except where specifically noted.

have changed from the preclinical modification ICD-9 version to the current 2013 version of ICD-10-CM:

ICD-9

413   **Angina pectoris**

ICD-9-CM

411.1   **Intermediate coronary syndrome—(includes unstable angina)**

413.0   **Angina decubitus**

413.1   **Prinzmetal angina**

413.9   **Other and unspecified angina pectoris—(includes angina of effort and stenocardia)**

ICD-10 and ICD-10-CM

All diseases of the circulatory system appear under the letter "I" in ICD-10.

I20.0   **Unstable angina**

I20.1   **Angina pectoris with documented spasm—(includes Prinzmetal angina)**

I20.8   **Other forms of angina pectoris—(includes angina of effort and stenocardia)**

I20.9   **Angina pectoris, unspecified**

No new codes have been added to the ICD-10 entries for angina pectoris in ICD-10-CM at the time of this publication.

ICD Structure

WHO published ICD-10 in three volumes: an index, an instructional manual, and a tabular list. ICD-10-CM will be published in two volumes: an index and a tabular list.

Volume 1: Tabular List

Volume 1 contains the listing of alphanumeric codes. The same hierarchical organization of ICD-9 applies to ICD-10: all codes with the same first three characters have common traits. Each character beyond three adds more specificity. In ICD-9-CM, valid codes can contain anywhere from three to five digits. However, ICD-10-CM for use in the United States has been expanded with valid codes containing anywhere from three to seven characters. In some instances, the final character may be an alpha character, not a number. In some cases, the use of a "reserve" subclassification (identified as an "X") has been incorporated into codes that continue with greater specificity beyond the fifth character to allow for built-in expansion within that established level of specificity. For example:

H83.3 Noise effects on inner ear
      Acoustic trauma of inner ear
      Noise-induced hearing loss of inner ear

    H83.3X Noise effects on inner ear

        H83.3X1 Noise effects on right inner ear

        H83.3X2 Noise effects on left inner ear

        H83.3X3 Noise effects on inner ear, bilateral

        H83.3X9 Noise effects on inner ear, unspecified ear

☞ KEY POINT

In ICD-10-CM, all codes and descriptions appear in bold font in the text.

The same ICD-9-CM hierarchical organization is at work in ICD-10-CM notes and instructions. When a note appears under a three-character category code, it applies to all codes within that category. For example, see the instructional note under category W22. The instructional notes at the category level apply to codes within the entire W22 category.

Instructions under a specific code apply only to that single code. For example, see the Excludes1 note under code W22.041, which applies only to code W22.041.

W22 **Striking against or struck by other objects**

> *EXCLUDES 1* *striking against or struck by object with subsequent fall (W18.09)*

> The appropriate 7th character is to be added to each code from category W22.
>
> **A** **initial encounter**
> **D** **subsequent encounter**
> **S** **sequela**

W22.0 **Striking against stationary object**

> *EXCLUDES 1* *striking against stationary sports equipment (W21.8)*

W22.01 **Walked into wall**

W22.02 **Walked into lamppost**

W22.03 **Walked into furniture**

W22.04 **Striking against wall of swimming pool**

W22.041 **Striking against wall of swimming pool causing drowning and submersion**

> *EXCLUDES 1* *drowning and submersion while swimming without striking against wall (W67)*

W22.042 **Striking against wall of swimming pool causing other injury**

W22.09 **Striking against other stationary object**

The following is an example of the tabular listing in ICD-10, for international use.

Other Disorders of the Skin and Subcutaneous Tissue (L80–L99)

L80 **Vitiligo**

L81 **Other disorders of pigmentation**

> *EXCLUDES 1* *birthmark NOS (Q82.5)*
> *naevus—see Alphabetic Index*
> *Peutz-Jeghers syndrome (Q85.8)*

L81.0 **Postinflammatory hyperpigmentation**

L81.1 **Chloasma**

L81.2 **Freckles**

L81.3 **Café au lait spots**

L81.4 **Other melanin hyperpigmentation**
Lentigo

L81.5 **Leukoderma, not elsewhere classified**

L81.6 **Other disorders of diminished melanin formation**

L81.7 **Pigmented purpuric dermatosis**
Angioma serpiginosum

L81.8 **Other specified disorders of pigmentation**
Iron pigmentation
Tattoo pigmentation

L81.9 **Disorder of pigmentation, unspecified**

 KEY POINT

When an instructional note appears under a three-character category code, it applies to all codes within that category. However, an instructional note under a specific code applies only to that single

---

L82 **Seborrhoeic keratosis**
Dermatosis papulosa nigra
Leser-Trélat disease

L83 **Acanthosis nigricans**
Confluent and reticulated papillomatosis

L84 **Corns and callosities**
Callus
Clavus

The following example shows how the tabular list looks in ICD-10-CM for use in the United States.

Notice the separation of exclusion notes into two separate types: Excludes 1 and Excludes 2.

Other Disorders of the Skin and Subcutaneous Tissue (L80–L99)

L80 **Vitiligo**
EXCLUDES 2 *vitiligo of eyelids (H02.73-)*
vitiligo of vulva (N90.8)

L81 **Other disorders of pigmentation**
EXCLUDES 1 *birthmark NOS (Q82.5)*
Peutz-Jeghers syndrome (Q85.8)
EXCLUDES 2 *nevus—see Alphabetic Index*

L81.0 **Postinflammatory hyperpigmentation**

L81.1 **Chloasma**

L81.2 **Freckles**

L81.3 **Café au lait spots**

L81.4 **Other melanin hyperpigmentation**
Lentigo

L81.5 **Leukoderma, not elsewhere classified**

L81.6 **Other disorders of diminished melanin formation**

L81.7 **Pigmented purpuric dermatosis**
Angioma serpiginosum

L81.8 **Other specified disorders of pigmentation**
Iron pigmentation
Tattoo pigmentation

L81.9 **Disorder of pigmentation, unspecified**

L82 **Seborrheic keratosis**
INCLUDES dermatosis papulosa nigra
Leser-Trélat disease
EXCLUDES 2 *seborrheic dermatitis (L21.-)*

L82.0 **Inflamed seborrheic keratosis**

L82.1 **Other seborrheic keratosis**
Seborrheic keratosis NOS

L83 **Acanthosis nigricans**
Confluent and reticulated papillomatosis

L84 **Corns and callosities**
Callus
Clavus

Coding Guidelines/Instructional Manual

ICD-10 is published in three volumes, yet volume 2, the instructional manual for ICD-10, will not be used in the United States for morbidity coding. Instead, the NCHS will continue to post current versions of the official ICD-10-CM coding guidelines on the NCHS website. The NCHS will continue to release the official ICD-10-CM on CD, and private publishers will produce the ICD-10-CM books. The Cooperating Parties (CMS, NCHS, AHA, and

KEY POINT

"Excludes" notes are expanded in ICD-10 to clarify priority of code assignment and to provide guidance.

KEY POINT

The current version of ICD-10-CM, code mappings, and coding guidelines are posted on the NCHS website: http://www.cdc.gov/nchs/icd/icd10cm.htm.

AHIMA) will continue to release updated versions of the official ICD-10-CM coding guidelines to accompany the code updates. These updated guidelines will be posted to the NCHS website. Updates are expected to be revised regularly (usually annually) by the Cooperating Parties, as were the ICD-9-CM guidelines. Additionally, these guidelines will be published in the *AHA Coding Clinic for ICD-10-CM*.

Section I of the draft official ICD-10-CM guidelines address ICD-10-CM conventions, the general rules for use of the ICD-10-CM classification system, independent of the guidelines. These conventions include instructional notes and other features inherent to the index and tabular sections, which universally apply to all health care settings.

See chapter 2 of this publication for further information on ICD-10-CM coding conventions.

Refer to the "ICD-10-CM Draft Official Guidelines for Coding and Reporting" in appendix A of this book for additional information.

Alphabetic Index

The alphabetic index provides a listing of the codes in the tabular list. As in the ICD-9-CM index, terms in the ICD-10 index are found alphabetically, by diagnosis. A code for a supernumerary nipple would be accessed by looking under "Supernumerary," then "nipple(s)." The following example shows how the alphabetic index appears in ICD-10-CM:

Alphabetical Index to Diseases and Nature of Injury

Supernumerary (congenital)
    aortic cusps Q23.8
    auditory ossicles Q16.3
    bone Q79.8
    breast Q83.1
    carpal bones Q74.0
    cusps, heart valve NEC Q24.8
        aortic Q23.8
        mitral Q23.2
        pulmonary Q22.3
    digit(s) Q69.9
    ear (lobule) Q17.0
    fallopian tube Q50.6
    finger Q69.0
    hymen Q52.4
    kidney Q63.0
    lacrimonasal duct Q10.6
    lobule (ear) Q17.0
    mitral cusps Q23.2
    muscle Q79.8
    nipple(s) Q83.3
    organ or site not listed—*see* Accessory
    ossicles, auditory Q16.3
    ovary Q50.31
    oviduct Q50.6
    pulmonary, pulmonic cusps Q22.3
    rib Q76.6
        cervical or first (syndrome) Q76.5
    roots (of teeth) K00.2
    spleen Q89.09
    tarsal bones Q74.2
    teeth K00.1
    testis Q55.29
    thumb Q69.1
    toe Q69.2
    uterus Q51.2
    vagina Q52.1
    vertebra Q76.49

 KEY POINT

The alphabetic index in ICD-10-CM functions similarly to the alphabetic index in ICD-9-CM, as the initial point of reference for proper code selection. Always refer to the tabular list to complete accurate code assignment.

ICD-10 Code Structure

All codes in ICD-10 and ICD-10-CM are alphanumeric as opposed to the strictly numeric characters in the main classification of ICD-9-CM. Of the 26 available letters, all but the letter U are used, which is reserved for additions and changes that may need to be incorporated in the future or for classification difficulties that may arise between revisions. Codes for terrorism were created after September 11, 2001, within the framework of ICD-10 and ICD-9-CM. They have been incorporated into ICD-9-CM since 2002 and proposed for implementation in ICD-10 as U codes for terrorism and have not officially been adopted by WHO. If the codes are to be adopted, they will be identified as U.S. codes by an asterisk to distinguish them from official ICD codes.

In ICD-10-CM, external causes due to acts of terrorism are classified to code category Y38. This category includes seven-character codes that identify injuries resulting from acts of terrorism, defined as "the unlawful use of force or violence against persons or property to intimidate or coerce a government, the civilian population, or any segment thereof, in furtherance of political or social objective." An additional code from category Y92 should be assigned to specify place of occurrence. The seventh character reports the encounter as A (Initial encounter), D (Subsequent encounter), or S (Sequela).

Y 38   Terrorism

> **NOTE** These codes are for use to identify injuries resulting from the unlawful use of force or violence against persons or property to intimidate or coerce a Government, the civilian population, or any segment thereof, in furtherance of political or social objective
>
> Use additional code for place of occurrence (Y92.-)
>
> The appropriate 7th character is to be added to each code from category Y38.
>
> **A   initial encounter**
> **D   subsequent encounter**
> **S   sequela**

The code structures of ICD-9-CM and ICD-10-CM are similar in that each classification system is maintained to be as congruent with the other as possible, pending transition. As ICD-9-CM expands its classification and code structure, ICD-10-CM is similarly expanded and maintained.

Though the use of alpha characters I and O may be confused with numbers 1 and Ø, coders should remember that the first character in ICD-10-CM is *always* a letter. The second character is a numeral, followed by either a numeral or alpha character in the third character space. Codes may also contain an alpha character in the seventh character position or a reserve subclassification, denoted as "X."

ICD-9-CM

Diseases of Arteries, Arterioles, and Capillaries (44Ø–449)

44Ø	**Atherosclerosis**
441	**Aortic aneurysm and dissection**
442	**Other aneurysm**
443	**Other peripheral vascular disease**
444	**Arterial embolism and thrombosis**
445	**Atheroembolism**
446	**Polyarteritis nodosa and allied conditions**

447	Other disorders of arteries and arterioles
448	Disease of capillaries
449	Septic arterial embolism

ICD-10-CM

Diseases of Arteries, Arterioles and Capillaries (I70–I79)

I70	Atherosclerosis
I71	Aortic aneurysm and dissection
I72	Other aneurysm
I73	Other peripheral vascular diseases
I74	Arterial embolism and thrombosis
I75	Atheroembolism
I76	Septic arterial embolism
I77	Other disorders of arteries and arterioles
I78	Diseases of capillaries
I79	Disorders of arteries, arterioles and capillaries in diseases classified elsewhere

ICD-10 Category Restructuring

The review of the different diseases and how they are classified in ICD-9 resulted in the restructuring of some of the categories in ICD-10.

ICD-9-CM

In ICD-9-CM, a fifth digit in categories 433 and 434 identifies whether cerebral infarction is present. The three-digit category description identifies the condition to general anatomic sites as precerebral or cerebral. The fourth-digit subclassifications either further specify type of occlusion (434) or anatomic site (433).

> The following fifth-digit subclassification is for use with category 433:
> | 0 | without mention of cerebral infarction |
> | 1 | with cerebral infarction |

| 433 | Occlusion and stenosis of precerebral arteries |
| | 433.2 | Vertebral artery |

ICD-10

In ICD-10, category I63 includes occlusion and stenosis of cerebral and precerebral arteries, resulting in cerebral infarction.

I63	Cerebral infarction
	I63.0	Cerebral infarction due to thrombosis of precerebral arteries
	I63.1	Cerebral infarction due to embolism of precerebral arteries
	I63.2	Cerebral infarction due to unspecified occlusion or stenosis of precerebral arteries
	I63.3	Cerebral infarction due to thrombosis of cerebral arteries
	I63.4	Cerebral infarction due to embolism of cerebral arteries
	I63.5	Cerebral infarction due to unspecified occlusion or stenosis of cerebral arteries
	I63.6	Cerebral infarction due to cerebral venous thrombosis, nonpyogenic
	I63.8	Other cerebral infarction
	I63.9	Cerebral infarction, unspecified

ICD-10-CM

In ICD-10-CM, further data granularity is incorporated to identify the affected artery (specific anatomic site) and laterality (left, right, or unspecified).

I63.0	**Cerebral infarction due to thrombosis of precerebral arteries**	
	I63.00	**Cerebral infarction due to thrombosis of unspecified precerebral artery**
	I63.01	**Cerebral infarction due to thrombosis of vertebral artery**
		I63.011	**Cerebral infarction due to thrombosis of right vertebral artery**
		I63.012	**Cerebral infarction due to thrombosis of left vertebral artery**
		I63.019	**Cerebral infarction due to thrombosis of unspecified vertebral artery**

KEY POINT

E codes of ICD-9-CM become V codes, W codes, X codes, and Y codes in ICD-10. ICD-9-CM's V codes become Z codes in ICD-10.

ICD-10-CM Codes

V03.10XA	Pedestrian on foot injured in collision with car, pick-up truck or van in traffic accident, initial encounter
W52.XXXS	Crushed, pushed or stepped on by crowd or human stampede, sequelae
X37.0XXA	Hurricane, initial encounter
Y65.2	Failure in suture or ligature during surgical operation
Z80.49	Family history of malignant neoplasm of other genital organs

GENERAL ORGANIZATION OF ICD-10

In ICD-10, a chapter may encompass more than one letter and more than one chapter may share a letter.

- Chapter 2—Neoplasms (C00–D49)
- Chapter 3—Diseases of the Blood and Blood-Forming Organs and Certain Disorders Involving the Immune Mechanism (D50–D89)

Organizational Changes

The tabular list comprises 21 chapters versus the 17 main chapters and two supplementary classifications (V and E codes) for ICD-9-CM. As in ICD-9-CM, many of the chapters classify diseases of an organ or system. Others are devoted to specific types of conditions grouped according to etiology or nature (e.g., neoplasms, referred to in ICD-10 as "special group" chapters). Three chapters do not fall into either of these categories.

KEY POINT

The three chapters that do not fall into either the body system or the "special groups" are: "Symptoms, Signs and Abnormal Clinical and Laboratory Findings, Not Elsewhere Classified"; "External Causes of Morbidity"; and "Factors Influencing Health Status and Contact with Health Services."

The revision of a chapter's title may have occurred for a variety of reasons. For example, the term "Complications of…" has been removed from the title of the pregnancy chapter as a number of categories in this chapter describe uncomplicated deliveries.

ICD-9-CM

Classification of Diseases and Injuries

1. **Infectious and Parasitic Diseases (001–139)**
2. **Neoplasms (140–239)**
3. **Endocrine, Nutritional and Metabolic Diseases, and Immunity Disorders (240–279)**
4. **Diseases of the Blood and Blood-Forming Organs (280–289)**
5. **Mental, Behavioral, and Neurodevelopmental Disorders (290–319)**
6. **Diseases of the Nervous System and Sense Organs (320–389)**
7. **Diseases of the Circulatory System (390–459)**
8. **Diseases of the Respiratory System (460–519)**
9. **Diseases of the Digestive System (520–579)**
10. **Diseases of the Genitourinary System (580–629)**
11. **Complications of Pregnancy, Childbirth, and the Puerperium (630–679)**
12. **Diseases of the Skin and Subcutaneous Tissue (680–709)**
13. **Diseases of the Musculoskeletal System and Connective Tissue (710–739)**
14. **Congenital Anomalies (740–759)**
15. **Certain Conditions Originating in the Perinatal Period (760–779)**
16. **Symptoms, Signs, and Ill-Defined Conditions (780–799)**

17. **Injury and Poisoning (800–999)**

Supplementary Classification of Factors Influencing Health Status and Contact with Health Services (V01–V91)

Supplementary Classification of External Causes of Injury and Poisoning (E000–E999)

ICD-10-CM

Classification of Diseases and Injuries

1. **Certain Infectious and Parasitic Diseases (A00–B99)**
2. **Neoplasms (C00–D49)**
3. **Diseases of the Blood and Blood-Forming Organs and Certain Disorders Involving the Immune Mechanism (D50–D89)**
4. **Endocrine, Nutritional and Metabolic Diseases (E00–E89)**
5. **Mental, Behavioral, and Neurodevelopmental Disorders (F01–F99)**
6. **Diseases of the Nervous System (G00–G99)**
7. **Diseases of the Eye and Adnexa (H00–H59)**
8. **Diseases of the Ear and Mastoid Process (H60–H95)**
9. **Diseases of the Circulatory System (I00–I99)**
10. **Diseases of the Respiratory System (J00–J99)**
11. **Diseases of the Digestive System (K00–K95)**
12. **Diseases of the Skin and Subcutaneous Tissue (L00–L99)**
13. **Diseases of the Musculoskeletal System and Connective Tissue (M00–M99)**
14. **Diseases of the Genitourinary System (N00–N99)**
15. **Pregnancy, Childbirth and the Puerperium (O00–O9A)**
16. **Certain Conditions Originating in the Perinatal Period (P00–P96)**
17. **Congenital Malformations, Deformations and Chromosomal Abnormalities (Q00–Q99)**
18. **Symptoms, Signs and Abnormal Clinical and Laboratory Findings, Not Elsewhere Classified (R00–R99)**
19. **Injury, Poisoning and Certain Other Consequences of External Causes (S00–T88)**
20. **External Causes of Morbidity (V00–Y99)**
21. **Factors Influencing Health Status and Contact with Health Services (Z00–Z99)**

In contrast to ICD-10-CM, ICD-10 contains the following additional chapter:

22. **Codes for Special Purposes (U00–U99)**

Chapter 20, the "External Causes of Morbidity" and chapter 21, "Factors Influencing Health Status and Contact with Health Services," are no longer considered to be supplementary, but are a part of the core classification.

Certain chapter titles have undergone revisions in ICD-10-CM. For example, the term "certain" is added to the title of chapter 1, "Infectious and Parasitic Diseases" to stress the fact that localized infections are classified with the diseases of the pertinent body system. The title of the ICD-9-CM chapter of congenital anomalies is expanded to include "Congenital Malformations, Deformations and Chromosomal Abnormalities."

There also is a rearrangement of the chapter order from ICD-9-CM to ICD-10-CM. This includes expanding the number of categories for disorders of the immune mechanism and placing them with diseases of the blood and blood-forming organs. In ICD-9-CM, these disorders are included with

KEY POINT

One major difference in ICD-10-CM is that codes will have complete descriptions rather than relying on the hierarchy.

"Endocrine, Nutritional and Metabolic Diseases and Immunity Disorders." The chapters for "Diseases of the Genitourinary System," "Pregnancy, Childbirth and the Puerperium," "Certain Conditions Originating in the Perinatal Period," and "Congenital Malformations, Deformations and Chromosomal Abnormalities" are placed sequentially in ICD-10-CM.

Also, some conditions are reassigned to a different chapter due to advances in medical technology that have led to insights into the origins of those conditions. For example, in ICD-9-CM, gout is classified to chapter 3, "Endocrine, Nutritional and Metabolic Diseases and Immunity Disorders," and in ICD-10-CM, it is classified to chapter 13, "Diseases of the Musculoskeletal System and Connective Tissue." See chapter 4 for more information on disease reclassifications.

NEW FEATURES TO ICD-10-CM

There are a number of new features to ICD-10-CM with which users will need to become familiar. These additions provide clarity and facilitate proper use of the classification.

Code Description Clarity

In ICD-9-CM, often the user must review the description of the category in order to determine the complete intent of the subcategory or subclassification. One needs to review the title of the category to understand the meaning of the code. In ICD-10-CM, the subcategory titles are usually complete, with the exception of some codes in the neoplasm and health circumstances sections.

ICD-9-CM

Typically, in ICD-9-CM, codes are presented in this fashion:

451   **Phlebitis and thrombophlebitis**

     451.0   **Of superficial vessels of lower extremities**

ICD-10-CM

In ICD-10-CM, most codes have complete descriptions:

I80   **Phlebitis and thrombophlebitis**

     I80.0   **Phlebitis and thrombophlebitis of superficial vessels of lower extremities**

         I80.03   **Phlebitis and thrombophlebitis of superficial vessels of lower extremities, bilateral**

Postprocedural Disorders

Categories for postprocedural disorders specific to a particular body system have been created at the end of each body system chapter. There has been no change to the classification of those situations in which postprocedural conditions are not specific to a particular body system, such as postoperative hemorrhage. These are found in ICD-10-CM, chapter 19, "Injury, Poisoning and Certain Other Consequences of External Causes," which is compatible to ICD-9-CM.

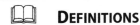

DEFINITIONS

iatrogenic. Adversely induced in the patient; caused by medical treatment.

QUICK TIP

Keep an eye out for the term "iatrogenic" as physicians may use it to describe a postprocedural disorder.

ICD-9-CM

In ICD-9-CM, complications specific to the digestive system are not located under one category.

564   Functional digestive disorders, not elsewhere classified

   564.2   Postgastric surgery syndromes

   564.3   Vomiting following gastrointestinal surgery

   564.4   Other postoperative functional disorders

569   Other disorders of intestine

   569.6   Colostomy and enterostomy complications

       569.60   Colostomy and enterostomy complications, unspecified

       569.61   Infection of colostomy or enterostomy

       569.62   Mechanical complication of colostomy and enterostomy

       569.69   Other complication

   997.4   Digestive system complications

ICD-10-CM

In ICD-10 and ICD-10-CM, complications specific to the digestive system are located under category K91, with specific fourth- and fifth-character subclassifications. The fourth-character subclassifications for category K91 include:

K91   Intraoperative and postprocedural complications and disorders of digestive system, not elsewhere classified

   K91.0   Vomiting following gastrointestinal surgery

   K91.1   Postgastric surgery syndromes

   K91.2   Postsurgical malabsorption, not elsewhere classified

   K91.3   Postprocedural intestinal obstruction

   K91.5   Postcholecystectomy syndrome

   K91.6   Intraoperative hemorrhage and hematoma of a digestive system organ or structure complicating a procedure

   K91.7   Accidental puncture and laceration of a digestive system organ or structure during a procedure

   K91.8   Other intraoperative and postprocedural complications and disorders of digestive system

Notes

The 10th revision contains some changes to instructional notes as well. At the beginning of each chapter, "excludes" notes are expanded to provide guidance on the hierarchy of chapters and to clarify the priority of code assignment.

ICD-10-CM

The following excludes note, found in chapter 14, indicates the priority of the "special group" chapters over the genitourinary system chapter.

Diseases of the Genitourinary System (N00–N99)

EXCLUDES 2   *certain conditions originating in the perinatal period (P04–P96)*
certain infectious and parasitic diseases (A00–B99)
complications of pregnancy, childbirth and the puerperium (O00–O9A)
congenital malformations, deformations and chromosomal abnormalities (Q00–Q99)
endocrine, nutritional and metabolic diseases (E00–E88)
injury, poisoning and certain other consequences of external causes (S00–T88)
neoplasms (C00–D49)
symptoms, signs and abnormal clinical and laboratory findings, not elsewhere classified (R00–R94)

 KEY POINT

"Excludes" notes are expanded in ICD-10 to clarify priority of code assignment and to provide guidance.

ICD-10-CM Blocks

After the appropriate includes and excludes notes, each chapter starts with a list of the subchapters, "code families" or "blocks" of three-character categories. These blocks provide an overview of the structure of the chapter.

For example, the blocks for chapter 14 are:

N00–N08	**Glomerular diseases**
N10–N16	**Renal tubulo-interstitial diseases**
N17–N19	**Acute kidney failure and chronic kidney disease**
N20–N23	**Urolithiasis**
N25–N29	**Other disorders of kidney and ureter**
N30–N39	**Other diseases of the urinary system**
N40–N53	**Diseases of male genital organs**
N60–N65	**Disorders of breast**
N70–N77	**Inflammatory diseases of female pelvic organs**
N80–N98	**Noninflammatory disorders of female genital tract**
N99	**Intraoperative and postprocedural complications and disorders of genitourinary system, not elsewhere classified**

SIGNIFICANT CHANGES TO ICD-10

Historically, three chapters in particular have had significant structural changes in the manner in which codes are "blocked" or grouped into sections and, therefore, classified:

- Chapter 5—Mental, Behavioral, and Neurodevelopmental Disorders
- Chapter 19—Injury, Poisoning and Certain Other Consequences of External Causes
- Chapter 20—External Causes of Morbidity

Because major changes were made to these chapters, field-testing took place in a number of countries. In addition, WHO depended on technical support from specific groups in the revision. For example, the Nordic Medical Statistics Committee (NOMESCO) and the WHO Global Steering Committee on the Development of Indicators for Accidents had a major influence on the revision of the classification of injuries and external causes.

Chapter 5. Mental, Behavioral, and Neurodevelopmental Disorders

Chapter 5 has undergone a number of revisions. The title changed from "Mental Disorders" in ICD-9-CM, to "Mental and Behavioral Disorders" in ICD-10. Recent updates standardized chapter titles for both ICD-9-CM and ICD-10-CM to "Mental, Behavioral, and Neurodevelopmental Disorders," to more accurately represent classification content.

Next, the number of subchapters was expanded from three to 11.

ICD-9-CM

Chapter 5. Mental Disorders (290–319)

Psychoses (290–299)

Neurotic Disorders, Personality Disorders, and Other Nonpsychotic Mental Disorders (300–316)

Intellectual Disabilities (317–319)

ICD-10

Chapter 5. Mental and Behavioural Disorders

F00–F09	Organic, including symptomatic, mental disorders
F10–F19	Mental and behavioural disorders due to psychoactive substance use
F20–F29	Schizophrenia, schizotypal and delusional disorders
F30–F39	Mood [affective] disorders
F40–F48	Neurotic, stress-related and somatoform disorders
F50–F59	Behavioural syndromes associated with physiological disturbances and physical factors
F60–F69	Disorders of adult personality and behaviour
F70–F79	Mental retardation
F80–F89	Disorders of psychological development
F90–F98	Behavioural and emotional disorders with onset usually occurring in childhood and adolescence
F99	Unspecified mental disorder

With this expansion, ICD-10 arranges specific disorders differently than they were in ICD-9-CM, and the clinical detail is also expanded.

ICD-10-CM

Chapter 5. Mental, Behavioral, and Neurodevelopmental Disorders

F01–F09	Mental disorders due to known physiological conditions
F10–F19	Mental and behavioral disorders due to psychoactive substance use
F20–F29	Schizophrenia, schizotypal, delusional, and other non-mood psychotic disorders
F30–F39	Mood [affective] disorders
F40–F48	Anxiety, dissociative, stress-related, somatoform and other nonpsychotic mental disorders
F50–F59	Behavioral syndromes associated with physiological disturbances and physical factors
F60–F69	Disorders of adult personality and behavior
F70–F79	Intellectual disabilities
F80–F89	Pervasive and specific developmental disorders
F90–F98	Behavioral and emotional disorders with onset usually occurring in childhood and adolescence
F99	Unspecified mental disorder

In the development of ICD-10-CM, some of the block titles and ranges within these chapters have been changed. For example:

 FOR MORE INFO

ICD-10-CM includes additional revisions to the categories for drug-induced mental and behavioral disorders due to psychoactive substance use.

ICD-9-CM

The ninth revision includes codes for a certain number of conditions that are drug induced.

292   **Drug-induced mental disorders**

     292.0   **Drug withdrawal**

     292.1   **Drug induced psychotic disorders**

         292.11   **Drug induced psychotic disorder with delusions**

         292.12   **Drug induced psychotic disorder with hallucinations**

     292.2   **Pathological drug intoxication**

     292.8   **Other specified drug induced mental disorders**

         292.81   **Drug induced delirium**

         292.82   **Drug induced persisting dementia**

         292.83   **Drug induced persisting amnestic disorder**

         292.84   **Drug induced mood disorder**

         292.85   **Drug induced sleep disorders**

         292.89   **Other**

     292.9   **Unspecified drug-induced mental disorder**

ICD-10

In ICD-10, a number of categories are available to specify the drug-induced mental and behavioral disorders due to psychoactive substance use. In addition, there are 10 fourth-character subdivisions to use with these categories to identify the specific mental and behavioral disorder, such as withdrawal state (.3) or withdrawal state with delirium (.4).

Mental and Behavioural Disorders Due to Psychoactive Substance Use (F10–F19)

F10	**Mental and behavioural disorders due to use of alcohol**
F11	**Mental and behavioural disorders due to use of opioids**
F12	**Mental and behavioural disorders due to use of cannabinoids**
F13	**Mental and behavioural disorders due to use of sedatives or hypnotics**
F14	**Mental and behavioural disorders due to use of cocaine**
F15	**Mental and behavioural disorders due to use of other stimulants, including caffeine**
F16	**Mental and behavioural disorders due to use of hallucinogens**
F17	**Mental and behavioural disorders due to use of tobacco**
F18	**Mental and behavioural disorders due to use of volatile solvents**
F19	**Mental and behavioural disorders due to multiple drug use and use of other psychoactive substances**

ICD-10-CM

ICD-10-CM includes additional revisions to this subchapter: Three other fourth-character subdivisions (except F17) identify abuse (.1), dependence (.2), or unspecified use (.9). Fifth- and sixth-character subdivisions further specify the state of the mental and behavioral disorder, such as intoxication, intoxication with delirium, psychotic disorder with hallucinations, remission, or withdrawal.

Mental and behavioral disorders due to psychoactive substance use (F10–F19)

F10	Alcohol related disorders
F11	Opioid related disorders
F12	Cannabis related disorders
F13	Sedative, hypnotic, or anxiolytic related disorders
F14	Cocaine related disorders
F15	Other stimulant related disorders
F16	Hallucinogen related disorders
F17	Nicotine dependence
F18	Inhalant related disorders
F19	Other psychoactive substance related disorders

Chapter 19. Injury, Poisoning, and Certain Other Consequences of External Causes

The axis of classification for chapter 19, "Injury, Poisoning and Certain Other Consequences of External Causes" (chapter 17, "Injury and Poisoning," in ICD-9-CM) changed from "type of injury" and "site of injury" in ICD-9-CM to "body region" and "type of injury" in ICD-10.

ICD-9-CM

"Fractures" is the first subchapter in the "Injury and Poisoning" chapter of ICD-9-CM. The breakdown is then by site (e.g., vault of skull, base of skull).

Chapter 17. Injury and Poisoning

Fractures (800–829)

Fracture of Skull (800–804)

800	Fracture of vault of skull
801	Fracture of base of skull
802	Fracture of face bones
803	Other and unqualified skull fractures
804	Multiple fractures involving skull or face with other bones

ICD-10

Chapter 19 in ICD-10 is a large chapter. It spans two letters, S00–T88. The S codes cover different injury types in relation to a particular, single body region, and the T codes cover injuries to unspecified or multiple body regions, poisonings, burns, frostbite, complications of care, and other consequences of external causes. The chapter, "Injury, Poisoning and Certain Other Consequences of External Causes" describes injuries to the head (the body region) and then breaks down the injury by type, (e.g., superficial injury of head, open wound of head).

Chapter 19. Injury, Poisoning and Certain Other Consequences of External Causes

Injuries to the Head (S00–S09)

S00	Superficial injury of head
S01	Open wound of head
S02	Fracture of skull and facial bones

S03	**Dislocation, sprain and strain of joints and ligaments of head**
S04	**Injury of cranial nerve**
S05	**Injury of eye and orbit**
S06	**Intracranial injury**
S07	**Crushing injury of head**
S08	**Traumatic amputation of part of head**
S09	**Other and unspecified injuries of head**

Categories SØ3 and SØ8 have undergone title changes in ICD-10-CM:

S03	**Dislocation and sprain of joints and ligaments of head**
S08	**Avulsion and traumatic amputation of part of head**

Chapter 20. External Causes of Morbidity and Mortality

The chapter for external causes of morbidity and mortality also has been changed in a number of ways. In ICD-9-CM, the supplementary classification of external causes of injury and poisoning (E codes) is found at the end of the tabular list. In ICD-10, these codes follow chapter 19, "Injury, Poisoning and Certain Other Consequences of External Causes," and consist of categories VØØ–Y99. In addition, the transport accidents section of the external causes chapter has been completely revised and extended with blocks of categories identifying the victim's mode of transport.

ICD-9-CM

In ICD-9-CM, the main axis is whether the event was a traffic or nontraffic accident.

**Supplementary Classification of External Causes
of Injury and Poisoning (E800–E999)**

Railway accidents (E800–E807)

Motor vehicle traffic accidents (E810–E819)

Motor vehicle nontraffic accidents (E820–E825)

Other road vehicle accidents (E826–E829)

ICD-10

In ICD-10 and ICD-10-CM, the main axis is the injured person's mode of transport. For land transport accidents, categories VØ1–V89, the vehicle of which the injured person is an occupant, or pedestrian status, is identified in the first two characters since it is perceived as the essential issue for prevention purposes. In ICD-10-CM, an additional category, VØØ, identifies pedestrian conveyance accidents due to falls, collisions with stationary objects, or other accidents not occurring with land transport vehicles.

Chapter 2Ø. External Causes of Morbidity and Mortality (VØ1–Y98)

V01–X58	**Accidents**
V01–V99	**Transport accidents**
V01–V09	**Pedestrian injured in transport accident**
V10–V19	**Pedal cyclist injured in transport accident**
V20–V29	**Motorcycle rider injured in transport accident**
V30–V39	**Occupant of three-wheeled motor vehicle injured in transport accident**

DEFINITIONS

classification. The systematic arrangement, based on established criteria, of similar entities. ICD-10 is a disease classification. The particular criterion on which the arrangement is based is called the axis of classification. The primary axis of the disease classification as a whole is by anatomy. Other axes have been used, such as etiology and morphology.

V40–V49	Car occupant injured in transport accident
V50–V59	Occupant of pick-up truck or van injured in transport accident
V60–V69	Occupant of heavy transport vehicle injured in transport accident
V70–V79	Bus occupant injured in transport accident
V80–V89	Other land transport accidents
V90–V94	Water transport accidents
V95–V97	Air and space transport accidents
V98–V99	Other and unspecified transport accidents

Another change to this chapter is to the codes for sequelae of external causes. Previously, late-effect codes for external causes were located in various subchapters throughout the supplementary classification. In ICD-10, all late effects for each intent (e.g., accidents, suicide, etc.) have been brought together in a block (subchapter), "Sequelae of External Causes of Morbidity and Mortality" (Y85–Y89). In ICD-10-CM, these are identified by the use of the alpha extensor for sequelae ("S") added to the code.

ICD-9-CM

E929	Late effects of accidental injury
E959	Late effects of self-inflicted injury
E969	Late effects of injury purposely inflicted by other person
E977	Late effects of injuries due to legal intervention
E989	Late effects of injury, undetermined whether accidentally or purposely inflicted
E999	Late effect of injury due to war operations and terrorism

ICD-10

Sequelae of External Causes of Morbidity and Mortality (Y85–Y89)

Y85	Sequelae of transport accidents
Y86	Sequelae of other accidents
Y87	Sequelae of intentional self-harm, assault and events of undetermined intent
Y88	Sequelae with surgical and medical care as external cause
Y89	Sequelae of other external causes

ICD-10-CM

T47.7X2S	Poisoning by emetics, intentional self-harm, sequela
T48.995S	Adverse effect of other agents primarily acting on the respiratory system, sequela
V43.51S	Car driver injured in collision with sport utility vehicle in traffic accident, sequela
V90.02S	Drowning and submersion due to fishing boat overturning, sequela
W55.01S	Bitten by cat, sequela
Y04.0S	Assault by unarmed brawl or fight, sequela

 DEFINITIONS

late effect. Abnormality, dysfunction, or other residual condition produced after the acute phase of an illness, injury, or disease is over. There is no time limit on when late effects can appear.

MODIFICATION OF ICD-10

At the International Conference for the Tenth Revision of the International Classification of Diseases, a recommendation was made that World Health Organization (WHO) should endorse the concept of an updating process between revisions. Prior to this time there was no provision for updating the ICD between revisions. In October 1997, a mechanism was finalized to put an update process into operation. The nine WHO collaborating centers for classification of diseases and an update reference committee have been identified as coordinators and reviewers of proposed updates. With a timeline for issuance of amendments established, one should expect to see modifications to ICD-10 coming from the secretariat at WHO.

History of the Modification

In May of 1994, the Centers for Disease Control and Prevention published an ICD-10 request for proposal (RFP). The contract sought the answer to the following questions:

- Is ICD-10 such a significant improvement over ICD-9-CM for morbidity classification that it should be implemented in the United States?

- Are there any codes or concepts in ICD-9-CM that have not been and should be included in ICD-10?

To answer these questions, the RFP required the contractor to perform an in-depth analysis addressing the following issues and to present recommendations in a report:

- Strengths and weaknesses of ICD-10 as compared with ICD-9-CM for data collection on:
    - risk factors
    - severity of illness
    - primary care encounters
    - preventive health requirements
    - any other topics important to morbidity, as opposed to mortality, reporting
- Compatibility of the ICD-10 and ICD-9-CM codes for diagnosis, health status (V codes), and external cause (E codes)

- Ease of use of the ICD system

- Adaptability to computerized patient records

- Identification and review of improvements

- Review of and recommendations for change in the tabular notes

- Alternatives to the dagger/asterisk for morbidity application (this system helps identify secondary diagnoses)

- Review of the tabular section and index with an emphasis on whether the category assignments, which are based on mortality, remain appropriate for morbidity

- If the categories are different between ICD-9-CM and ICD-10, determination of what the impact would be on trend analysis

 FOR MORE INFO

The WHO collaborating center for classification of diseases for the United States is the National Center for Health Statistics, 6525 Belcrest Road, Hyattsville, Maryland 20872.

In September 1994, the Center for Health Policy Studies (CHPS) was awarded the contract to perform the in-depth evaluation of ICD-10. Phase 1 of the contract consisted of describing how significant the modifications to ICD-10 were expected to be and, if made, how such revisions would impact comparability between the two systems. Any problems identified were to be accompanied by solutions. The development of a revised alphabetic index and crosswalk between ICD-9-CM and ICD-10-CM was also a part of phase 1.

Phase 1

The contractor formed the Technical Advisory Panel (TAP) to perform the evaluation. The 20 members came from the health care and coding community. They included federal members from the Agency for Health Care Policy and Research (CMS and NCHS), nonfederal members from the hospital and physician environment, and classification experts. After evaluating ICD-10, CHPS provided the following goals for a clinical modification of ICD-10:

- Return to the level of specificity implemented in ICD-9-CM

- Facilitate alphabetic index use to assign codes

- Modify code titles and language to enhance consistency with accepted U.S. clinical practice

- Modify the dagger and asterisk codes

- Remove codes unique to mortality coding and those designed for the needs of emerging nations

- Remove procedure codes included with diagnosis codes

- Remove "multiple codes"

In answer to the main questions posed in the evaluation contract, CHPS indicated that ICD-10 is not a significant improvement over ICD-9-CM for morbidity classification, and that a clinical modification should be implemented in the United States that would include the codes or concepts lacking in ICD-10.

Phase 2

Phase 2 consisted of further refinement of the clinical modification based on the draft created under the evaluation study. Since WHO holds a copyright on ICD-10, there are specific rules regarding changes. WHO requirements include the following:

- Title changes cannot alter the meaning of the category or code.

- There must be limited modifications to the three- and four-character codes.

During this phase, ICD-10 was looked at from the standpoint of creating codes for ambulatory and managed-care encounters, clinical decision making, and outcomes research. This phase also involved a review by physician groups and others to ensure clinical accuracy. The reviewers for this phase included the following:

- American Academy of Pediatrics

- American Academy of Neurology

- American College of Obstetricians and Gynecologists

- American Urological Association

- National Association of Children's Hospitals and Related Institutions
- American Burn Association
- The Burn Foundation
- ANSI Z16.2 Workgroup
- American Academy of Dermatology
- CDC Diabetes Education Program
- National Center for Injury Prevention and Control
- National Center for Infectious Diseases
- National Center for Chronic Disease Prevention and Health Promotion
- Veterans Administration's National Diabetes Program

 DEFINITIONS

residual category. Place for classifying a specified form of a condition that does not have its own specific subdivision.

During phase 2, focused reviews were performed. This examination included the evaluation of residual categories to decide if further specificity was needed. An analysis also was made of previous ICD-9-CM coordination and maintenance committee recommendations where adoption was not possible due to ICD-9-CM space limitations.

Phase 3

The third phase involved a review of the public comments on the proposed ICD-10-CM released to the public in the winter of 1997. More than 1,200 comments from more than 20 organizations were received. Phase 3 reviewers included the American Academy of Ophthalmology, American Academy of Orthopaedic Surgeons, Johns Hopkins Injury Center, and Pennsylvania Head Injury Center.

As a result of these three phases, there were thousands of clinical modifications made to ICD-10.

Fourth-, Fifth-, Sixth-, and Seventh-Character Addition

To be able to have the desired specificity, fifth, sixth, and seventh characters were added throughout the classification. These characters may identify such things as more specificity about a disorder, whether the patient's condition exists on the right or left side, the trimester in which the patient is experiencing problems, and whether the encounter was initial, subsequent, or with sequela. The following is an example of added specificity at the fifth character:

ICD-10

P78.8 Other specified perinatal digestive system disorders

ICD-10-CM

P78.8 Other specified perinatal digestive system disorders
P78.81 Congenital cirrhosis (of liver)
P78.82 Peptic ulcer of newborn
P78.89 Other specified perinatal digestive system disorders

A sample of the trimester specified with a sixth character follows:

ICD-10

O99.0 **Anemia complicating pregnancy, childbirth and the puerperium**

ICD-10-CM

O99.0 **Anemia complicating pregnancy, childbirth and the puerperium**

    O99.01 **Anemia complicating pregnancy**

        O99.011 **Anemia complicating pregnancy, first trimester**

        O99.012 **Anemia complicating pregnancy, second trimester**

        O99.013 **Anemia complicating pregnancy, third trimester**

        O99.019 **Anemia complicating pregnancy, unspecified trimester**

The following examples demonstrate laterality at the sixth-character level and the encounter status in the seventh character:

ICD-10

S72 **Fracture of femur**

    S72.0 **Fracture of neck of femur**

        S72.00 **Closed fracture of neck of femur**

ICD-10-CM

S72 **Fracture of femur**

    S72.0 **Fracture of head and neck of femur**

        S72.00 **Fracture of unspecified part of neck of femur**

            S72.001 **Fracture of unspecified part of neck of right femur**

                S72.001A **Fracture of unspecified part of neck of right femur, initial encounter for closed fracture**

                S72.001B **Fracture of unspecified part of neck of right femur, initial encounter for open fracture type I or II**

                S72.001C **Fracture of unspecified part of neck of right femur, initial encounter for open fracture type IIIA, IIIB, or IIIC**

                S72.001D **Fracture of unspecified part of neck of right femur, subsequent encounter for closed fracture with routine healing**

                S72.001E **Fracture of unspecified part of neck of right femur, subsequent encounter for open fracture type I or II with routine healing**

                S72.001F **Fracture of unspecified part of neck of right femur, subsequent encounter for open fracture type IIIA, IIIB, or IIIC with routine healing**

                S72.001G **Fracture of unspecified part of neck of right femur, subsequent encounter for closed fracture with delayed healing**

                S72.001H **Fracture of unspecified part of neck of right femur, subsequent encounter for open fracture type I or II with delayed healing**

S72.001J	Fracture of unspecified part of neck of right femur, subsequent encounter for open fracture type IIIA, IIIB, or IIIC with delayed healing
S72.001K	Fracture of unspecified part of neck of right femur, subsequent encounter for closed fracture with nonunion
S72.001M	Fracture of unspecified part of neck of right femur, subsequent encounter for open fracture type I or II with nonunion
S72.001N	Fracture of unspecified part of neck of right femur, subsequent encounter for open fracture type IIIA, IIIB, or IIIC with nonunion
S72.001P	Fracture of unspecified part of neck of right femur, subsequent encounter for closed fracture with malunion
S72.001Q	Fracture of unspecified part of neck of right femur, subsequent encounter for open fracture type I or II with malunion
S72.001R	Fracture of unspecified part of neck of right femur, subsequent encounter for open fracture type IIIA, IIIB, or IIIC with malunion
S72.001S	Fracture of unspecified part of neck of right femur, sequela

INCORPORATION OF COMMON SUBCLASSIFICATIONS

In ICD-10, fourth- and fifth-character subdivisions were often provided for optional use. In ICD-10-CM these subdivisions are incorporated into the code listing, thus making them a required component of the code's use. In addition, full code titles are adopted in ICD-10-CM to provide a clear understanding of the code's meaning.

ICD-10

S52   Fracture of forearm

The following subdivisions are provided for optional use in a supplementary character position where it is not possible or not desired to use multiple coding to identify fracture and open wound; a fracture not indicated as closed or open should be classified as closed.

0	closed
1	open

EXCLUDES   *fracture at wrist and hand level (S62.-)*

S52.0   Fracture of upper end of ulna
Coronoid process
Elbow NOS
Monteggia's fracture-dislocation
Olecranon process
Proximal end

ICD-10-CM

S52 Fracture of forearm

> **NOTE** A fracture not identified as displaced or nondisplaced should be coded to displaced.
>
> A fracture not designated as open or closed should be coded to closed.
>
> The open fracture designations are based on the Gustilo open fracture classification.

> **EXCLUDES 1** *traumatic amputation of forearm (S58.-)*

> **EXCLUDES 2** *fracture at wrist and hand level (S62.-)*

The appropriate 7th character is to be added to each code from category S52.

- **A** initial encounter for closed fracture
- **B** initial encounter for open fracture type I or II
- **C** initial encounter for open fracture type IIIA, IIIB, or IIIC
- **D** subsequent encounter for closed fracture with routine healing
- **E** subsequent encounter for open fracture type I or II with routine healing
- **F** subsequent encounter for open fracture type IIIA, IIIB, or IIIC with routine healing
- **G** subsequent encounter for closed fracture with delayed healing
- **H** subsequent encounter for open fracture type I or II with delayed healing
- **J** subsequent encounter for open fracture type IIIA, IIIB, or IIIC with delayed healing
- **K** subsequent encounter for closed fracture with nonunion
- **M** subsequent encounter for open fracture type I or II with nonunion
subsequent encounter for open fracture type IIIA, IIIB, or IIIC with nonunion
- **P** subsequent encounter for closed fracture with malunion
- **Q** subsequent encounter for open fracture type I or II with malunion
- **R** subsequent encounter for open fracture type IIIA, IIIB, or IIIC with malunion
- **S** sequela

S52.0 Fracture of upper end of ulna
Fracture of proximal end of ulna

> **EXCLUDES 2** *fracture of elbow NOS (S42.40-)*
> *Fractures of shaft of ulna (S52.2-)*

S52.00 Unspecified fracture of upper end of ulna

- **S52.001** Unspecified fracture of upper end of right ulna
- **S52.002** Unspecified fracture of upper end of left ulna
- **S52.009** Unspecified fracture of upper end of unspecified ulna

S52.01 Torus fracture of upper end of ulna

The appropriate 7th character is to be added to all codes in subcategory S52.01

- **A** initial encounter for closed fracture
- **D** subsequent encounter for fracture with routine healing
- **G** subsequent encounter for fracture with delayed healing
- **K** subsequent encounter for fracture with nonunion
- **P** subsequent encounter for fracture with malunion
- **S** sequela

- **S52.011** Torus fracture of upper end of right ulna
- **S52.012** Torus fracture of upper end of left ulna
- **S52.019** Torus fracture of upper end of unspecified ulna

---

KEY POINT

The modifications to ICD-10 will provide the detail required for morbidity coding in the United States, thereby meeting the goal for more comprehensive and qualitative patient data for all uses and users.

Laterality

In the past, there have been proposals to the ICD-9-CM coordination and maintenance committee to add laterality codes (i.e., right, left, or bilateral). This has been done in ICD-10-CM; however, ICD-10-CM does not add laterality in all cases. Many codes affected by this modification are found in the neoplasm and injury chapters.

ICD-10

C56   Malignant neoplasm of ovary

ICD-10-CM

C56   Malignant neoplasm of ovary
Use additional code to identify any functional activity

C56.0   Malignant neoplasm of right ovary

C56.1   Malignant neoplasm of left ovary

C56.9   Malignant neoplasm of ovary, unspecified side

Trimester Specificity Obstetrical Coding

Neither ICD-9 nor ICD-10 expands the codes in the "Pregnancy, Childbirth and the Puerperium" chapter to specify circumstances surrounding the pregnancy. In ICD-9-CM, a fifth-digit subdivision denotes the current episode of care. The episode of care is defined as the encounter in which the patient is receiving care, whether delivery occurred during that encounter, or an antepartum or postpartum condition is being treated without delivery occurring during that episode of care. The fifth digits from ICD-9-CM were not adopted for ICD-10-CM. Instead, the last character in the code reports the patient's trimester. Because certain obstetric conditions or complications occur at only one point in the obstetric period, not all codes will include all three trimesters or a character to describe the trimester at all.

ICD-10

O60   Preterm labour
Onset (spontaneous) of labour before 37 completed weeks of gestation.

ICD-10-CM

O60   Preterm labor
INCLUDES onset (spontaneous) of labor before 37 completed weeks of gestation
EXCLUDES1 false labor (O47.0-)
threatened labor NOS (O47.0-)

O60.0   Preterm labor without delivery

O60.00   Preterm labor without delivery, unspecified trimester

O60.02   Preterm labor without delivery, second trimester

O60.03   Preterm labor without delivery, third trimester

Expansion of Alcohol and Drug Codes

Although ICD-10 had already made major changes to chapter 5, "Mental and Behavioural Disorders," analysis of the codes for disorders due to alcohol and drug use has resulted in further modifications. The ICD-10 codes were reviewed for ways to better describe these disorders due to psychoactive substance use.

The result is the identification of the effects of use (e.g., abuse and dependence) at the fourth-character level, the specific aspects to the use (e.g., withdrawal), at

---

 CLINICAL NOTE

The first trimester is the period of pregnancy from the first day of the last normal menstrual period through the completion of 13 weeks of gestation. The second trimester is the period of pregnancy from the beginning of the 14th through the 27th completed week of gestation. The third trimester is the period of pregnancy from the beginning of the 28th week until delivery.

DEFINITIONS

trimester. Period of three months.

---

the fifth-character level, and some of the manifestations (e.g., delirium), at the sixth-character level.

ICD-10

F10.-   Mental and behavioural disorders due to use of alcohol
- .0   Acute intoxication
- .1   Harmful use
- .2   Dependence syndrome
- .3   Withdrawal state
- .4   Withdrawal state with delirium
- .5   Psychotic disorder
- .6   Amnesic syndrome
- .7   Residual and late-onset psychotic disorder
- .8   Other mental and behavioural disorders
- .9   Unspecified mental and behavioural disorder

ICD-10-CM

F10   Alcohol related disorders

Use additional code for blood alcohol level, if applicable (Y90.-)

F10.1   Alcohol abuse

> **EXCLUDES 1**   alcohol dependence (F10.2-)
> alcohol use, unspecified (F10.9-)

F10.10   Alcohol abuse, uncomplicated

F10.12   Alcohol abuse with intoxication

> **F10.120   Alcohol abuse with intoxication, uncomplicated**
>
> **F10.121   Alcohol abuse with intoxication delirium**
>
> **F10.129   Alcohol abuse with intoxication, unspecified**

F10.14   Alcohol abuse with alcohol-induced mood disorder

F10.15   Alcohol abuse with alcohol-induced psychotic disorder

> **F10.150   Alcohol abuse with alcohol-induced psychotic disorder with delusions**
>
> **F10.151   Alcohol abuse with alcohol-induced psychotic disorder with hallucinations**
>
> **F10.159   Alcohol abuse with alcohol-induced psychotic disorder, unspecified**

F10.18   Alcohol abuse with other alcohol-induced disorders

> **F10.180   Alcohol abuse with alcohol-induced anxiety disorder**
>
> **F10.181   Alcohol abuse with alcohol-induced sexual dysfunction**
>
> **F10.182   Alcohol abuse with alcohol-induced sleep disorder**
>
> **F10.188   Alcohol abuse with other alcohol-induced disorder**

F10.19   Alcohol abuse with unspecified alcohol-induced disorder

---

KEY POINT

In ICD-10-CM, the sixth character may identify:
- Trimester
- Laterality
- Certain manifestations

Expansion of Injury Codes

To further enhance the restructuring of chapter 19, "Injury, Poisoning and Certain Other Consequences of External Causes," ICD-10-CM will provide codes to further specify the type and site of the injury. Also, as mentioned previously, subdivisions have been incorporated into the code listing, thus making them a required component of the code's use.

KEY POINT

Health care providers will need to be educated on the additional details required to be documented in the medical record in order to code injuries. For example, with the reporting of laterality, providers will need to document where the injury occurred.

ICD-10

S51   Open wound of forearm

> **EXCLUDES 1**   *open wound of wrist and hand (S61.-)*
> *traumatic amputation of forearm (S58.-)*

S51.Ø   Open wound of elbow

ICD-10-CM

S51   Open wound of elbow and forearm

> Code also any associated wound infection

> **EXCLUDES 1**   *open fracture of elbow and forearm (S52.- with open fracture 7th character)*
> *traumatic amputation of elbow and forearm (S58.-)*

> **EXCLUDES 2**   *open wound of wrist and hand (S61.-)*

> The appropriate 7th character is to be added to each code from category S51.
>
> **A   initial encounter**
> **D   subsequent encounter**
> **S   sequela**

S51.Ø   Open wound of elbow

S51.ØØ   Unspecified open wound of elbow

S51.ØØ1   Unspecified open wound of right elbow

S51.ØØ2   Unspecified open wound of left elbow

S51.ØØ9   Unspecified open wound of unspecified elbow

S51.Ø1   Laceration without foreign body of elbow

S51.Ø11   Laceration without foreign body of right elbow

S51.Ø12   Laceration without foreign body of left elbow

S51.Ø19   Laceration without foreign body of unspecified elbow

S51.Ø2   Laceration with foreign body of elbow

S51.Ø21   Laceration with foreign body of right elbow

S51.Ø22   Laceration with foreign body of left elbow

S51.Ø29   Laceration with foreign body of unspecified elbow

S51.Ø3   Puncture wound without foreign body of elbow

S51.Ø31   Puncture wound without foreign body of right elbow

S51.Ø32   Puncture wound without foreign body of left elbow

S51.Ø39   Puncture wound without foreign body of unspecified elbow

S51.Ø4   Puncture wound with foreign body of elbow

S51.Ø41   Puncture wound with foreign body of right elbow

S51.Ø42   Puncture wound with foreign body of left elbow

S51.Ø49   Puncture wound with foreign body of unspecified elbow

	S51.05	**Open bite of elbow**
		Bite of elbow NOS

EXCLUDES 1 *superficial bite of elbow (S50.36, S50.37)*

	S51.051	**Open, bite, right elbow**
	S51.052	**Open bite, left elbow**
	S51.059	**Open bite, unspecified elbow**

S51.8 Open wound of forearm

EXCLUDES 2 *open wound of elbow (S51.0-)*

S51.80 Unspecified open wound of forearm

S51.801 **Unspecified open wound of right forearm**

S51.802 **Unspecified open wound of left forearm**

S51.809 **Unspecified open wound of unspecified forearm**

Combination Codes

A combination code is a single code used to classify two diagnoses, or a diagnosis with an associated manifestation or complication. Combination codes may be identified by subterm entries in the alphabetic index or by instructional notes in the tabular list. Assign only the combination code that fully identifies the diagnostic conditions documented. Multiple coding should not be used when combination codes clearly identify all of the elements documented in the diagnostic statement. Alternately, if a combination code does not adequately describe the nature of the associated manifestation or complication, an additional code should be assigned.

ICD-10

K50 Crohn's disease [regional enteritis]
INCLUDES granulomatous enteritis
EXCLUDES 1 *ulcerative colitis (K51.-)*

K50.0 Crohn's disease of small intestine
Crohn's disease [regional enteritis] of:
duodenum
ileum
jejunum
Ileitis
regional
terminal
EXCLUDES *with Crohn's disease of both large and small intestine (K50.8)*

ICD-10-CM

K50 Crohn's disease [regional enteritis]
INCLUDES granulomatous enteritis
EXCLUDES 1 *ulcerative colitis (K51.-)*
Use additional code to identify manifestations, such as:
pyoderma gangrenosum (L88)

K50.0 Crohn's disease of small intestine
Crohn's disease [regional enteritis] of duodenum
Crohn's disease [regional enteritis] of ileum
Crohn's disease [regional enteritis] of jejunum
Regional ileitis
Terminal ileitis
EXCLUDES 1 *Crohn's disease of both small and large intestine (K50.8-)*

K50.00 Crohn's disease of small intestine without complications

K50.01 Crohn's disease of small intestine with complications

K50.011 **Crohn's disease of small intestine with rectal bleeding**

✔ QUICK TIP

The Uniform Hospital Discharge Data Set defines that this definition of principal diagnosis applies only to inpatients in acute, short-term, general hospitals.

📖 DEFINITIONS

principal diagnosis. Condition established after study to be chiefly responsible for occasioning the admission of the patient to the hospital for care.

K50.012	Crohn's disease of small intestine with intestinal obstruction
K50.013	Crohn's disease of small intestine with fistula
K50.014	Crohn's disease of small intestine with abscess
K50.018	Crohn's disease of small intestine with other complication
K50.019	Crohn's disease of small intestine with unspecified complications

Combination of Dagger and Asterisk Codes

In ICD-9 and ICD-10, WHO provides a classification scheme in which certain disease entities may be classified twice: once according to etiology, or cause of the disease, and once according to its manifestations or symptoms. The coder can choose to use one code or the other. In ICD-9-CM and ICD-10-CM, this dual classification was eliminated. In certain ICD-10-CM classifications, the manifestation is merged with the etiology codes.

ICD-10

A02.2†	Localized salmonella infections
	Salmonella:
	Arthritis+ (M01.3*)
	Meningitis+ (G01*)
	Osteomyelitis+ (M90.2*)
	Pneumonia+ (J17.0*)
	Renal tubulo-interstitial disease+ (N16.0*)

ICD-10-CM

A02.2	Localized salmonella infections
A02.20	Localized salmonella infection, unspecified
A02.21	Salmonella meningitis
A02.22	Salmonella pneumonia
A02.23	Salmonella arthritis
A02.24	Salmonella osteomyelitis
A02.25	Salmonella pyelonephritis
	Salmonella tubulo-interstitial nephropathy
A02.29	Salmonella with other localized infection

Movement of Categories

The ICD-10-CM reviewers identified the need to move additional disease categories from one chapter to another as the types of conditions grouped under the ICD-10 category were better classified elsewhere.

ICD-10

Diseases of the Digestive System (K00–K93)

| K07 | Dentofacial anomalies [including malocclusion] |
| K10 | Other diseases of jaw |

ICD-10-CM

Diseases of the Musculoskeletal System and Connective Tissue (M00–M99)

| M26 | Dentofacial anomalies [including malocclusion] |
| M27 | Other diseases of jaws |

CODING AXIOM

Both ICD-9 and ICD-10 provide the dual classification scheme in which certain disease entities may be classified twice: once according to etiology of the disease and once according to its manifestations. This is called the dagger and asterisk system.

Expansion of Postoperative Complication Codes

Building on ICD-10's feature of adding codes for postprocedural disorders to particular body system chapters, NCHS expands ICD-10-CM further by deactivating codes found in chapter 19, "Injury, Poisoning and Certain Other Consequences of External Causes," and adding these conditions to the body system chapters.

ICD-10

T81.0	**Haemorrhage and haematoma complicating a procedure, not elsewhere classified**
T81.2	**Accidental puncture and laceration during a procedure, not elsewhere classified**

ICD-10-CM

K91.6   **Intraoperative hemorrhage and hematoma of a digestive system organ or structure complicating a procedure**

> **EXCLUDES 1**   *intraoperative hemorrhage and hematoma of a digestive system organ or structure due to accidental puncture and laceration during a procedure (K91.7-)*

    K91.61   **Intraoperative hemorrhage and hematoma of a digestive system organ or structure complicating a digestive system procedure**

    K91.62   **Intraoperative hemorrhage and hematoma of a digestive system organ or structure complicating other procedure**

K91.7   **Accidental puncture and laceration of a digestive system organ or structure during a procedure**

    K91.71   **Accidental puncture and laceration of a digestive system organ or structure during a digestive system procedure**

    K91.72   **Accidental puncture and laceration of a digestive system organ or structure during other procedure**

Deactivated Codes

To meet data-gathering goals desired by the federal government for coding in the United States, some codes that are valid in ICD-10 have been deactivated for ICD-10-CM. These codes fall into several categories that are considered by NCHS and CMS to be highly unspecified. To maintain international data-gathering requirements, deactivated ICD-10 codes cannot be reassigned in ICD-10-CM.

For example, the ICD-10 codes T81.0 and T81.2 have been deactivated in ICD-10-CM. In previous updates, a notation was placed into the tabular list for deactivated codes. Beginning with the 2009 update, this notation was removed from the tabular list sections where codes T81.0 and T81.2 were previously included in the ICD-10-CM classification. However, the following is an example of such a notation as listed in the 2011 update:

T00–T06   **deactivated**
> *Code to individual injuries.*

Recent revisions to ICD-10-CM, including the 2012 and 2013 draft classifications, do not contain separate notations for deactivated codes. Instead, the deactivated codes are removed from the code set. Code deletions are noted on the ICD-10-CM Tabular List of Diseases and Injuries Addenda for each effective year.

 KEY POINT

Not all codes in ICD-10 are available in ICD-10-CM. Some are deactivated by NCHS to meet federal data-gathering goals.

Encounter for Procedure Codes

Some ICD-10 codes actually identify a procedure, rather than a disease or health status. These codes were reviewed and a determination was made to either deactivate them, or in some instances to revise the category title. For example:

ICD-10

Z23 Need for immunization against single bacterial diseases

Z24 Need for immunization against certain single viral diseases

Z25 Need for immunization against other single viral diseases

Z26 Need for immunization against other single infectious diseases

Z27 Need for immunization against combinations of infectious diseases

Z28 Immunization not carried out

Z29 Need for other prophylactic measures

ICD-10-CM

Z23 **Encounter for immunization**
    Code first any routine childhood examination
    NOTE procedure codes are required to identify the types of immunizations given

Z24 deactivated

Z25 deactivated

Z26 deactivated

Z27 deactivated

Z28 **Immunization not carried out and underimmunization status**

Z29 deactivated

Categories Z24–Z27 and Z29 have been deactivated and category Z23 has been retitled. Current revisions to the ICD-10-CM draft do not contain any notation of the deactivation status.

Highly Nonspecific Codes

ICD-10 includes codes for "multiple" injuries. In ICD-10-CM, these nonspecific multiple codes have been deactivated. Coders will, instead, be expected to report multiple, individual codes to describe specific injuries.

ICD-10

S30.7 Multiple superficial injuries of abdomen, lower back and pelvis

S49.7 Multiple injuries of shoulder and upper arm

ICD-10-CM

S30.7 deactivated

S49.7 deactivated

Other codes providing overly generalized information have also been deleted, such as:

A16 Respiratory tuberculosis, not confirmed bacteriologically or histologically

For the purpose of tracking disease and health-related issues in the United States, codes associated with conditions in which the death occurs without contact with medical authorities are not appropriate for U.S. reporting. These codes, used in mortality reporting for ICD-10, have been deleted in ICD-10-CM. Some examples include:

 KEY POINT

Current revisions to ICD-10-CM do not contain notations of deactivated code status. Instead, the deactivated code is simply removed from the classification. Consult the current ICD-10-CM Tabular List of Disease and Injuries Addenda for any recent code deletions.

R95 Sudden infant death syndrome

R98 Unattended death

S18 Traumatic amputation at neck level

Notes

In addition to the analysis of the codes themselves, the notes in ICD-10 were reviewed. Many of the clinical modifications reflect the addenda to both systems as published over the years, while others were added as new codes to ICD-10-CM.

ICD-10

C34 Malignant neoplasm of bronchus and lung

ICD-10-CM

This excludes note was added because of the addition of codes C46.50–C46.52 for Kaposi's sarcoma of the lung.

C34 Malignant neoplasm of bronchus and lung

> **EXCLUDES 1** *Kaposi's sarcoma of lung (C46.5-)*

ICD-10

D05 Carcinoma in situ of breast

> **EXCLUDES** *carcinoma in situ of skin of breast (D04.5)*
> *melanoma in situ of breast (skin) (D03.5)*

ICD-10-CM

The note for Paget's disease is found in ICD-9-CM.

D05 Carcinoma in situ of breast

> **EXCLUDES 1** *carcinoma in situ of skin of breast (D04.5)*
> *melanoma in situ of breast (skin) (D03.5)*
> *Paget's disease of breast or nipple (C50.-)*

DISCUSSION QUESTIONS

1. What are some reasons for clinically modifying ICD-10 in the United States?

   _____

   _____

   _____

   _____

2. Iatrogenic illnesses have been relocated in ICD-10-CM. Where do they now occur?

   _____

   _____

   _____

   _____

3. How are dagger and asterisk codes handled in ICD-10-CM?

_____

_____

_____

_____

4. What are three reasons why ICD-10 codes would be deactivated in ICD-10-CM?

_____

_____

_____

_____

Chapter 3:
ICD-10-CM Coding Conventions

With an understanding of the overall clinical modifications made to ICD-10, it is time to build on that knowledge and examine the conventions of the ICD-10-CM system. While many of the rules remain the same, others are new, expanded, or have been deleted. These rules must be understood to be accurately applied and to correctly assign a code from ICD-10-CM.

Both the tabular list, volume 1, and the alphabetic index, volume 2, contain conventions. Some rules are unique to one volume or the other. For example, the "excludes" note is found only in the tabular list. Other conventions are found in both volumes, such as the use of the term "with" to indicate certain codes that have been provided for diseases in combination.

Prior to reviewing the various conventions, this chapter will provide an explanation of the overall arrangement of ICD-10-CM. Chapter 2 introduced the contents of ICD-10-CM, while this chapter focuses on the general order of each volume. Note that the 10th revision of ICD is based on the concepts and structure of the 9th revision of ICD. These are not separate classification systems; ICD-10-CM is the "next generation" of the ICD-CM classification. It may be helpful to think of ICD-10-CM as a "version 10.0" of the ICD system.

Coding guidelines for ICD-10-CM need to be carefully reviewed as part of any orientation and training program. Coders will need to be as well versed in the application of the guidelines for the new system as they were with coding guidelines for ICD-9-CM. Guidelines for coding and reporting with ICD-10-CM appear on the official government version of ICD-10-CM and on the National Center for Health Statistics (NCHS) website: http://www.cdc.gov/nchs/icd/icd10cm.htm.

ICD-10-CM coding guidelines mainly follow logic similar to ICD-9-CM coding guidelines. However, there are some significant differences that correlate to the increased granularity afforded by this new coding system. For example:

- Pre-existing complications from diabetes in a post pancreas transplant patient are classified to codes from the diabetes categories in order to describe the complications.

- Classification of intrauterine death and stillbirth differs from ICD-9-CM. Codes O36.4 Maternal care for intrauterine death, or O02.1 Missed abortion (early intrauterine death) before 20 completed weeks of gestation), are used on the maternal record only. Code P95 Stillbirth, is used on the baby's record only.

- Many manifestations associated with a disease process are included in the code, thereby minimizing, or sometimes eliminating, the need for dual coding. For example:
    - Angina can now be reported with atherosclerotic heart disease using a single code, negating complex sequencing instructions.

 OBJECTIVES

In this chapter, you will learn:

- The general arrangement of ICD-10-CM
- The conventions in the tabular list and alphabetic index of ICD-10-CM
- How these conventions compare and contrast to ICD-9-CM
- How to use these conventions for assigning an ICD-10-CM code

 KEY POINT

The "ICD-10-CM Draft Official Guidelines for Coding and Reporting" for 2013 can be downloaded at the following URL: http://www.cdc.gov/nchs/icd/icd10cm.htm.

– Crohn's disease of the large intestine with intestinal obstruction is reported with a single code.

It is necessary to keep current with the guidelines as they are updated. Coders need to review all sections of the guidelines to fully understand all of the rules and instructions necessary to ensure appropriate code selection. There are no codes for procedures in ICD-10-CM. Procedures are coded with the procedure classification appropriate for the setting in which the procedure occurred, such as those codes in the ICD-10-PCS or CPT coding systems.

AXIS OF CLASSIFICATION

ICD-10-CM is an arrangement of similar entities encounter, diseases, and other conditions on the basis of specific criteria. Diseases can be arranged in a variety of ways: according to etiology, anatomy, or severity. The particular criterion chosen is called the axis of classification.

Anatomy is the primary axis of classification of ICD-10-CM. Thus, there are chapters entitled "Diseases of the Circulatory System" and "Diseases of the Genitourinary System." ICD-10-CM employs other axes as well, such as etiology, as in the chapter, "Certain Infectious and Parasitic Diseases."

Different axes are used in classifying different diseases within the same chapters. The choice is based upon the most important aspects of the disease from both a statistical and clinical point of view. For example:

- Pneumonia: etiology or cause of the pneumonia

- Malignant neoplasm: site

- Cardiac arrhythmia: type

- Leukemia: morphology

ARRANGEMENT OF THE TABULAR LIST

The tabular list consists of chapters, subchapters, three-character categories, four-character subcategories, and five-, six-, and seven-character subdivisions.

Chapters and Subchapters

As mentioned earlier, the chapter order in ICD-10-CM is not necessarily the same as in lCD-9-CM. Disorders of the immune mechanism in ICD-10-CM are found with diseases of the blood and blood-forming organs. In ICD-9-CM these disorders are included with endocrine, nutritional, and metabolic diseases. Chapters for diseases of the genitourinary system; pregnancy, childbirth, and the puerperium; certain conditions originating in the perinatal period; and congenital malformations, deformations, and chromosomal abnormalities are placed consecutively in ICD-10 and are the same in ICD-10-CM.

The ICD-10-CM classification is divided into 21 chapters. The chapter title describes general content contained within the chapter. The code range describes the extent of the chapter; for example, chapter 7, "Diseases of the Eye and Adnexa (H00–H59)."

Chapters may encompass more than one letter. For example, chapter 1, "Certain Infectious and Parasitic Diseases," contains code categories A00–B99. Similarly, letters may be shared across chapters. For example, chapter 7, "Diseases of the Eye and Adnexa" contains code categories H00–H59 and chapter 8, "Diseases of the Ear and Mastoid Process," contains code categories H60–H95.

Chapters are subdivided into subchapters or "blocks" containing code categories that classify closely related conditions. Each chapter begins with a summary of its subchapters to provide an overview of the classification structure at that level.

The title describes the content of the subchapter with the code range describing the extent of the subchapter; for example, "Disorders of vitreous body and globe (H43–H44)."

Three-Character Category

Although ICD-10-CM codes are composed of three to seven alphanumeric characters, the first character is always alphabetic. All letters are used except for the letter U, which is reserved for future additions and changes. In general, the first three code characters contain one letter, followed by two numbers, such as:

A00   **Cholera**

However, recent revisions to certain classifications have resulted in exceptions, whereby the initial alphabetic character is followed by one number, with a subsequent alphabetic character. These exceptions include, but are not limited to:

- Chapter 2, category C4A, between C43 and C44

  C4A   **Merkel cell carcinoma**

- Chapter 2, categories C7A and B, between C75 and C76

  C7A   **Malignant neuroendocrine tumors**
  C7B   **Secondary neuroendocrine tumors**

- Chapter 13, category M1A, between M08 and M10

  M1A   **Chronic gout**

- Chapter 15, category O9A, following O99

  O9A   **Maternal malignant neoplasms, traumatic injuries and abuse classifiable elsewhere but complicating pregnancy, childbirth and the puerperium**

Three-character categories are the essential subdivisions of the disease classification. The disease classification begins with category A00 and ends with Z99. Not all letters of the alphabet or all numbers at the second and third positions have been used.

Three-character categories may represent a single disease entity or may represent a group of homogenous or closely related conditions. The three-character category title describes the general content of the category. For example, category K55 provides codes for a number of vascular disorders of the intestines, while category R64 is very specific to the condition cachexia.

K55   **Vascular disorders of intestine**
R64   **Cachexia**

Generally the sequence of the categories within a block begins with categories that have specific titles, and progresses to categories with less specific titles. The next-to-the-last three-character category in a series is called the "residual" three-character category. This is the one used for "other specified disease." For example:

Hernia (K40–K46)

K40	**Inguinal hernia**
K41	**Femoral hernia**
K42	**Umbilical hernia**
K43	**Ventral hernia**
K44	**Diaphragmatic hernia**
K45	**Other abdominal hernia**
K46	**Unspecified abdominal hernia**

Three-character category K45 is the residual category for abdominal hernias.

There are three-character categories that have not been subdivided. These unsubdivided three-character categories describe a disease that needs no further specificity. For example:

L22 **Diaper dermatitis**
  INCLUDES Diaper erythema
  Diaper rash
  Psoriasiform diaper rash

The majority of three-character categories are subdivided into four-character subcategories. Whenever a three-character category has been subdivided, the three-character level code is considered an invalid code and cannot be used. A fourth-character subcategory (and perhaps a fifth-, sixth-, or seventh-character subdivision) is required for a valid code. Each character beyond the first three characters provides greater specificity. For example, category K35 cannot stand alone as the code for acute appendicitis. A fourth character 2, 3, or 8 must be used. For example:

K35	**Acute appendicitis**
K35.2	**Acute appendicitis with generalized peritonitis**
K35.3	**Acute appendicitis with localized peritonitis**
K35.8	**Other and unspecified acute appendicitis**

Four-Character Subcategory

Four-character subcategories are the subdivisions of three-character categories, and define the axis of classification by describing the site, etiology, manifestation, or stage of the disease classified to the three-character category. A four-character subcategory consists of a three-character category code, plus a decimal, and an additional number or character. The fourth character is usually a number; however, exceptions may exist, such as:

- Chapter 13, subcategory M79.A between M79.7 and M79.8

  M79.A **Nontraumatic compartment syndrome**

The axes of the subdivisions vary according to the nature of the condition or conditions included within the three-character category. For example, the subdivisions may describe the stages of the disease (i.e., acute, subacute,

 KEY POINT

Some three-character code groupings stand alone as the valid code for the condition. Do not "zero fill" these codes, as that makes them invalid. Valid codes in ICD-10-CM may have three, four, five, six, or seven characters.

chronic), the sites of the disease (upper end, shaft, etc.), or the causes of the disease (Streptococcus, rhinovirus, etc.). For example:

N70   Salpingitis and oophoritis
    N70.0   Acute salpingitis and oophoritis
        N70.01   Acute salpingitis
        N70.02   Acute oophoritis
        N70.03   Acute salpingitis and oophoritis
    N70.1   Chronic salpingitis and oophoritis
        Hydrosalpinx
        N70.11   Chronic salpingitis
        N70.12   Chronic oophoritis
        N70.13   Chronic salpingitis and oophoritis
    N70.9   Salpingitis and oophoritis, unspecified
        N70.91   Salpingitis, unspecified
        N70.92   Oophoritis, unspecified
        N70.93   Salpingitis and oophoritis, unspecified

Four-character subcategories within a three-character category progress in terms of specificity. Often the next-to-the-last four-character subdivision, identified by the fourth character .8, is the residual category ("other specified") and is the place to classify a specified form of a condition that does not have its own subdivision.

The last four-character subcategory is used for coding the unspecified form (site, cause, etc.) of the condition. Generally this four-character subcategory is identified by the fourth character .9. For example:

G50   Disorders of trigeminal nerve
    <u>INCLUDES</u>   disorders of 5th cranial nerve
    G50.0   Trigeminal neuralgia
        Syndrome on paroxysmal facial pain
        Tic douloureux
    G50.1   Atypical facial pain
    G50.8   Other disorders of trigeminal nerve
    G50.9   Disorder of trigeminal nerve, unspecified

Often four-character subcategories are themselves further subdivided to provide even greater specificity. Whenever a four-character subcategory has been subdivided, that four-character code grouping cannot stand alone as the code for the disease to be encoded. The following example of an unsubdivided four-character subcategory shows that code O15.1 can be assigned as the code for eclampsia in labor. The subdivided four-character subcategory O15.0, however, cannot be used as the code for eclampsia in pregnancy. A fifth character must be used. For example:

O15   Eclampsia
    <u>INCLUDES</u>   convulsions following conditions in O10-14 and O16
    O15.0   Eclampsia in pregnancy
        O15.00   Eclampsia in pregnancy, unspecified trimester
        O15.02   Eclampsia in pregnancy, second trimester
        O15.03   Eclampsia in pregnancy, third trimester
    O15.1   Eclampsia in labor
    O15.2   Eclampsia in the puerperium

DEFINITIONS

clinical manifestation. Display or disclosure of signs and symptoms of an illness.

O15.9   Eclampsia, unspecified as to time period
Eclampsia NOS

To retain the same degree of specificity present in ICD-10-CM, manifestations of diseases are identified in the same fashion as in ICD-9-CM. Below are two ways to identify the diseases, each followed separately by an example.

Example 1

As individual five-character subdivisions of the four-character subcategories to represent the etiology of the disease.

A02.2   Localized salmonella infections

A02.20   Localized salmonella infection, unspecified

A02.21   Salmonella meningitis

A02.22   Salmonella pneumonia

A02.23   Salmonella arthritis

A02.24   Salmonella osteomyelitis

A02.25   Salmonella pyelonephritis

A02.29   Salmonella with other localized infection

Example 2

As an additional code assigned whenever a three-character category or four-character subcategory is followed by an instructional note to "code first underlying condition." The code for the condition first represents the etiology of the diseases, while the secondary code represents the manifestation of the disease.

The World Health Organization (WHO) does not allow manifestations in the primary tabulation of causes for morbidity and mortality. Consequently, the manifestation code never appears as a first-listed diagnosis. For example:

H42   Glaucoma in diseases classified elsewhere
Code first underlying condition, such as:
amyloidosis (E85.-)
aniridia (Q13.1)
Lowe's syndrome (E72.03)
Reiger's anomaly (Q13.81)
specified metabolic disorder (E70-E88)
EXCLUDES 1   *glaucoma (in):*
diabetes mellitus (E08.39, E09.39, E10.39, E11.39, E13.39)
onchocerciasis (B73.02)
syphilis (A52.71)
tuberculous (A18.59)

In order to assign fourth or fifth digits in ICD-9-CM, the coder is referred back to a previous page, section, or chapter header. ICD-10-CM has made every attempt to provide the full code title for all codes, decreasing reliance on cross-references and, therefore, decreasing the margin for error due to incomplete or invalid code assignment.

Five-, Six-, and Seven-Character Subclassifications

In ICD-9-CM, there are never more than five digits to a code. In ICD-10-CM, there are five-, six-, and seven-character codes. For example:

ICD-9-CM

882   Open wound of hand except finger(s) alone

882.0   Without mention of complication

882.1   Complicated

GENERAL INFO

The code examples provided are intended for academic purposes to illustrate the differences between ICD-9-CM and ICD-10-CM. They are not intended to represent direct mappings, except where specifically noted.

882.2   With tendon involvement

ICD-10-CM

S61.4   Open wound of hand

    S61.40   Unspecified open wound of hand

        S61.401   Unspecified open wound of right hand

        S61.402   Unspecified open wound of left hand

        S61.409   Unspecified open wound of unspecified hand

    S61.41   Laceration without foreign body of hand

        S61.411   Laceration without foreign body of right hand

        S61.412   Laceration without foreign body of left hand

        S61.419   Laceration without foreign body of unspecified hand

Five- and six-character subdivisions are used in two ways: first, to provide specific codes for individual inclusion terms within a single four-character subcategory; second, to provide a second axis of classification for an entire three-character category or series of three-character categories. This second axis permits a different cross section of the condition than is provided by the four-character category.

Five- and six-character subclassifications are presented in their natural sequence. When they occur, seventh characters in ICD-10-CM are listed in a table and referenced in the instructions for that code.

If a code that requires a seventh character is not six characters in length, a placeholder "X" must be used to fill in the empty characters.

Seventh Characters

ICD-10-CM has incorporated the use of seventh characters to specify the encounter status for that episode of care, or to identify the status of the current condition under care for that specific encounter.

Certain categories require applicable seventh characters. A seventh character must always be submitted in the seventh character data field. If a code that requires a seventh character is less than six characters in length, placeholders of "X" must be used to fill the empty character spaces. If a seventh character is required, it must be assigned to all codes within the category or subcategory, or as otherwise instructed by the notations in the Tabular List.

S42.481G   Torus fracture of lower end of right humerus, subsequent encounter for delayed healing

T15.02XA   Foreign body in cornea, left eye, initial encounter

X75.XXXS   Intentional self-harm by explosive material, sequelae

X73.1XXA   Intentional self-harm by hunting rifle discharge, initial encounter

X95.01XA   Assault by airgun discharge, initial encounter

W22.042S   Striking against wall of swimming pool causing other injury, sequelae

Where applicable, an instructional note appears under the three-character category, or further divided subcategory, directing the coder to add a seventh character to each code within the category or subcategory. Every code must have one of these characters to be valid. The valid codes created by these required characters are not found listed individually within the tabular list under each subclassification level to which they apply. Instead, the coder must refer to the

 KEY POINT

Use of the fifth, sixth, or seventh character is not optional. If five-digit subclassifications appear in ICD-9-CM, they must be used. If five-, six-, or seven-character subclassifications appear in ICD-10-CM, they must be used.

instructional note and add the appropriate seventh character to the available code at its highest specification level within the category. For example:

S59   Other and unspecified injuries of elbow and forearm

> *EXCLUDES 2*   *other and unspecified injuries of wrist and hand (S69.-)*

> The appropriate 7th character is to be added to each code from subcategories S59.0, S59.1, and S59.2.
>
> **A   initial encounter for closed fracture**
> **D   subsequent encounter for fracture with routine healing**
> **G   subsequent encounter for fracture with delayed healing**
> **K   subsequent encounter for fracture with nonunion**
> **P   subsequent encounter for fracture with malunion**
> **S   sequela**

S59.0   Physeal fracture of lower end on ulna

> **S59.00   Unspecified physeal fracture of lower end of ulna**
>
> > **S59.001   Unspecified physeal fracture of lower end of ulna, right arm**
> >
> > **S59.002   Unspecified physeal fracture of lower end of ulna, left arm**
> >
> > **S59.009   Unspecified physeal fracture of lower end of ulna, unspecified arm**

Coma Scale

The convention of using seventh characters in ICD-10-CM for more granularity in coding has been implemented in a unique way within the coma subcategory to denote time. For example:

> The appropriate 7th character is to be added to each code R40.21-, R40.22-, and R40.23-.
>
> **0   unspecified time**
> **1   in the field [EMT or ambulance]**
> **2   at arrival to emergency department**
> **3   at hospital admission**
> **4   24 hours or more after hospital admission**

> > **R40.2121   Coma scale, eyes open, to pain, in the field**
> >
> > **R40.2222   Coma scale, best verbal response, incomprehensible words, at arrival to emergency department**
> >
> > **R40.2334   Coma scale, best motor response, abnormal, 24 hours or more after hospital admission**

Fetus Identification in Multiple Gestation

ICD-10-CM provides a specialized group of characters to be used in chapter 15, "Pregnancy, Childbirth and the Puerperium (O00–O9A)," to identify the fetus for which the code applies in multiple gestation pregnancies. These seventh-character codes are assigned under each category for which an instructional note specifies that the appropriate seventh character is required. For example:

> **0   not applicable or unspecified**
> **1   fetus 1**
> **2   fetus 2**
> **3   fetus 3**
> **4   fetus 4**
> **5   fetus 5**
> **9   other fetus**

Placeholder X

There are many ways that the hierarchal coding system of ICD-9-CM and ICD-10-CM provides an advantage over other types of coding systems. For collating data and statistical analysis, the hierarchical codes allow disease groups to be monitored easily. Coders using the system become familiar with these hierarchies easing the code look-up process. But despite the system's many advantages, there are disadvantages as well. Chief among the intrinsic disadvantages is the fixed space within each classification: there can only be 10 divisions of each code at the next level. The creation of an alpha first-character relieved much of the space problems for ICD-10-CM, providing 26 characters instead of 10, but there is still concern that medical advances could outstrip the room left in the coding system. In an effort to plan for these medical advances, some placeholders have been added to ICD-10-CM, allowing for additional detail to be added to the classification in the future. For example:

O45.8	**Other premature separation of placenta**	
O45.8X	**Other premature separation of placenta**	
	O45.8X1	**Other premature separation of placenta, first trimester**
	O45.8X2	**Other premature separation of placenta, second trimester**
	O45.8X3	**Other premature separation of placenta, third trimester**
	O45.8X9	**Other premature separation of placenta, unspecified trimester**

Note that the definition of O45.8 and O45.8X are exactly the same. The intent being, that if, in the future, there are causes of premature separation of the placenta that should be assigned unique codes, these causes would be assigned numbers that replace the "X" placeholder. Until then, coders are required to use the "X" as directed in the ICD-10-CM text, making it unacceptable to simply drop it.

If a code requiring a seventh character is not six characters in length, a placeholder "X" must be used to fill the empty character fields.

TABULAR LIST CONVENTIONS

The ICD-10-CM tabular list employs certain abbreviations, punctuations, symbols, and other conventions that must be clearly understood in order to use the classification system appropriately.

NEC and NOS

Two abbreviations are found in the tabular list: NEC and NOS. The abbreviation NEC means "not elsewhere classified" or "not elsewhere classifiable." NOS means "not otherwise specified."

As in ICD-9-CM, the abbreviation NEC represents "other specified" classifications. Codes titled "other" or "other specified" in the tabular list are reported when the information in the medical record provides detail for which a specific code does not exist.

In the tabular list, the phrase "not elsewhere classified" is applied to residual categories that do not appear in sequence with (i.e., immediately following) the pertinent specific categories. These residual categories are entitled "other specified." For example, K73 is the residual category for chronic hepatitis. This category is not immediate to the specific categories for forms of chronic hepatitis. The forms of the disease are assigned to various categories throughout the classification. An exclusion note in an NEC category directs the coder to certain types of the condition that are classified more appropriately elsewhere. For example:

K70   Alcoholic liver disease

K71   Toxic liver disease

K72   Hepatic failure, not elsewhere classified

K73   Chronic hepatitis, not elsewhere classified
> **EXCLUDES 1** *alcoholic hepatitis (chronic) (K70.1-)*
> *drug-induced hepatitis (chronic) (K71.-)*
> *granulomatous hepatitis (chronic) NEC (K75.3)*
> *reactive, nonspecific hepatitis (chronic) (K75.2)*
> *viral hepatitis (chronic) (B15–B19)*

The abbreviation NOS is equivalent to "unspecified." The term is assigned when the documentation does not provide sufficient detail to assign a more specific code. Double check the medical record for information about the condition before selecting an NOS code.

The term "bronchitis" alone means the same as "bronchitis, unspecified" or "bronchitis NOS." For example:

J40   Bronchitis, not specified as acute or chronic
> **INCLUDES** bronchitis NOS
> catarrhal bronchitis
> bronchitis with tracheitis NOS
> tracheobronchitis NOS

A term without an essential modifier is the unspecified form of the condition, though there are exceptions. Unqualified terms can be classified to a three-character category for a more specific type of condition. For example, "mitral stenosis" is a common descriptor used as a diagnosis. ICD-10-CM assumes the cause to be rheumatic, whether or not "rheumatic" is included in the diagnosis. For example:

Index
Stenosis, stenotic
    Mitral (chronic) (inactive) (valve) I05.0

Tabular

I05   Rheumatic mitral valve diseases
> **INCLUDES** conditions classifiable to both I05.0 and I05.2-I05.9, whether
> specified as rheumatic or not

   I05.0   Rheumatic mitral stenosis

{ } Braces
ICD-9-CM uses braces to enclose a series of terms, each of which is modified by the word(s) following the brace. However, in ICD-10-CM no braces are used. For example:

ICD-9-CM

Code 560.9 includes obstruction, occlusion, stenosis, or stricture of intestine or colon.

KEY POINT

Code to the highest level of specificity allowed by the medical record documentation.

560.9   Unspecified intestinal obstruction
Enterostenosis

Obstruction
Occlusion
Stenosis
Stricture
} of intestine or colon

ICD-10-CM

K56.69   Other intestinal obstruction
Enterostenosis NOS
Obstructive ileus NOS
Occlusion of colon or intestine NOS
Stenosis of colon or intestine NOS
Stricture of colon or intestine NOS

Note that no braces were used to list the inclusion terms in K56.69.

[ ] Brackets

Brackets enclose synonyms, alternative wordings, or explanatory phrases in ICD-9-CM and ICD-10-CM. For example, Crohn's disease is defined by the phrase in brackets as regional enteritis.

K50   Crohn's disease [regional enteritis]

In ICD-9-CM, brackets are also used to enclose the fifth digits available for the fourth-digit subcategory. Since ICD-10-CM presents the five- and six-character subclassifications in their natural sequence, the use of brackets for this purpose is not necessary in ICD-10-CM.

In the index, bracketed codes indicate certain etiology/manifestation multiple coding and sequencing rules apply. The bracketed code is sequenced in addition to the preceding code. For example:

Myasthenia G70.9
  syndrome
    in
      neoplastic disease (*see also* Neoplasm) D49.9 *[G73.3]*
      pernicious anemia D51.0 *[G73.3]*

: Colon

ICD-9-CM employs colons in the tabular list following an incomplete term that needs one or more modifiers to assign the term for the given code. The colon is used for the term that has more than one possible essential modifier. In ICD-10-CM, colons appear in the tabular list after includes and excludes notes or other coding instruction such as "Note." Colons may also appear following an incomplete term that requires one or more of the terms following the colon to be documented to support code assignment. For example:

C22   Malignant neoplasm of liver and intrahepatic bile ducts
  EXCLUDES 1   *malignant neoplasm of biliary tract NOS (C24.9)*
                secondary malignant neoplasm of liver and intrahepatic bile duct (C78.7)
  Use additional code to identify:
    alcohol abuse and dependence (F10.-)
    hepatitis B (B16.-, B18.0–B18.1)
    hepatitis C (B17.1-, B18.2)

, Comma

Commas are found in both ICD-10-CM and ICD-9-CM for the same reasons. Words following a comma are often essential modifiers. For example, the term "postpartum" is an essential modifier and must be present in the statement for deep-vein thrombosis or pelvic thrombophlebitis to assign code O87.1.

O87.1   **Deep phlebothrombosis in the puerperium**
Deep-vein thrombosis, postpartum
Pelvic thrombophlebitis, postpartum

Commas also appear in code descriptions as essential modifiers:

O88.Ø11   Air embolism in pregnancy, first trimester

( ) Parentheses

In ICD-9-CM, parentheses enclose supplementary words that may be present or absent in the statement of a disease or procedure, but do not affect the code. Parentheses also enclose the categories included in a subchapter, and a code or code range listed in an excludes note. The same rules for parentheses apply to ICD-10-CM.

Nonessential modifiers usually appear in the three-character category that has been assigned the unspecified form of the disease modified. For example, the nonessential modifiers in the example below are: (acute), (chronic), (nonpuerperal), and (subacute).

N61   **Inflammatory disorders of breast**
Abscess (acute) (chronic) (nonpuerperal) of areola
Abscess (acute) (chronic) (nonpuerperal) of breast
Carbuncle of breast
Infective mastitis (acute) (subacute) (nonpuerperal)
Mastitis (acute) (subacute) (nonpuerperal) NOS

§ Section Mark

The section mark symbol in some versions of ICD-9-CM precedes a code to denote the placement of a footnote at the bottom of the page. The footnote applies to all subdivisions within that code. This symbol is not found in ICD-10-CM; rather, the subdivisions are listed in their natural sequence. For example:

ICD-9-CM

789   **Other symptoms involving abdomen and pelvis**

The following fifth-digit subclassification is to be used for codes 789.Ø, 789.3, 789.4, and 789.6:

Ø   **unspecified site**
1   **right upper quadrant**
2   **left upper quadrant**
3   **right lower quadrant**
4   **right lower quadrant**
5   **periumbilic**
6   **epigastric**
7   **generalized**
9   **other specified site**
multiple sites

§789.Ø   **Abdominal pain**

§   Requires fifth digit. Valid digits are in [brackets] under each code. See category 789 for codes and definitions.

ICD-10-CM

R10.1	**Pain localized to upper abdomen**	
	R10.10	**Upper abdominal pain, unspecified**
	R10.11	**Right upper quadrant pain**
	R10.12	**Left upper quadrant pain**
	R10.13	**Epigastric pain**

Inclusion Term, Includes Note

Inclusion terms and includes notes carry the same meaning in ICD-10-CM as they do in ICD-9-CM.

Since titles are not always self-explanatory, the tabular list contains "inclusion" terms to clarify the content (intent) of the chapter, subchapter, category, or subdivision to which the terms apply. These inclusion terms are listed below the code title and describe other conditions classified to that code, such as synonyms of the condition listed in the code title, or an entirely different condition. For example:

R71.8	**Other abnormality of red blood cells**
	Abnormal red-cell morphology NOS
	Abnormal red-cell volume NOS
	Anisocytosis
	Poikilocytosis

Inclusion notes appearing under chapter and subchapter titles provide general definitions to the content of that section. These notes apply to each category within the chapter or subchapter. For example:

Chapter 16. Certain Conditions Originating in the Perinatal Period (P00–P96)

NOTE These codes are for use when the listed maternal conditions are specified as the cause of confirmed morbidity or potential morbidity which have their origin in the perinatal period (before birth through the first 28 days after birth). Codes from these categories are also for use for newborns who are suspected of having an abnormal condition resulting from exposure from the mother or the birth process, but without signs or symptoms, and, which after examination and observation, is found not to exist. These codes may be used even if treatment is begun for a suspected condition that is ruled out.

Infections Specific to the Perinatal Period (P35–P39)

INCLUDES infections acquired in utero, during birth via the umbilicus, or during the first 28 days after birth

Inclusion notes appearing under three-, four-, and five-character codes may define or provide a list of specific terms applicable to that category, and, if subdivided, to each subdivision.

The inclusion note appearing under the three-character category Q60 applies to all codes beneath it:

Q60	**Renal agenesis and other reduction defects of kidney**
	INCLUDES congenital absence of kidney
	congenital atrophy of kidney
	infantile atrophy of kidney
Q60.0	**Renal agenesis, unilateral**
Q60.1	**Renal agenesis, bilateral**
Q60.2	**Renal agenesis, unspecified**
Q60.3	**Renal hypoplasia, unilateral**

KEY POINT

Many of the alternative names found in the alphabetic index are not listed as inclusion terms in the tabular list. To code accurately, the coder should consult the index and then verify the code found in the tabular list.

KEY POINT

The placement of instructional notes is important. Notes appearing at the beginning of chapters apply to all categories within the chapter. Notes appearing at the beginning of subchapters apply to all codes within the subchapter. Notes appearing at three-character categories apply to all four-, five-, six-, and seven-character codes within the various subdivisions.

Q60.4   **Renal hypoplasia, bilateral**

Q60.5   **Renal hypoplasia, unspecified**

Q60.6   **Potter's syndrome**

Notes

Throughout the tabular list in ICD-9-CM, notes describe the general content of the succeeding categories and provide instructions for using the codes. The same holds true for ICD-10-CM. For example:

G09   **Sequelae of inflammatory diseases of central nervous system**

> **NOTE**   Category G09 is to be used to indicate conditions whose primary classification is to G00–G08 as the cause of sequelae, themselves classifiable elsewhere. The "sequelae" include conditions specified as residuals.
>
> Code first condition resulting from (sequela) of inflammatory diseases of central nervous system

Excludes Notes

Exclusion notes always appear with the word "excludes."

The purpose of excludes notes is to guide readers to proper application of codes. In ICD-9-CM, there has been significant confusion regarding excludes notes. In ICD-9-CM, an excludes note may indicate that two codes are mutually exclusive, and are not to be reported together. For example, the excludes note with the code for male stress incontinence of urine excludes the code for female stress incontinence. These codes are mutually exclusive and would never be reported correctly together. However, the excludes note for 304.6 Other specified drug dependence, has a different role. This excludes note excludes tobacco (305.1) from the drugs identified by 304.6. Yet, it would be appropriate and correct to report both codes for a patient with a tobacco habit and a glue-sniffing habit.

Excludes notes have been expanded in ICD-10-CM so there is no confusion over the intent of the codes. The excludes notes in ICD-10-CM are labeled as a type 1 or 2 excludes note:

An Excludes 1 note indicates codes listed elsewhere that would never be used together. The two conditions are not the same, and are, in fact, mutually exclusive. It may also be referred to as a pure excludes note; meaning "not coded here." For example, Excludes 1 is used when two conditions cannot occur together, such as a congenital form versus an acquired form of the same condition.

An Excludes 2 note may be interpreted as "not included here." It indicates codes that may be reported together with the listed codes, if appropriate. This note is clarifying that the excluded condition is not considered part of the main code, and could be reported in addition to the main code.

General exclusions are found at the beginning of a chapter, block, or category title. For example:

Chapter 5. Mental, Behavioral, and Neurodevelopmental Disorders (F01–F99)

> **INCLUDES**   disorders of psychological development
>
> **EXCLUDES 2**   *symptoms, signs and abnormal clinical laboratory findings, not elsewhere classified (R00–R99)*

KEY POINT

The excludes notes in ICD-10-CM are labeled as a type 1 or 2 excludes note.

An "Excludes 1" note indicates codes listed elsewhere that would never be used together. The two conditions are not the same, and are, in fact, mutually exclusive.

An "Excludes 2" note indicates codes that may be reported together with the listed codes, if appropriate. This excludes note clarifies that the excluded condition is not considered part of the main code, and can be reported in addition to the main code.

An excludes note is a warning that the coder may be in the wrong category, so the excludes note should be read carefully when checking a code in the tabular list. Some excludes notes are warning that the two conditions are not the same and do not occur together. For example, the excludes note for three-character category Q16 shows that this is not the code for congenital deafness. That code is found in category H9Ø.

> **Q16   Congenital malformations of ear causing impairment of hearing**
> **EXCLUDES 1**   *congenital deafness (H90.-)*

Some excludes notes serve as a warning that the codes in that section do not include that particular condition and it may be appropriate to look elsewhere. The codes may or may not be appropriately used together. For example, the excludes note for three-character category T83 indicates that this code does not include, or specify, the failure or rejection of a transplanted organ. The correct code can be found in category T86.

> **T83   Complications of genitourinary prosthetic devices, implants and grafts**
> **EXCLUDES 2**   *failure and rejection of transplanted organs and tissues (T86.-)*

Certain categories represent diseases in combination, or the specific manifestation in combination, with the etiology. Exclusion notes in these cases instruct the coder not to use the code if the condition mentioned in the exclusion note is also present. Using both codes is inaccurate, redundant, and confusing. Examples: if the patient had cholecystitis and cholelithiasis, choose the appropriate code under category K8Ø.

> **K81   Cholecystitis**
> **EXCLUDES 1**   *cholecystitis with cholelithiasis (K80.-)*

If the patient has a mycobacterium infection of tuberculosis, choose the correct code from A15–A19 and not A31.

> **A31   Infection due to other mycobacteria**
> **EXCLUDES 2**   *leprosy (A30.-)*
> *tuberculosis (A15–19)*

Exclusion notes may reference the condition excluded. Sometimes, however, a condition may be so general that coding instructions are provided instead of a code reference. The absence of a code reference or coding instruction tells the coder that this is a "normal" condition, not to be coded at all. The following excludes note directs the coder to the alphabetic index. For example:

> **Z39.Ø   Encounter for care and examination immediately after delivery**
> Care and observation in uncomplicated cases when the delivery
> occurs outside a healthcare facility
> **EXCLUDES 1**   *care for postpartum complication—see Alphabetic Index*

"Code First" Note

The ICD-10-CM "code first" note tells the coder that two codes are necessary to describe the condition. The code first note appears within a category that describes the manifestation of a condition. The additional code (i.e., the one used first), describes the etiology of the condition. Code first notes may identify the additional code or examples of the additional code required, a range of codes, or instructions to code the underlying disease, or they may identify the causative drug or substance. Review the medical record prior to coding the underlying disease.

KEY POINT

Since general exclusion notes are not repeated, review the exclusion notes prior to final code selection.

Example 1

K87   Disorders of gallbladder, biliary tract and pancreas in diseases classified elsewhere

Code first underlying disease

EXCLUDES 1   *cytomegaloviral pancreatitis (B25.2)*
mumps pancreatitis (B26.3)
syphilitic gallbladder (A52.74)
syphilitic pancreas (A52.74)
tuberculosis of gallbladder (A18.83)
tuberculosis of pancreas (A18.83)

Example 2

F48.2   Pseudobulbar affect

Involuntary emotional expression disorder
Code first underlying cause, if known, such as:
   amyotrophic lateral sclerosis (G12.21)
   multiple sclerosis (G35)
   sequelae of cerebrovascular disease (I69.-)
   sequelae of traumatic intracranial injury (S06.-)

"Use Additional Code" Note

The "use additional code" notes common to both ICD-9-CM and ICD-10-CM carry the same meaning: a specific instruction to use an additional code to completely describe a condition. The additional code may identify the following:

- The cause of the disease:

  J02.8   Acute pharyngitis due to other specified organisms
  Use additional code (B95–B97) to identify infectious agent

- An associated condition

  F94.1   Reactive attachment disorder of childhood
  Use additional code to identify any associated failure to thrive or growth retardation

- The nature of the condition:

  O91   Infections of breast associated with pregnancy, the puerperium and lactation
  Use additional code to identify infection

Depending on the nature of the diagnosis and associated conditions documented, additional codes may be required for accurate and complete reporting. A note may indicate or otherwise suggest one or more potential conditions that may warrant additional codes. The phrase "such as" may be used to direct the coder to identify and report any associated manifestations, as well as providing an example. For example:

K50   Crohn's disease [regional enteritis]

INCLUDES   granulomatous enteritis
EXCLUDES 1   *ulcerative colitis (K51.-)*
Use additional code to identify manifestations, such as:
   pyoderma gangrenosum (L88)

 KEY POINT

"Code first" and "use additional code" notes may appear independently of each other, or to designate certain etiology/ manifestation paired codes. These instructions prompt the coder that an additional code should be reported to represent a complete diagnostic statement. A code title that specifies "in diseases classified elsewhere" specifically identifies manifestation codes that should never be reported alone, or as a first-listed diagnosis.

Typeface

Chapter and subchapter titles, three-character categories, and all valid codes and their titles, including those requiring seventh characters, are in bold typeface in the tabular list. Main terms in the alphabetic index are also in bold typeface.

Excludes, includes, use, and code first underlying notes, as well as all code groupings not used for primary tabulations of disease, are not bolded.

Terminology

The connective word "and" can be interpreted to mean "and/or" in the tabular list and the alphabetic index. The connective word "also" may indicate that the sites or conditions are included in the code (i.e., a combination code).

The preposition "with" in the alphabetic index references the code for diseases in combination. A "with" reference always follows the main term (or subterm) of reference (e.g., "with" appears as a subterm but not in strict alphabetical sequence).

.– Point Dash

A point dash (.–) replaces the list of options available at a level of specificity past the three-character category. It instructs the coder to turn to the category or subcategory referenced to review the subdivisions available for coding.

In ICD-10-CM, the following excludes note indicates the category JØ2 for a patient who has an acute sore throat. The point dash indicates the code is incomplete. An additional character completes the code. For example:

JØ3   **Acute tonsillitis**
> EXCLUDES 1 *acute sore throat (JØ2.-)*
> *hypertrophy of tonsils (J35.1)*
> *peritonsillar abscess (J36)*
> *sore throat NOS (JØ2.9)*
> *streptococcal sore throat (JØ2.Ø)*
> EXCLUDES 2 *chronic tonsillitis (J35.Ø)*

ARRANGEMENT OF THE ALPHABETIC INDEX

The alphabetic index in ICD-10-CM is divided into three sections, similar to ICD-9-CM. It consists of the main alphabetic "Index to Diseases and Injuries," the "Table of Drugs and Chemicals," and the "Index to External Causes."

The main section in the alphabetic index of ICD-10-CM contains alphabetically sequenced terms pertaining to diseases, syndromes, pathological conditions, injuries, and signs and symptoms as reasons to contact the health care provider. The alphabetic index is organized by main terms, printed in bold type for easy reference. Main terms identify disease conditions. For example, chronic tonsillitis is found under the main term "Tonsillitis."

Adjectives, such as "chronic" and "hereditary," and references to anatomic sites, such as "foot" and "kidney," appear as main terms with cross-references to "*see* condition." For example, "Chronic—*see* condition; Kidney—*see* condition."

Neoplasms are listed in the alphabetic index in two ways: by anatomic site and morphology. The list of anatomic sites is found in a table under the main term entry "Neoplasm, neoplastic." The table contains six columns: "Malignant

Primary," "Malignant Secondary," "Ca in situ," "Benign, Uncertain," and "Unspecified Behavior."

Histological terms for neoplasms, such as "Carcinoma," and "Adenoma," are listed as main terms in the alphabetic index with cross-references to the neoplasm table.

The alphabetically listed terms in the "Index of External Causes" describe the circumstances of an accident or act of violence (the underlying cause or means of injury). The main terms represent the type of accident or violent encounter (e.g., "assault," "collision"). The index includes terms for codes classified to VØØ–Y98, excluding drugs and chemicals.

The "Table of Drugs and Chemicals" is an extensive, but not exhaustive (new products are developed every day) resource containing a list of drugs, industrial solvents, corrosives, metals, gases, noxious plants, household cleaning products, pesticides, and other toxic agents that can be harmful. The table provides the diagnostic codes for poisoning by, and adverse effect of, these products—whether the poisoning is accidental (unintentional), an assault, self-inflicted, or if it is undetermined whether accidental or intentional.

ALPHABETIC INDEX CONVENTIONS

The extensive amount of information in ICD-10-CM requires a complete understanding of the conventions and rules established to accurately assign a code.

The NCHS has clinically modified the ICD-10 index developed by the World Health Organization. These modifications include adding entries for new fifth- and sixth-character subclassifications, and deleting entries for codes that do not apply to the clinical modification.

Main Term

The alphabetic index is organized by main terms printed in bold typeface for easy reference. Main terms describe disease conditions. For example, acute bronchitis is found under the main term "Bronchitis," and congestive heart failure is found under "Failure."

There are exceptions to the rule. Obstetric conditions are found under "Delivery," "Pregnancy," and "Puerperal," and under main terms for specific conditions such as "Labor" and "Vomiting."

Complications of medical and surgical procedures are indexed under "Complication" and under the terms relating to specific conditions, including "Dehiscence" and "Infection."

Late effects of certain conditions (e.g., cerebral infections, injuries, infectious diseases) are found under the main term "Sequelae" with a note to "see also condition."

The Z codes from chapter 21, "Factors Influencing Health Status and Contact with Health Services (ZØØ–Z99)," are found under main terms such as "Examination," "History," "Observation," "Problem," "Screening," "Status," or "Vaccination."

 KEY POINT

If a term describing a condition can be expressed in more than one form, all forms will appear in the main term entry. For example, "excess," "excessive," and "excessively" are listed together in the alphabetic index.

 KEY POINT

An essential modifier that is the sole essential modifier for a main term appears in the alphabetic index on the same line as the main term, separated by a comma. For example: Insufflation, fallopian Z31.41. "Fallopian" is an essential modifier, and the only essential modifier of the main term "insufflation."

MODIFIERS

Main terms in the alphabetic index may be followed by nouns or adjectives that further describe them. These descriptors are called modifiers, and there are two types: essential modifiers and nonessential modifiers.

Essential modifiers are descriptors that affect code selection for a given diagnosis, due to the axis of classification. For coding purposes, these modifiers describe essential differences in the site, etiology, or clinical type of disease. All terms must be present in the diagnosis to code according to the category modified.

ICD-10-CM

In the ICD-10-CM index, the axis of classification for pneumonia is etiology or cause. "Aspiration," "pneumococcal," and "viral" are essential modifiers of pneumonia. Each term describes a different cause that requires a different code. As such, separate subterm entries exist for each subclassification code.

The modifiers must be present in the diagnosis to assign these codes. For example:

Pneumonia J18.9

Aspiration pneumonia J69.0

Pneumococcal pneumonia J13

Viral pneumonia J12.9

Main terms with multiple essential modifiers present each modifier on a separate line in a list indented below the main term. These multiple essential modifiers are called "subterms." For example, "allergic," "cluster," and "drug-induced" are essential modifiers for the main term "Headache." Each appears as a subterm under "Headache." For example:

Headache R51
    allergic NEC G44.89
    cluster G44.009
    drug-induced NEC G44.40

Subterms may also be modified by other essential modifiers. In the alphabetic index they are further indented. For example, "visual" is an essential modifier of the main term "Disorder." "Cortex" is an essential modifier of the subterm "visual," and "blindness" is an essential modifier of the main term "Disorder" and subterms "visual" and "cortex." For example:

Disorder
    visual
        cortex
            blindness H47.619
                left brain H47.612
                right brain H47.611

Nonessential modifiers do not affect code selection for a given diagnosis, due to the axis of classification. Nonessential modifiers appear as parenthetical terms following the words they modify. For example, etiology is the axis of classification for pneumonia. The terms "acute," "double," and "septic" are nonessential modifiers since they describe conditions other than the cause of pneumonia. The code for "pneumonia" is J18.9 despite the absence or presence of any of the nonessential modifiers. For example:

 KEY POINT

Nonessential modifiers may be present or absent for the diagnosis to be coded. Either way, the code remains the same.

Pneumonia (acute) (double) (migratory) (purulent) (septic) (unresolved)J18.9

Nonessential modifiers may follow subterms in the alphabetic index. For example:

Murmur (cardiac) (heart) (organic) R01.1
    aortic (valve)—*see* Endocarditis, aortic

Abbreviations

In the alphabetic index the abbreviation NEC, "not elsewhere classified," serves as a warning regarding ill-defined terms. The code is assigned only if a review of the code choices does not yield a more appropriate code for the condition.

NEC following "Granuloma, foreign body (in soft tissue)" indicates that M60.20 may not be the correct code or subcategory for classifying a foreign body granuloma. Before assigning the NEC code for a given diagnosis, first scan all available subterms to determine whether there is another more specific entry. This ensures that the most appropriate code is assigned.

In this case, NEC references the residual category for a condition (e.g., the category for "other specified" forms of soft tissue foreign body granulomas). After scanning subterms in the index, the coder may be directed to a specified subcategory, such as for skin or subcutaneous tissue, L92.3, or to a more appropriate code within the NEC subcategory.

An index entry may also appear as "specified NEC." This convention ensures that the correct code will be chosen although the term to be coded does not appear in the index. For example:

Granuloma
    foreign body (in soft tissue) NEC M60.20
        shoulder region M60.21-
        skin L92.3
        specified site NEC M60.28
        subcutaneous tissue L92.3

Cross-References

In the alphabetic index, cross-references direct the coder to other possible main terms or sources for information pertaining to a term or its synonyms.

There are two types of cross-references: "— *see*" and "(*see also*)."

In ICD-10-CM, *"see"* directs the coder to another term in the index that provides more complete information. It is also used with anatomical site main entries to prompt the coder that the index is organized by condition. For example, the cross-reference *"see"* indicates that the term "hardening of arteries" is coded to "arteriosclerosis."

Hardening
    artery — *see* Arteriosclerosis

Similarly, the cross-reference directs the coder to a specific cardiovascular condition affecting the heart. For example:

Heart — *see* condition

CODING AXIOM

In ICD-10-CM, as in ICD-9-CM, always locate the code in the alphabetic index first; then confirm the code choice in the tabular section.

KEY POINT

Review the alphabetic index for cross-references and notes prior to confirming in the tabular list. Notes at the beginning of main terms may not be repeated.

The cross-reference *"see also"* prompts the use of another main term for additional information than what is listed under the first term selected. For example:

Necrosis, necrotic (ischemic) (*see also* Gangrene)

Modifiers under "necrosis" are not definitive. Modifiers that apply to "necrosis" may be the same as those for "gangrene." If the modifier cannot be found under "necrosis," the cross-reference instructs to "(*see also* Gangrene)."

Notes

The omission of the notes that were common in ICD-9-CM is new to the ICD-10-CM index. Because the information in the notes section of the ICD-9-CM index is repeated in the tabular section of ICD-9-CM, it may have been considered redundant. Editors may also have felt that to retain the notes in the index encouraged coders to code from the index—a practice discouraged by experienced coders concerned with maintaining data integrity.

Etiology and Manifestation of Disease

Both the etiology and the manifestation of the disease for certain conditions must be coded.

"Code first" and "use additional code" notations are used as sequencing rules in the classification for certain codes. Some of these codes are etiology/manifestation pairings that require mandatory multiple coding; whereas, other codes may occur independently or be reported alone, as appropriate. Bracketed codes in the index indicate the presence of manifestation codes, which must be sequenced in addition to the preceding code. In this example, the diagnosis of myasthenia syndrome in neoplastic disease requires two codes for complete representation of the condition. Along with the cross-reference, the index lists code D49.9 followed by bracketed code G73.3. In the tabular list, code G73.3 is listed in italicized font, with "in diseases classified elsewhere" listed in the code title. An instructional note prompts to "code first underlying disease." This designates a manifestation code that must be sequenced and reported secondary to the etiological condition.

> **Myasthenia** G70.9
>   syndrome
>   in
>   diabetes mellitus — *see* E09–E13 with .44
>   neoplastic disease (*see also* Neoplasm) D49.9 *[G73.3]*
>   pernicious anemia D51.0 *[G73.3]*
>   thyrotoxicosis E05.90 *[G73.3]*
>   with thyroid storm E05.91 *[G73.3]*

ICD-10-CM coding conventions include two types of etiology/manifestation codes, those that specify "in disease classified elsewhere" in the code title, and others that do not.

For example, code H42 includes "in diseases classified elsewhere" in the code description/title:

> **H42   Glaucoma in diseases classified elsewhere**
>   Code first underlying condition

Code G13.0 is also a manifestation code, but it does not have "in diseases classified elsewhere" in the code description/title.

G13.0 **Paraneoplastic neuromyopathy and neuropathy**
Code first underlying neoplasm

The phrase "use additional code" identifies an etiology code, whereas the phrase "code first" identifies a manifestation code. Follow sequencing instruction in the text.

DISCUSSION QUESTIONS

1. What is meant by "axis of classification"? Please give examples of some axes.

   _____

   _____

   _____

   _____

2. Explain the rules surrounding the use of parentheses in the tabular section and index to diseases.

   _____

   _____

   _____

   _____

3. Why should a coder use caution when selecting a code designated as NEC or NOS?

   _____

   _____

   _____

   _____

4. How are seventh characters used in the classification? Give an example.

   _____

   _____

   _____

   _____

5. Discuss the two types of excludes notes and how each is different.

   _____

   _____

   _____

   _____

Chapter 4:
ICD-10-CM Code Book Chapters

This chapter provides a review and analysis of the changes to individual chapters within certain classification blocks or three-character code categories. While not every revision or change has been identified for each chapter, the highlights provided here assist in ensuring that ICD-10-CM coding is performed accurately, in accordance with coding conventions and with the current draft "ICD-10-CM Draft Official Guidelines for Coding and Reporting" available at the time of publication.

With any revision to a classification, changes are made for specific reasons. Overall, conditions classified in ICD-10-CM have been grouped in a way that is most appropriate for general epidemiological purposes and the evaluation of health care.

Specific reasons for changes to the contents of the chapters include the intent to:

- Increase clinical detail about a specific disorder

- Reclassify diseases in accordance with current advances in clinical science and technologies

- Report recently identified diseases, (i.e., since the last revision)

- Accommodate the required detail of a group of diseases

- Make effective use of available space

In general, conditions have been moved as a group within a chapter and individual conditions have been reclassified. For example, certain disorders of the immune mechanism were expanded and the category group was moved to "Diseases of the Blood and Blood-forming Organs." In ICD-9-CM, these disorders are included with "Endocrine, Nutritional, and Metabolic Diseases."

CHAPTER 1. CERTAIN INFECTIOUS AND PARASITIC DISEASES (AØØ–B99)

This chapter includes diseases due to infective organisms, including communicable diseases and diseases of suspected infectious origin. Additionally, conditions classifiable to this chapter include those that are generally recognized as communicable or transmissible. Although ICD-10-CM includes many infectious disease classifications specific to affected anatomic site, certain other infections are classified to other chapters. These conditions include congenitally acquired infections (chapter 16), influenza (chapter 10), postoperative infections (classified by body system), infections complicating pregnancy and delivery (chapter 15), and traumatic wound infections (chapter 19). Codes classifiable to this chapter are mutually exclusive from the same condition classifiable elsewhere. For example, enterocolitis due to *Clostridium difficile* is classified to AØ4.7 instead of K52.9 Noninfective gastroenteritis and colitis, unspecified. The alphabetic index lists a specific code for this condition as identified by causal organism. When confirmed by the tabular list, the text does not prompt the coder to assign an additional code. By contrast, certain infections classified elsewhere require an additional code to specify the causal organism. Instructional notes in the tabular list prompt the coder that an additional code is necessary. In these cases, the appropriate code from B95–B97 Bacterial and viral infectious agents, is assigned. Instructions in this chapter include:

- Single codes used to identify the disease or condition. For example:

  A46   Erysipelas

- Combination codes that identify both the condition and causal organism or causal organism, manifestation, and/or affected anatomic site. For example:

  A08.11   Acute gastroenteropathy due to Norwalk agent

- Multiple coding: Certain conditions require more than one code in order to report in its entirety. These conditions may identify infections etiology and manifestations classified elsewhere, or single conditions that require more than one code, but are not part of the etiology/manifestation combination. Conventions in the text prompt for the use of additional codes, when needed, or for specific sequencing of codes. "Code first" and "use additional code" notations are used as sequencing rules in the classification for certain codes. Some of these codes are etiology/manifestation pairings that require multiple coding in specific sequence, whereas, other codes may occur independently or be reported alone, as appropriate. For example:

Example 1

Etiology/manifestation coding (multiple coding, in specific sequence):

Diagnosis: Infectious endocarditis in Q fever

A78   Q fever

I39   *Endocarditis and heart valve disorders in diseases classified elsewhere*
   Code first underlying disease, such as:
   Q fever (A78)

In example 1, code I39 is identified as a manifestation code by the phrase "in diseases classified elsewhere" in the code title and the instructional note "code first underlying disease." Manifestation codes can never be reported alone, or as the first-listed diagnosis.

Note that throughout the classification, certain codes may list the instructional notation "code first" (the underlying disease or condition), yet may not be identified as manifestation codes. In these cases, the condition may occur independently and, thus, be reported alone.

Example 2

Conditions requiring multiple codes to report in their entirety, yet are not part of the etiology/manifestation convention:

Diagnosis: HIV disease with disseminated histoplasmosis capsulati

B20   Human immunodeficiency virus [HIV] disease

B39.3   Disseminated histoplasmosis capsulate

In example 2, code B39.3 Disseminated histoplasmosis capsulati, is not identified as a manifestation code. It is not a manifestation condition, because it may occur independently, even though it is often associated with other underlying diseases (including AIDS). Manifestation codes in

ICD-10-CM may be identified by the phrase "in diseases classified elsewhere" in the code title. These codes cannot be sequenced first or reported alone. A manifestation code may not have "in diseases classified elsewhere" in the title. In such cases, there will be a "use additional code" note at the etiology code and a "code first" note at the manifestation code. Follow the sequencing rules in the text.

Category B39 Histoplasmosis, lists the following instructions, which apply to all codes with the category, including code B39.3:

B39   Histoplasmosis
Code first associated AIDS (B20)
Use additional code for any associated manifestations, such as:
    endocarditis (I39)
    meningitis (G02)

Chapter 1 contains 22 code families represented by the first characters "A" and "B." The coding families classified to chapter 1 are:

A00–A09	**Intestinal infectious diseases**
A15–A19	**Tuberculosis**
A20–A28	**Certain zoonotic bacterial diseases**
A30–A49	**Other bacterial diseases**
A50–A64	**Infections with a predominantly sexual mode of transmission**
A65–A69	**Other spirochetal diseases**
A70–A74	**Other diseases caused by chlamydiae**
A75–A79	**Rickettsioses**
A80–A89	**Viral infections of the central nervous system**
A90–A99	**Arthropod-borne viral fevers and viral hemorrhagic fevers**
B00–B09	**Viral infections characterized by skin and mucous membrane lesions**
B10	**Other human herpesviruses**
B15–B19	**Viral hepatitis**
B20	**Human immunodeficiency virus [HIV] disease**
B25–B34	**Other viral diseases**
B35–B49	**Mycoses**
B50–B64	**Protozoal diseases**
B65–B83	**Helminthiases**
B85–B89	**Pediculosis, acariasis and other infestations**
B90–B94	**Sequelae of infectious and parasitic diseases**
B95–B97	**Bacterial, viral and other infectious agents**
B99	**Other infectious diseases**

ICD-10-CM Subchapter Restructuring

After reviewing different disease categories, the developers of ICD-10 restructured some of their groupings to bring together those groups that were related by cause. For example, the ICD-9-CM subchapter, "Syphilis and Other Venereal Diseases," has been rearranged, and the subchapter "Rickettsioses and other Arthropod-borne Diseases" has been split into two separate subchapters in ICD-10-CM.

CODING AXIOM

Follow the instructions in the alphabetic index and tabular list carefully to ensure accurate code assignment and sequencing.

QUICK TIP

Consider indexing the main term "Infection" when the organism is specified, but not indexed under the main term.

KEY POINT

The term "certain" has been added to the title of chapter 1, "Infectious and Parasitic Diseases," to stress the fact that localized infections are classified to other chapters, with the diseases of the pertinent body system.

ICD-9-CM

080–088   Rickettsioses and other arthropod-borne diseases

090–099   Syphilis and other venereal diseases

100–104   Other spirochetal diseases

ICD-10-CM

A50–A64   Infections with a predominantly sexual mode of transmission

A65–A69   Other spirochetal diseases

A75–A79   Rickettsioses

A90–A99   Arthropod-borne viral fevers and hemorrhagic fevers

Section and Category Title Changes

As the examples above illustrate, a number of category and subchapter titles have been revised in chapter 1. Titles were changed to better reflect the content, which was often necessary when specific types of diseases were given their own block, a new category was created, or an existing category was redefined. For example, the ICD-9-CM classification for "Late Effects" has been retitled in ICD-10-CM to "Sequelae."

ICD-9-CM Section	ICD-10-CM Block
090–099 Syphilis and Other Venereal Diseases	A50–A64 Infections with a Predominately Sexual Mode of Transmission
137–139 Late Effects of Infectious and Parasitic Diseases	B90–B94 Sequelae of Infectious and Parasitic Diseases

ICD-9-CM Category	ICD-10-CM Category
046 Slow virus infections and prion diseases of central nervous system	A81 Atypical virus infections of central nervous system

Organizational Adjustments

When comparing ICD-9-CM to ICD-10-CM, many codes have been added, deleted, combined, and relocated to other sections. These changes include:

- ICD-9-CM code 034.0 Streptococcal sore throat, has been moved in ICD-10-CM to chapter 10, "Diseases of the Respiratory System."

- Human immunodeficiency virus disease followed the subchapter, "Other Bacterial Diseases," in ICD-9-CM, whereas it now follows the subchapter for viral hepatitis in ICD-10-CM.

- ICD-10 code for opportunistic mycoses, B48.7, has been deleted in ICD-10-CM. The conditions that would have been classified to this code have been moved to B48.8. See the following examples from ICD-9-CM, ICD-10, and ICD-10-CM:

ICD-9-CM

118   Opportunistic mycoses

ICD-10

B48.7 Opportunistic mycoses

Mycoses caused by fungi of low virulence that can establish an infection only as a consequence of factors such as the presence of debilitating disease or the administration of immunosuppressive and other therapeutic agents or radiation therapy. Most of the causal fungi are normally saprophytic in soil and decaying vegetation.

ICD-10-CM

Note: Code B48.7 has been deleted in ICD-10-CM.

> **B48.8** **Other specified mycoses**
> Adiaspiromycosis
> Infection of tissue and organs by Alternaria
> Infection of tissue and organs by Dreschlera
> Infection of tissue and organs by Fusarium
> Infection of tissue and organs by saprophytic fungi NEC

- Fifth-character designations to indicate the method of tuberculosis identification have been eliminated. See the following table for a comparison.

ICD-9-CM		ICD-10-CM	
011.40	TB Fibrosis lung confirm unsp	A15.0	Tuberculosis of lung
011.41	TB Fibrosis lung exam not done	A15.0	Tuberculosis of lung
011.42	TB Fibrosis lung exam unknown	A15.0	Tuberculosis of lung
011.43	TB Fibrosis lung tubercle bacilli, by microscopy	A15.0	Tuberculosis of lung

- New codes have been created where needs have been identified for unique codes to facilitate reporting. ICD-9-CM did not provide a separate code for septicemia due to *Enterococcus*. As such, a code has been added to ICD-10-CM to classify this disorder. See comparison below:

ICD-9-CM		ICD-10-CM	
038.8	Other specified septicemias	A41.81	Sepsis due to Enterococcus

- ICD-10-CM requires etiology/manifestation code assignment for certain infectious diseases and associated manifestations formerly reported by a single code in ICD-9-CM. These conditions include complications of ornithosis (*Chlamydia psittaci*) and histoplasmosis infections. See example below:

ICD-9-CM		ICD-10-CM	
115.01	Histoplasma capsulatum meningitis	B39.4	Histoplasmosis capsulati unspecified
		G02	Meningitis in other infx & parasitic dz classified elsewhere

Chapter 1 Coding Guidance

Human Immunodeficiency Virus

Code B20 Human immunodeficiency virus [HIV] disease, includes acquired immune deficiency syndrome (AIDS), AIDS-related complex (ARC) and HIV infection, symptomatic. This code is assigned for all subsequent encounters once a patient has developed an HIV-related illness or associated symptoms. Report code B20, as the first-listed diagnosis for patient encounters for HIV-related conditions. Assign additional codes to identify all manifestations of HIV infection, as documented. For example:

Diagnosis: Multiple cutaneous Kaposi's sarcoma lesions in HIV disease

B20 Human immunodeficiency virus [HIV] disease
Use additional code(s) to identify all manifestations of HIV infection

C46.0 Kaposi's sarcoma of skin
Code first any human immunodeficiency virus [HIV] disease (B20)

Patient encounters for conditions unrelated to HIV disease are coded and sequenced with the unrelated condition (e.g., illness or injury) as the first-listed diagnosis, followed by code B20 and other reportable secondary diagnoses. For example:

Diagnosis: Patient with symptomatic HIV disease admitted for surgical treatment of acute cholecystitis with cholelithiasis

K80.00 Calculus of gallbladder with acute cholecystitis without obstruction

B20 Human immunodeficiency virus [HIV] disease

Code B20 excludes:

- Asymptomatic human immunodeficiency virus [HIV] infection status (Z21): assign when the patient is without HIV or AIDS symptoms, but has been determined HIV positive.

- HIV disease complicating pregnancy, childbirth and the puerperium (O98.7-): chapter 15 codes take sequencing priority. Assign the appropriate O98.7 code, followed by the appropriate code for the HIV disease or status.

- Exposure to HIV virus (Z20.6): assign to report contact with, or exposure to the HIV virus in the absence of positive evidence of transmission.

- Inconclusive serologic evidence of HIV (R75): assign for patients with inconclusive HIV serology, but no definitive diagnosis or manifestations of the illness.

Infectious Agent

Categories B95–B97 identify the infectious agents in conditions classified elsewhere. Certain infections are classified to other chapters, but do not identify the causal infectious agent (organism). In these cases, it is necessary to use an additional code from chapter 1 to identify the organism. An instructional note is found at the infection code to prompt that an additional code should be assigned. For example:

Diagnosis: Urinary tract infection due to *Escherichia coli*

N39.0 Urinary tract infection, site not specified
Use additional code (B95–B97), to identify infectious agent

B96.2 Escherichia coli [E. coli] as the cause of diseases classified elsewhere

Resistant infections

It is important to code and report all infections documented as antibiotic resistant. An instructional note has been added to the beginning of chapter 1, which instructs the coder to assign the appropriate category Z16 Infection with drug resistant microorganisms code, following the appropriate infection code all such cases. For example:

Diagnosis: Antimycobacterial-resistant primary pulmonary tuberculosis

A15.Ø   **Tuberculosis of lung**

Z16.341   **Resistance to single antimycobacterial drug**

Note: Code Z16.341 includes resistance to antimycobacterial drug "NOS"; if multiple drug resistance is not specified, classification defaults to the single drug resistance code.

Instructions for reporting Methicillin resistant *Staphylococcus aureus* (MRSA) infections contain the following main points:

- Do not assign separate codes for the type of infection (B95.62) and the MRSA organism (Z16.11) if a combination diagnosis code includes both the causal organism and drug resistance. For example:

J15.212   **Pneumonia due to Methicillin resistant Staphylococcus aureus**

In this example, the code description includes both the causal organism (*Staphylococcus aureus*) and drug resistance status (Methicillin-resistance)

- MRSA infections that are not classified with combination codes require separate reporting of the causal organism and drug-resistance status. For example:

T81.4   **Infection following a procedure**

B95.62   **Methicillin resistant Staphylococcus aureus infection as the cause of diseases classified elsewhere**

Z16.11   **Resistance to penicillins**

In this example, code T81.4 does not specify either the organism or the drug resistance status. Separate codes are required to report the diagnosis in entirety.

- Assign code Z22.322 Carrier or suspected carrier of MRSA, to report MRSA colonization status.

- Assign code Z22.321 Carrier or suspected carrier of MSSA, for patients documented as Methicillin susceptible *Staphylococcus aureus* (MSSA) colonization.

- Simultaneous MRSA colonization and active, documented MRSA infection requires two codes. Code the nature or manifestation of the active MRSA infection as described in the documentation. Assign code Z22.322 to specify carrier status.

Sepsis and Septicemia

Sepsis may be caused by the invasion of toxins, which may include bacteria, fungi, viruses, and other organisms, into the blood stream. As such, classification may vary depending on the nature of the organism. For example, when consulting the alphabetic index under the main term "Sepsis," note the following:

Sepsis (generalized) (unspecified organism) A41.9
    Bacillus anthracis A22.7
    Brucella (*see also* Brucellosis) A23.9
    candidal B37.7
    Erysipelothrix (rhusiopathiae)(erysipeloid) A26.7
    extraintestinal yersiniosis A28.2
    herpesviral BØØ.7

Code category A41 Other sepsis, lists multiple exclusions for specific systemic (septic) infections more appropriately classified elsewhere. Similarly, site-specific or organ-specific sepsis should not be coded as a systemic sepsis. Instructional notes at the beginning of category A41 direct the coder to sequence first sepsis due to other circumstances, such as postprocedural sepsis (T81.4) and sepsis occurring during labor (O75.3).

Coding instructions for sepsis, severe sepsis, and septic shock provide guidance for accurate reporting of the severity, nature, cause, and conditions associated with systemic infection. The number and sequence of codes required vary according to the circumstances of the condition and encounter. These key concepts include:

- Assign the appropriate code for the underlying systemic infection.

- Sepsis of unknown type or causal organism is reported with A41.9 Sepsis, unspecified.

- Report a code from subcategory R65.2 only when the diagnosis of severe sepsis or associated acute organ dysfunction has been documented.

- Severe sepsis requires a minimum of two codes: one for the underlying systemic infection first, followed by an appropriate code from subcategory R65.2 Severe sepsis.

- Assign additional codes for any associated acute organ dysfunction (e.g., renal failure, respiratory failure) when coding severe sepsis.

- Septic shock indicates the presence of severe sepsis. For all cases of septic shock, report the code for the underlying systemic infection *first*, followed by R65.21 Severe sepsis with septic shock or code T81.12 Postprocedural septic shock. For example:

  Diagnosis: Severe gram-negative sepsis with acute respiratory failure

A41.50	**Gram-negative sepsis, unspecified**
R65.20	**Severe sepsis without septic shock**
J96.00	**Acute respiratory failure**

- Postprocedural sepsis requires provider documentation (linkage) of the relationship between the surgery or procedure and the infection. Do not assume a causal relationship in absence of supportive documentation.

- Septic shock cannot be assigned as a first-listed or principal diagnosis. Instead, sequence first the systemic infection or precipitating complication.

  Refer to the "ICD-10-CM Draft Official Guidelines for Coding and Reporting" in appendix A of this book for additional information.

Level of Detail in Coding

As in ICD-9-CM, diagnosis codes are to be used and reported to the highest level of specificity available. ICD-10-CM provides, in the majority of cases, an exponentially increased level of specificity than ICD-9-CM. In chapter 1, this code expansion is intended to facilitate identification of specific types of causal organisms, or other indicators of severity. For example:

ICD-9-CM		ICD-10-CM	
036.2	Meningococcemia	A39.2	Acute meningococcemia
		A39.3	Chronic meningococcemia
		A39.4	Meningococcemia unspecified
038.0	Streptococcal septicemia	A40.0	Sepsis due to Streptococcus Group A
		A40.1	Sepsis due to Streptococcus Group B
		A40.3	Sepsis due to Streptococcus Pneumoniae
		A40.8	Other streptococcal sepsis
		A40.9	Streptococcal sepsis unspecified

Combination Codes

Certain infectious disease classifications have been expanded in ICD-10-CM to facilitate identification of secondary disease processes, specific manifestations, or associated complications. As such, code to the highest level of specificity as documented in the record. Consult the instructions in the text to determine whether additional codes are necessary to report the associated conditions or manifestations. For example:

ICD-9-CM		ICD-10-CM	
002.0	Typhoid fever	A01.00	Typhoid fever unspecified
		A01.01	Typhoid meningitis
		A01.02	Typhoid fever with heart involvement
		A01.03	Typhoid pneumonia
		A01.04	Typhoid arthritis
		A01.05	Typhoid osteomyelitis
		A01.09	Typhoid fever with other complications

Diagnosis: Acute typhoid cholecystitis

A01.09   Typhoid fever with other complications

In this example, the alphabetic index directs the coder to assign one code. The index lists "Typhoid, cholecystitis (current)" as A01.09. Similarly, "Cholecystitis, typhoidal" is listed as A01.09. There are no further instructions in the tabular list to assign additional codes.

Late Effects (Sequelae)

ICD-10-CM classifies late effect conditions or "sequelae" to categories B90–B94. These codes identify that a residual condition remains or is due to a previous illness or injury after the acute phase has resolved. There is no time limit restricting the reporting of late effect codes. Residual conditions may occur months or years following the causal condition. Two codes, sequenced in the following order, are often required: the condition resulting from the sequela is sequenced first, followed by the appropriate late effect code.

There are two sequencing exceptions: 1) a Tabular List instruction note that indicates the sequela code is first, followed by the manifestation(s) code(s); or 2) the sequela code has a fourth, fifth, or sixth character that includes the manifestation(s).

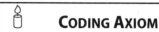

CODING AXIOM

An additional code from category B95–B97 Bacterial and viral infectious agents, is not necessary when the causal organism is specified in the code title (description).

CODING AXIOM

Human Immunodeficiency Virus (HIV) Infections

Review the coding guidelines (C.1.a) and notes at the category levels of the ICD-10-CM text.

CODING AXIOM

Sequela of Infectious and Parasitic Diseases

Sequelae include residual conditions (late effects) of diseases classifiable elsewhere, of which the disease itself is no longer present.

Code chronic current infections to the active infectious disease, as appropriate.

Sequelae codes are NOT used to report chronic infections.

CODING AXIOM

Bacterial and Viral Infectious Agents

Report codes B95–B97 as additional codes to identify the infectious agent (organism) in diseases classified elsewhere. In general, the instructional note "Use additional code" prompts the coder that an additional code is necessary if the causal organism or agent is known.

Chapter 1 Coding Exercises

Assign the appropriate ICD-10-CM diagnosis codes for all reportable diagnoses, excluding external causes of morbidity (VØØ–Y99):

Answers to coding exercises are listed in the back of the book.

1. Acute *E. coli* cystitis _____

   _____

2. Coxsackie enteritis _____

   _____

3. Bell's palsy as late effect of Lyme disease _____

   _____

4. Sequelae of poliomyelitis, secondary kyphoscoliosis of thoracic spine

   _____

   _____

5. AIDS-related encephalopathy _____

   _____

6. HIV infection status _____

   _____

7. Septicemia due to systemic progression of *Pseudomonas aeruginosa* urinary tract infection _____

   _____

8. Severe pneumococcal septicemia due to pneumococcal pneumonia, with SIRS and acute kidney failure _____

   _____

9. Methicillin-resistant *S. aureus* septicemia _____

   _____

Chapter 1 Coding Scenarios

Assign the appropriate ICD-10-CM diagnosis codes for all reportable diagnoses, excluding external causes of morbidity (VØØ–Y99).

Answers to coding exercises are listed in the back of the book.

1. An otherwise healthy 26-year-old female presents to the emergency department with fever, an erythematous, pruritic rash on her face, trunk and limbs, painful bilateral joint pain and swelling of the hands, wrists, and knees. Past medical history is noncontributory. The patient stated that her 5-year-old child had a similar mild rash two weeks ago, but did not appear ill or complain of joint pain. A blood test was obtained to rule out the presence of suspected parvovirus antibodies. Test results were positive for immunoglobulin M (IgM) antibody to parvovirus B19, confirming a suspected clinical diagnosis consistent with recent parvovirus infection. The patient was placed on rest, hydrated, and given ibuprofen (800mg) with resolution fever. She was advised that the joint pain should resolve in a couple weeks. The patient was also advised to rest, restrict activities, and follow up with her physician if symptoms worsen.

    Diagnosis: Arthritis due to Parvovirus B19 infection

    _____

    _____

2. A 42-year-old patient with a two-year history of AIDS was admitted with fever, nonproductive cough, pleuritic chest pain, and shortness of breath. He stated a history of progressive weight loss and fatigue throughout the 30 days preceding admission. Diagnostic imaging was positive for pulmonary infiltrates. Sputum was positive for *Pneumocystis jiroveci*. The patient was placed on supplemental oxygen therapy, prednisone, and pentamidine isethionate. The patient showed marked improvement within 48 hours of admission and was discharged home with instructions and a prescription to continue oral pentamidine isethionate for 14 days.

    Diagnosis: Pneumocystis jiroveci pneumonia

    _____

    _____

3. A 53-year-old diabetic male sustained a deep laceration to the left proximal thumb with a chef's knife while deboning poultry in the kitchen of a local restaurant. He placed a dishtowel over the cut to stop the bleeding, and then wrapped the finger in a gauze bandage. Approximately 48 hours after the initial injury, he replaced the bandage. A couple days later, when he removed the bandage, the cut had become red and swollen. Upon seeking care for the wound, his physician cleaned the wound and prescribed a broad-spectrum antibiotic. However, the patient failed to complete the dosage when the wound began to improve. Approximately five days after stopping the antibiotic, he developed fatigue, malaise, and tachycardia. Within 24 hours from the onset of symptoms, he presented to the emergency department at his local hospital with progressively worsening fever, chills, tachycardia, lethargy, and confusion. Upon admission, his fever was 104 degrees, blood pressure 88/60 mm Hg, respiratory rate 22, and pulse 110. The patient was determined to be in shock, likely of septic origin based on the evaluation of the infected wound present on examination, and recent history. Blood chemistry revealed a BUN of 54 g/dl and creatinine of 1.8 mg/dl. Blood cultures grew gram-negative rods identified as *E. coli*. The patient was admitted to ICU, placed on intravenous ciprofloxacin at 400 mg IV q12h and mechanical ventilation for the associated acute respiratory failure. The patient responded well to treatment and was discharged in improved condition with favorable prognosis.

Diagnosis: *E. coli* septicemia

_____

_____

Chapter 2. Neoplasms (CØØ–D49)

This chapter contains 21 code families represented by the first characters "C" and "D." The letter D is also shared with chapter 3, "Diseases of the Blood and Blood-Forming Organs and Certain Disorders Involving the Immune System." The code families classified to chapter 2 are:

CØØ–C14	Malignant neoplasm of lip, oral cavity and pharynx
C15–C26	Malignant neoplasm of digestive organs
C3Ø–C39	Malignant neoplasm of respiratory and intrathoracic organs
C4Ø–C41	Malignant neoplasm of bone and articular cartilage
C43–C44	Melanoma and other malignant neoplasms of skin
C45–C49	Malignant neoplasms of mesothelial and soft tissue
C5Ø	Malignant neoplasm of breast
C51–C58	Malignant neoplasm of female genital organs
C6Ø–C63	Malignant neoplasms of male genital organs
C64–C68	Malignant neoplasm of urinary tract
C69–C72	Malignant neoplasms of eye, brain and other parts of central nervous system
C73–C75	Malignant neoplasm of thyroid and other endocrine glands
C7A	Malignant neuroendocrine tumors
C7B	Secondary neuroendocrine tumors
C76–C8Ø	Malignant neoplasms of ill-defined, secondary and unspecified sites
C81–C96	Malignant neoplasms of lymphoid, hematopoietic and related tissue
DØØ–DØ9	In situ neoplasms
D1Ø–D36	Benign neoplasms, except benign neuroendocrine tumors
D3A	Benign neuroendocrine tumors
D37–D48	Neoplasms of uncertain behavior, polycythemia vera and myelodysplastic syndromes
D49	Neoplasms of unspecified behavior

This chapter includes classifications for neoplasms by behavior and anatomic site. The term "neoplasm" may be translated from its Greek origin as new (neo) growth (plasm). The classification for neoplasms of unspecified behavior includes the terms "growth NOS," and "new growth NOS." However, for classification purposes, the term "mass" is not synonymous with "neoplasm" or "tumor," and is classified elsewhere as a disorder or symptom of the affected anatomic site. Neoplasms (i.e., tumors) are abnormal growths or masses of tissue that may vary in biological behavior or "morphology." To ensure accurate coding and reporting, it is important to understand the distinctions between the behavior categories. ICD-10-CM classifies neoplasms in the same manner as ICD-9-CM, as:

- **Malignant (primary or secondary)**: indicates the presence of cancer; tumors that have the potential for invasion of other bodily tissues for deleterious effect.

- **Carcinoma in situ:** describes neoplastic cells or tumors confined to the point of origin that are undergoing malignant changes, without invasion of surrounding normal tissue.

- **Benign:** describes neoplastic cells or tumors that do not invade adjacent structures or spread to other distant anatomic sites. However, they may cause certain potentially harmful effects, due to displacement of or pressure on adjacent tissues or structures. Excision of the tumor often characteristically "cures" its adverse effects.

- **Uncertain behavior:** is used when diagnosis of behavior is not possible. Certain factors, such as intermediate stages of tissue change may necessitate additional testing and further diagnostic study. These codes indicate a neoplasm undergoing the process of a determination for which a definitive diagnosis has not yet been established.

- **Unspecified behavior:** is used when neither behavior of the tumor nor morphology is specified in the diagnostic statement. A patient referral to another medical care site for further diagnostic studies is commonplace with these diagnoses. These diagnosis codes are common in the outpatient setting to report a working diagnosis.

As in ICD-9-CM, the alphabetic index includes the ICD-10-CM Neoplasm Table that lists code assignments for neoplasms by anatomic site. Each anatomic site is displayed vertically, corresponding to six vertical columns that contain site-specific codes by neoplasm behavior. The remainder of the alphabetic index also contains morphological terms and cross-references as guidance for neoplasm classification. For example:

> **Fibroma** (*see also* Neoplasm, connective tissue, benign)
> ameloblastic, *see* Cyst, calcifying odontogenic
> cementifying, *see* Neoplasm, bone, benign
> **Fibrosarcoma** (*see also* Neoplasm, connective tissue, malignant)
> ameloblastic C41.4
> upper jaw (bone) C41.0

Although the description of a neoplasm often indicates the appropriate classification column in the alphabetic index (e.g., malignant, benign), the remainder of the index should be consulted to verify the classification, or to clarify ambiguous or absent terminology. It is imperative, however, as in ICD-9-CM, to consult the tabular list to confirm the code. In ICD-10-CM, codes listed with a dash (-) following the code require a fifth character to specify laterality. Codes lacking the required characters are incomplete and, therefore, invalid. For example:

> **Carcinoma** (malignant) (*see also* Neoplasm, malignant, by site)
> ceruminous C44.29-

Default code C44.29- is an incomplete code that represents a range of possible classifications. A code is invalid if it is not coded to the full number of required characters. The dash (-) indicates that additional digits are required. The tabular list provides the complete list of valid codes classified to the C44.29 subcategory as:

> **C44.29** **Other specified malignant neoplasm of skin of ear and external auricular canal**
> **C44.291** **Other specified malignant neoplasm of skin of unspecified ear and external auricular canal**
> **C44.292** **Other specified malignant neoplasm of skin of right ear and external auricular canal**
> **C44.299** **Other specified malignant neoplasm of skin of left ear and auricular canal**

Section, Category, and Code Title Changes

As the examples above illustrate, a number of category and subchapter titles have been revised in chapter 2. Titles were changed to better reflect the content, which was often necessary when specific types of neoplasms were given their own block, a new category was created, or an existing category was redefined.

ICD-9-CM		ICD-10-CM	
141	Malignant neoplasm of tongue	C01	Malignant neoplasm of base of tongue
		C02	Malignant neoplasm of other and unspecified parts of tongue
148.1	Malignant neoplasm, pyriform sinus	C12	Malignant neoplasm of pyriform sinus

In the example above, a separate three-character code was created in ICD-10-CM to classify malignant neoplasm of pyriform sinus. Previously, this neoplasm was classified within ICD-9-CM category 148 Malignant neoplasm of hypopharynx.

At the subcategory level, the codes for the cervical, thoracic, and abdominal sites for malignant neoplasm of the esophagus have been revised in ICD-10-CM. Certain codes and descriptions have been reclassified in order to streamline and consolidate the classification for consistency. For example, note the reclassification of malignant esophageal neoplasms:

ICD-9-CM

150	Malignant neoplasm of esophagus
150.0	Cervical esophagus
150.1	Thoracic esophagus
150.2	Abdominal esophagus
150.3	Upper third of esophagus
150.4	Middle third of esophagus
150.5	Lower third of esophagus
150.8	Other specified part
150.9	Esophagus, unspecified

ICD-10-CM

C15	Malignant neoplasm of esophagus
C15.3	Malignant neoplasm of upper third of esophagus
C15.4	Malignant neoplasm of middle third of esophagus
C15.5	Malignant neoplasm of lower third of esophagus
C15.8	Malignant neoplasm of overlapping sites of esophagus
C15.9	Malignant neoplasm of esophagus, unspecified

In general, however, ICD-10-CM chapter 2 has undergone significant expansion to increase the specificity of code classifications. Many conditions previously classified in ICD-9-CM have either been given unique classifications, or have been further specified by type, anatomic site and laterality.

Code expansion by neoplasm type, site or histology:

ICD-9-CM		ICD-10-CM	
155.0	Malignant neoplasm of liver, primary	C22.0	Liver cell carcinoma
		C22.1	Intrahepatic bile duct carcinoma
		C22.2	Hepatoblastoma
		C22.3	Angiosarcoma of liver
		C22.4	Other sarcomas of liver
		C22.7	Other specified carcinomas of liver
		C22.8	Malignant neoplasm of liver, primary unsp as to type

Code expansion by anatomic site:

ICD-9-CM		ICD-10-CM	
209.31	Merkel cell carcinoma of face	C4A.0	Merkel cell ca of lip
		C4A.10	Merkel cell ca unspecified eyelid incl. canthus
		C4A.11	Merkel cell ca right eyelid incl. canthus
		C4A.12	Merkel cell ca left eyelid incl. canthus
		C4A.20	Merkel cell ca unspecified ear & ext auricular canal
		C4A.21	Merkel cell ca right ear & ext auricular canal
		C4A.22	Merkel cell ca left ear & ext auricular canal
		C4A.30	Merkel cell ca of unspecified parts of face
		C4A.31	Merkel cell ca nose
		C4A.39	Merkel cell ca of other parts of face
209.35	Merkel cell carcinoma of trunk	C4A.51	Merkel cell ca anal skin
		C4A.52	Merkel cell ca skin breast
		C4A.59	Merkel cell ca other part of trunk
211.3	Benign neoplasm colon	D12.0	Benign neoplasm of cecum
		D12.1	Benign neoplasm of appendix
		D12.2	Benign neoplasm of ascending colon
		D12.3	Benign neoplasm of transverse colon
		D12.4	Benign neoplasm of descending colon
		D12.5	Benign neoplasm of sigmoid colon
		D12.6	Benign neoplasm of colon, unspecified

Code expansion by anatomic site/laterality:

ICD-9-CM		ICD-10-CM	
162.3	Malignant neo UL bronchus or lung	C34.10	Malig neo up lobe bronch/lung unsp side
		C34.11	Malig neoplsm upper lobe right bronchus/lung
		C34.12	Malig neoplsm upper lobe left bronchus/lung

ICD-9-CM		ICD-10-CM	
174.1	Malignant neo central portion breast	C50.111	Malig neoplsm central portion R female breast
		C50.112	Malig. neoplsm central portion L female breast
		C50.119	Malig neoplsm central portion Unsp female breast

Organizational Adjustments

When comparing ICD-9-CM to ICD-10-CM, some codes have been added, deleted, combined, and moved. The codes for malignant neoplasm of retroperitoneum and peritoneum were in the subchapter, "Malignant Neoplasm of Digestive Organs and Peritoneum (150–159)," in ICD-9-CM. These codes have been moved in ICD-10-CM to the subchapter section, "Malignant Neoplasms of Mesothelial and Soft Tissue (C45–C49)."

ICD-9-CM

Malignant Neoplasm of Digestive Organs and Peritoneum (150–159)

150	Malignant neoplasm of esophagus
151	Malignant neoplasm of stomach
152	Malignant neoplasm of small intestine, including duodenum
153	Malignant neoplasm of colon
154	Malignant neoplasm of rectum, rectosigmoid junction, and anus
155	Malignant neoplasm of liver and intrahepatic bile ducts
156	Malignant neoplasm of gallbladder and extrahepatic bile ducts
157	Malignant neoplasm of pancreas
158	Malignant neoplasm of retroperitoneum and peritoneum
159	Malignant neoplasm of other and ill-defined sites within the digestive organs and peritoneum

ICD-10-CM

Malignant Neoplasms of Mesothelial and Soft Tissue (C45–C49)

C45	Mesothelioma
C46	Kaposi's sarcoma
C47	Malignant neoplasm of peripheral nerves and autonomic nervous system
C48	Malignant neoplasm of retroperitoneum and peritoneum
C49	Malignant neoplasm of other connective and soft tissue

Concurrent with changes to ICD-9-CM, alphanumeric category codes were added to the neoplasm chapter in 2010 to provide unique classifications for neuroendocrine tumor. These changes have been accommodated in ICD-10-CM classifications according to morphology (e.g., malignant, benign). In these alphanumeric code categories, the third character is a letter.

C7A   **Malignant neuroendocrine tumors**

Code also any associated multiple endocrine neoplasia [MEN] syndromes (E31.2-)

Use additional code to identify any associated endocrine syndrome, such as: carcinoid syndrome (E34.0)

EXCLUDES 2   *malignant pancreatic islet cell tumors (C25.4)*

Merkel cell carcinoma (C4A.-)

   C7A.0   **Malignant carcinoid tumors**

     C7A.00   **Malignant carcinoid tumor of unspecified site**

     C7A.01   **Malignant carcinoid tumors of the small intestine**

       C7A.010   **Malignant carcinoid tumor of the duodenum**

       C7A.011   **Malignant carcinoid tumor of the jejunum**

       C7A.012   **Malignant carcinoid tumor of the ileum**

       C7A.019   **Malignant carcinoid tumor of the small intestine, unspecified portion**

Chapter 2 Coding Guidance

ICD-10-CM chapter 2 contains classifications for all malignant neoplasms, in-situ, uncertain or unspecified neoplasms and most benign neoplasms. Certain benign neoplasms, such as certain polyps (e.g., colon, cervix uteri, adenoid) are classified to the specific body system chapters. In general, coding advice for the classification of neoplasms in ICD-10-CM parallels that of ICD-9-CM, with one significant exception.

Encounter for Complication Associated with a Neoplasm

In most cases, encounters for treatment of complications of a neoplasm (e.g., dehydration, pain) are reported with the complication sequenced first, followed by the appropriate neoplasm code. However, when the neoplasm complication is anemia, an exception is made. In these cases, when the patient encounter is for management of the anemia associated with the malignancy and the treatment is focused on the anemia, the *malignancy* code is sequenced as the first-listed diagnosis followed by code D63.0 Anemia in neoplastic disease. This exception is in opposition to ICD-9-CM guidelines for the same scenario. For example:

> **Diagnosis:** Patient with hepatocellular carcinoma is admitted for treatment of severe cancer-related anemia

> **C22.0**   **Liver cell carcinoma**

> **D63.0**   **Anemia in neoplastic disease**

Note that when an encounter is for the management of anemia associated with an adverse effect of cancer therapy, and the treatment is focused on the anemia, sequence the appropriate *anemia* code first, followed by the appropriate adverse effect and neoplasm code.

As mentioned above, coding advice for the classification of neoplasms in ICD-10-CM parallels that of ICD-9-CM. Key concepts are described below.

General Neoplasm Coding and Sequencing

When coding conditions associated with neoplasms, a code for the neoplasm must also be reported, as appropriate. In general, neoplasms are sequenced according to the circumstances of the encounter:

- If treatment is directed at the malignancy, sequence the malignancy first.

  Exception: Encounters for therapy require the appropriate Z51.- listed first.

- If the treatment of a patient with an existing primary malignancy is focused on a secondary neoplasm (metastatic site), the secondary neoplasm is sequenced first.

- Complications of neoplasms are sequenced first if the treatment is focused on the complication.

  Exception: Encounters for treatment of neoplasm-related anemia require the neoplasm to be sequenced first in ICD-10-CM, followed by code D63.0 Anemia in neoplastic disease.

  For complications associated with neoplasm related therapies, sequencing is determined by the circumstances of the encounter. See the discussion on encounters for therapy on page 84.

- Complications resulting from the surgical treatment of a neoplasm require the complication to be sequenced first.

- Primary malignancies previously excised, for which there is no treatment, and no evidence of any existing malignancy, are reported with the appropriate code from category Z85 Personal history of malignant neoplasm. Primary malignancies previously excised, but still under treatment require coding and reporting of the primary malignancy code.

- Sequencing of pathological fractures are determined by the circumstances of admission and focus of treatment. The condition requiring the focus of treatment is sequenced first.

- Neoplasms of overlapping boundaries of one or more contiguous sites are reported with a fourth character .8 overlapping sites. For example:

  Diagnosis: Sarcoma of the left lower back and buttock

  C49.8   **Malignant neoplasm of overlapping sites of connective and soft tissue**

  Exception: Multiple malignant noncontiguous tumors may represent separate primary sites. In such case, assign separately classifiable codes for each site of primary occurrence. If the documentation is unclear, physician clarification may be necessary to assist in accurate code assignment.

Neoplasm-Related Pain

Specific sequencing guidelines exist for the reporting of neoplasm-related pain. When reporting neoplasm related pain, it is not necessary to assign an additional code to report the anatomic site of the pain.

Report code G89.3 Neoplasm related pain (acute)(chronic) for pain specified as related, associated or due to a malignancy, whether primary or secondary. This code may be reported as the first-listed code when the reason for the encounter is for pain control or management. Code also the underlying neoplasm. For example:

  Diagnosis: Encounter for pain control, primary prostate cancer metastatic to bone

  G89.3   **Neoplasm related pain (acute) (chronic)**

  C79.51   **Secondary malignant neoplasm of bone**

  C61   **Malignant neoplasm of prostate**

Exception: When the reason for the encounter is management of the neoplasm and neoplasm-related pain is documented and treated, code G89.3 may be reported as an additional diagnosis. For example:

Diagnosis: Patient admitted for treatment of dehydration, he has bone metastasis from primary cancer and chronic, stable neoplasm-related pain

E86.Ø	Dehydration
C79.51	Secondary malignant neoplasm of bone
G89.3	Pain, neoplasm related
C61	Malignant neoplasm of prostate

Encounters for Therapy

Code sequencing practices to report encounters for antineoplastic chemotherapy (Z51.11), antineoplastic immunotherapy (Z51.12), and antineoplastic radiation therapy (Z51.Ø) vary depending upon the circumstances of the encounter:

- **Encounters for therapy.** These encounters are reported with the appropriate encounter for therapy (Z51) code listed first, followed by the code for the neoplasm. Assign additional codes to report additional sites or complications, as appropriate.

- **Associated surgery.** Patient care episodes involving the surgical removal or treatment of a neoplasm followed by adjunct therapy during the same encounter are reported with the neoplasm code assigned as the first-listed diagnosis.

- **Encounters solely for therapy.** These encounters are reported with the appropriate Z51 subcategory code as the first-listed diagnosis. If multiple therapies are provided during a single encounter, these codes may be sequenced according to the circumstances of care or treatment, in any sequence.

- **Encounters for therapy during which a patient develops complications (e.g., dehydration, nausea, and vomiting).** These encounters are reported with the appropriate Z51 subcategory code listed first to report the circumstances necessitating the encounter, followed by additional codes to describe the complications. For example:

Diagnosis: Encounter for radiation therapy and initiation of chemotherapy for breast cancer, right upper outer quadrant, metastatic to axillary nodes, developed nausea with vomiting

Z51.Ø	Encounter for antineoplastic radiation therapy
Z51.11	Encounter for antineoplastic chemotherapy
C5Ø.411	Malignant neoplasm of upper-outer quadrant of right female breast
C77.3	Secondary and unspecified malignant neoplasm of axilla and upper limb lymph nodes
R11.2	Nausea with vomiting, unspecified

- **Adverse effects.** When an encounter is for management of an adverse effect of cancer therapy, sequence the appropriate *complication or condition* code first, followed by the adverse effect code, and lastly, the code for the malignant neoplasm. For example:

Diagnosis: Fever and chills due to adverse effect of chemotherapy, carcinoma of pancreas

R50.9   **Drug induced fever**

T45.1X5A **Adverse effect of antineoplastic and immunosuppressive drugs, initial encounter**

C25.9   **Malignant neoplasm of pancreas, unspecified**

Malignant Neoplasm in a Pregnant Patient

Codes from chapter 15, "Pregnancy, Childbirth and the Puerperium," take precedence over codes classifiable to other chapters, and are always sequenced first. Report the appropriate code from subcategory O9A.1- Malignant neoplasm complicating pregnancy, childbirth and the puerperium first, followed by a chapter 2 code to identify the type of neoplasm. For example:

Diagnosis: Postgestational choriocarcinoma

O9A.13   **Malignant neoplasm complicating the puerperium**

C58   **Malignant neoplasm of placenta**

Melanoma

It is necessary to reference the alphabetic index when coding melanoma. The Neoplasm Table includes the cross-reference "see Melanoma" under the main term "Neoplasm, neoplastic" and subterm "melanoma." Additionally, no codes are provided for reference with the subterm "melanoma" in the Neoplasm Table. It is incorrect to code melanoma to "Neoplasm, primary site, skin, NEC" unless specifically directed to do so by coding conventions in the text. Therefore, consult the alphabetic index under the main term "Melanoma" and the appropriate subterm for the type or anatomic site. Note that melanoma in situ is classified to category D03. The alphabetic index provides cross-references for certain histological types of melanoma that are classified elsewhere. For example:

Melanoma (malignant) C43.9
    acral lentiginous, malignant—*see* Melanoma, skin, by site
    amelanotic—*see* Melanoma, skin, by site
    balloon cell—*see* Melanoma, skin, by site
    in
        giant pigmented nevus—*see* Melanoma, skin, by site
        Hutchinson's melanotic freckle—*see* Melanoma, skin, by site
    in situ D03.9
        abdominal wall D03.59
        ala nasi D03.39
        ankle D03.7-

Refer to the "ICD-10-CM Draft Official Guidelines for Coding and Reporting" in appendix A of this book for additional information.

Chapter 2 Coding Exercises

Assign the appropriate ICD-10-CM diagnosis codes for all reportable diagnoses, excluding external causes of morbidity (VØØ–Y99).

Answers to coding exercises are listed in the back of the book.

1. Adenocarcinoma of rectum _____

    _____

2. Fibroadenoma of the breast _____

    _____

3. Malignant carcinoid tumor of the jejunum _____

    _____

4. Multiple secondary metastatic mesentery carcinoid tumors _____

    _____

5. Acute exacerbation of chronic myeloid leukemia _____

    _____

6. Hodgkin lymphoma of intrathoracic lymph nodes _____

    _____

7. Encounter for chemotherapy, carcinoma of ovary _____

    _____

8. Adenocarcinoma of the prostate with metastasis to bone _____

    _____

9. Malignant neoplasm of endocervix and exocervix _____

    _____

10. Intraductal carcinoma in situ of the right breast _____

    _____

Chapter 2 Coding Scenarios

Assign the appropriate ICD-10-CM diagnosis codes for all reportable diagnoses, excluding external causes of morbidity (VØØ–Y99).

Answers to coding exercises are listed in the back of the book.

1. A 62-year-old female presents for initiation of antineoplastic immunotherapy and chemotherapy following surgical resection of primary upper-outer carcinoma of the left breast.

    _____

    _____

2. A 57-year-old male is admitted to observations status with severe nausea and vomiting due to adverse effects of chemotherapy for oat cell carcinoma of the right upper lobe of the lung.

    _____

    _____

3. A 60-year-old male presents for radiation therapy of adenocarcinoma of the prostate with metastasis to the pelvic bone.

   _____

   _____

4. A 48-year-old female presents with a recent history of progressive episodes of nausea, vomiting, and right upper quadrant (RUQ) abdominal pain. She is five years status post resection of colorectal carcinoma. Workup reveals metastatic liver cancer from her previously resected primary sigmoid colon cancer._____

   _____

5. A 68-year-old patient presents for treatment of biopsy-confirmed metastatic carcinoid lesions of the liver from her coexisting primary transverse carcinoid tumor of the cecum. _____

   _____

6. A patient presents with suspicious neoplastic lesions of the choroid. Due to the small size of the lesion, biopsy is contraindicated, as adequate sample is not possible at this time. _____

   _____

CHAPTER 3. DISEASES OF THE BLOOD AND BLOOD-FORMING ORGANS AND CERTAIN DISORDERS INVOLVING THE IMMUNE MECHANISM (D50–D89)

Chapter 3 contains seven code families represented by the first character "D." The letter is also shared with the previous chapter, "Neoplasms." The coding families classified to chapter 3 are:

D50–D53 Nutritional anemias

D55–D59 Hemolytic anemias

D60–D64 Aplastic and other anemias and other bone marrow failure syndromes

D65–D69 Coagulation defects, purpura and other hemorrhagic conditions

D70–D77 Other disorders of blood and blood-forming organs

D78 Intraoperative and postprocedural complications of the spleen

D80–D89 Certain disorders involving the immune mechanism

ICD-10-CM Category Restructuring

In ICD-9-CM, there were no subchapters within the chapter for diseases of blood and blood-forming organs. Blocks have since been added to this restructured chapter for ICD-10-CM. The arrangement of the various disorders, given the addition of these new blocks, has resulted in the restructuring of several categories.

ICD-9-CM

280 Iron deficiency anemias

281 Other deficiency anemias

282 Hereditary hemolytic anemias

283 Acquired hemolytic anemias

284 Aplastic anemia and other bone marrow failure syndromes

285 Other and unspecified anemias

286 Coagulation defects

287 Purpura and other hemorrhagic conditions

288 Diseases of white blood cells

289 Other diseases of blood and blood-forming organs

ICD-10-CM

Nutritional Anemias (D50–D53)

D50 Iron deficiency anemia

D51 Vitamin B12 deficiency anemia

D52 Folate deficiency anemia

D53 Other nutritional anemias

Category Title Changes

A number of category title revisions were made in chapter 3. Titles were changed to better reflect the categorical content. These revisions serve to bring the terminology of the classification into congruency with current medical practice. This was often necessary when specific types of diseases were reclassified, a new category was created, or an existing category was redefined.

 KEY POINT

In ICD-10-CM, the contents of chapters 3 and 4 are different than in ICD-9-CM. Immune disorder categories were expanded and included within classifications for diseases of the blood and blood-forming organs. Additionally, these classifications were resequenced to precede the endocrine, nutritional and metabolic disease chapter.

ICD-9-CM

281   **Other deficiency anemias**

    281.0   **Pernicious anemia**

    281.1   **Other vitamin B12 deficiency anemia**

    281.2   **Folate-deficiency anemia**

    281.3   **Other specified megaloblastic anemias not elsewhere classified**

    281.4   **Protein-deficiency anemia**

    281.8   **Anemia associated with other specified nutritional deficiency**

    281.9   **Unspecified deficiency anemia**

ICD-10-CM

D50   **Iron deficiency anemia**

D51   **Vitamin B12 deficiency anemia**

D52   **Folate deficiency anemia**

D53   **Other nutritional anemias**

    D53.0   **Protein deficiency anemia**

    D53.1   **Other megaloblastic anemias, not elsewhere classified**

    D53.2   **Scorbutic anemia**

    D53.8   **Other specified nutritional anemias**

    D59.9   **Nutritional anemia, unspecified**

Organizational Adjustments

When comparing ICD-9-CM to ICD-10-CM, some codes have been added, deleted, combined, and moved. For example, code block D80–D89 includes disorders of the immune mechanism that were previously classified to chapter 4, "Endocrine, Nutritional and Metabolic Diseases, and Immunity Disorders (240–279)," in ICD-9-CM. These adjustments serve to improve the organizational structure of the classification by allowing for greater ease in identification of the type of conditions classified to chapter 3.

For example, the code for chronic lymphadenitis, nonspecific mesenteric lymphadenitis, and unspecified lymphadenitis in ICD-9-CM were classified to the chapter on diseases of the blood and blood-forming organs. These conditions have been moved to the chapter for diseases of the circulatory system where they are best classified with other disorders of the lymphatic vessels and lymph nodes in ICD-10-CM.

ICD-9-CM

289   **Other diseases of blood and blood-forming organs**

    289.1   **Chronic lymphadenitis**

    289.2   **Nonspecific mesenteric lymphadenitis**

    289.3   **Lymphadenitis, unspecified, except mesenteric**

ICD-10-CM

I88   **Nonspecific lymphadenitis**

    I88.0   **Nonspecific mesenteric lymphadenitis**

    I88.1   **Chronic lymphadenitis, except mesenteric**

    I88.8   **Other nonspecific lymphadenitis**

    I88.9   **Nonspecific lymphadenitis, unspecified**

By contrast, the specific code for iron deficiency anemia secondary to inadequate dietary iron intake that was available in ICD-9-CM is deleted in ICD-10-CM.

The condition that would have been classified to this code will now be coded to the residual subcategory in ICD-10-CM.

ICD-9-CM

280.1 · **Iron deficiency anemia secondary to inadequate dietary iron intake**

ICD-10-CM

D50.8 **Other iron deficiency anemias**
Iron deficiency anemia due to inadequate dietary iron intake

Intraoperative and Postprocedural Complications of the Spleen (D78)

In ICD-10-CM, postoperative complications have been moved to procedure-specific body system chapters. Code category D78 includes both intraoperative and postprocedural complications of the spleen. Intraoperative complications include hemorrhage and hematoma complicating a procedure (D78.Ø), accidental puncture and laceration during a procedure (D78.1), and other complications of the spleen (D78.81). Postoperative complications include hemorrhage and hematoma following procedures on the spleen (D78.21), following other procedure (D78.22) and other postprocedural complications of spleen (D78.89). Code assignment is based on the provider's documentation of the relationship between the condition and the procedure.

Chapter 3 Coding Guidance

Official Guidelines

At the time of this publication, no official coding guidelines have been published for chapter 3 classification codes. To ensure accurate code assignment, apply the ICD-10-CM conventions and instructions within the ICD-10-CM text.

Level of Detail in Coding

As in ICD-9-CM, diagnosis codes are to be used and reported to the highest degree of specificity available. ICD-10-CM provides, in the majority of cases, an exponentially increased level of specificity than ICD-9-CM. In chapter 3, this code expansion is intended to facilitate identification of specific disease types that have become separately identifiable due to advances in medical technologies and updates of currently applicable clinical terminology. For example:

New ICD-10-CM codes have been created for specific diseases or disorders not previously identifiable with unique codes in ICD-9-CM.

ICD-9-CM		ICD-10-CM	
289.59	Other diseases of spleen	D73.Ø	Hyposplenism
		D73.3	Abscess of spleen
		D73.4	Cyst of spleen
		D73.5	Infarction of spleen

Classification codes for folate deficiency anemia have been expanded to distinguish between dietary, drug-induced deficiency and other causal factors.

ICD-9-CM		ICD-10-CM	
281.2	Folate-deficiency anemia	D52.0	Dietary folate deficiency anemia
		D52.1	Drug-induced folate deficiency anemia
		D52.8	Other folate deficiency anemias
		D52.9	Folate deficiency anemia, unspecified

Classification changes often occur to reflect advances in medical technology. For example, certain hemolytic anemias caused by enzyme deficiency have been separately classified in ICD-10-CM to further identify the absence of a specific enzyme.

ICD-9-CM		ICD-10-CM	
282.3	Other hemolytic anemias due to enzyme deficiency	D55.2	Anemia due to disorders of glycolytic enzymes
		D55.3	Anemia due to disorders of nucleotide metabolism
		D55.8	Other anemias due to enzyme disorders
		D55.9	Anemia due to enzyme disorder, unspecified

Combination Codes

Certain disease classifications have been expanded in ICD-10-CM to facilitate identification of secondary disease processes, specific manifestations, or associated complications. As such, code to the highest level of specificity as documented in the record. In chapter 3, sickle-cell crisis codes have been revised from a multiple coding convention requiring two codes to a combination code reportable by a single classification code. For example:

ICD-9-CM Multiple Coding

282.62   **Hb-SS disease with crisis**
Use additional code for type of crisis, such as:
    acute chest syndrome (517.3)
    splenic sequestration (289.52)

ICD-10-CM Combination Codes

D57.00   Hb-SS disease with crisis, unspecified
D57.01   Hb-SS disease with acute chest syndrome
D57.02   Hb-SS disease with splenic sequestration

Drug-Induced Conditions

Combination codes that include both the causal drug (e.g., benzodiazepines), and external cause (e.g., therapeutic use), replace the need for a separate external cause code. Conditions due to the therapeutic effects of drugs are coded with the condition indicating the nature of the adverse effect sequenced first. Instructional notes in the text direct the coder to assign the appropriate code from categories T36–50 in addition to the code for the specific manifestation or condition. Code section T36–T50 includes poisoning by, adverse effects of, and underdosing of drugs, medicaments and biological substances. Conditions due to the adverse effects of drugs in therapeutic use are classified with fifth or sixth character 5. For example:

ICD-10-CM

D52.1 Drug-induced folate deficiency anemia
> Use additional code for adverse effect, if applicable, to identify drug (T36–T50 with fifth or sixth character 5)

Diagnosis: Cycloserine-induced folate deficiency anemia, adverse effect in therapeutic use

D52.1   Drug-induced folate deficiency anemia

T37.1X5A Adverse effect of antimycobacterial drugs, initial encounter

Multiple Coding

Instructional notes appear throughout the text to provide sequencing instruction when more than one code is necessary to report the diagnosis in completion:

- **Code first/use additional code.** These notes direct the coder that although certain conditions may occur independently of each other, multiple codes may be necessary to report associated conditions or designate underlying cause, as appropriate. For example:

    > **D89.81   Graft-versus-host disease**
    > Code first underlying cause, such as:
    >> complications of transplanted organs and tissue (T86.-)
    >> complications of blood transfusion (T80.89)
    > Use additional code to identify associated manifestations, such as:
    >> desquamative dermatitis (L30.8)
    >> diarrhea (R19.7)
    >> elevated bilirubin (R17)
    >> hair loss (L65.9)

    Note: A sixth character is required to report GVHD by severity.

- **Etiology/manifestation coding.** ICD-10-CM *requires* the underlying condition to be sequenced first followed by the manifestation. Codes that may not be reported alone, or sequenced as a first-listed diagnosis may be identified by the phrase "In diseases classified elsewhere" in the code title. For example:

    > **D77   Other disorders of blood and blood-forming organs in diseases classified elsewhere**
    > Code first underlying disease, such as:
    >> amyloidosis (E85.-)

- **Code also.** This note alerts the coder that more than one code may be necessary to report the condition in its entirety. Code sequencing is discretionary. Factors that may determine sequencing include severity and reason for the encounter. For example:

    > **D61.82   Myelophthisis**
    > Leukoerythroblastic anemia
    > Myelophthisic anemia
    > Panmyelophthisis
    > Code also the underlying disorder, such as:
    >> malignant neoplasm of breast (C50.-)
    >> tuberculosis (A15.-)

Chapter 3 Coding Exercises

Assign the appropriate ICD-10-CM diagnosis codes for all reportable diagnoses, excluding external causes of morbidity (VØØ–Y99).

Answers to coding exercises are listed in the back of the book.

1. Dietary-induced folic acid deficiency anemia _____

   _____

2. Sickle-cell thalassemia crisis with splenic sequestration _____

   _____

3. Hb-C disease _____

   _____

4. Aplastic anemia due to adverse effects of antineoplastic chemotherapy

   _____

5. Pancytopenia _____

   _____

6. Secondary sideroblastic anemia in myelodysplastic syndrome _____

   _____

7. Toxic neutropenic fever _____

   _____

8. Hypogammaglobulinemia _____

   _____

9. Sarcoidosis of lung _____

   _____

Chapter 3 Coding Scenarios

Assign the appropriate ICD-10-CM diagnosis codes for all reportable diagnoses, excluding external causes of morbidity (V00–Y99).

Answers to coding exercises are listed in the back of the book.

1. A 14-year-old male presents with a history of congenital Gaucher disease and a two-month history of pallor, easy bruising, fatigue, and splenomegaly. CBC reveals thrombocytopenia. The physician diagnoses presenting symptoms as leukoerythroblastic anemia (myelophthisis).

   _____

   _____

2. A patient presents to the emergency department with epistaxis and purpura. She is five days post-transfusion and now presents with severe thrombocytopenia. Laboratory testing is positive for HPA-1a antibodies. The patient is admitted to the hospital and treated with intravenous immunoglobulin (IVIg) and corticosteroids.

   _____

   _____

3. A patient is admitted two months status post bone marrow transplant with cramping, lower abdominal pain, fever, diarrhea, and desquamative dermatitis. Skin biopsy revealed an increased presence of donor lymphocytes characteristic of acute graft-versus-host disease. The patient was placed on high-dose corticosteroids with marked improvement.

   _____

   _____

CHAPTER 4. ENDOCRINE, NUTRITIONAL AND METABOLIC DISEASES (E00–E89)

Chapter 4 contains 10 code families with the first character "E." The coding families classified to chapter 4 are:

E00–E07	**Disorders of thyroid gland**
E08–E13	**Diabetes mellitus**
E15–E16	**Other disorders of glucose regulation and pancreatic internal secretion**
E20–E35	**Disorders of other endocrine glands**
E36	**Intraoperative complications of endocrine system**
E40–E46	**Malnutrition**
E50–E64	**Other nutritional deficiencies**
E65–E68	**Overweight, obesity and other hyperalimentation**
E70–E88	**Metabolic disorders**
E89	**Postprocedural endocrine and metabolic complications and disorders, not elsewhere classified**

ICD-10-CM Category Restructuring

Certain disease categories have been restructured in ICD-10-CM. This was done to separate out particular disorders, or to create unique categories, where necessary. For example, in ICD-9-CM there is a subchapter for nutritional deficiencies (260–269), which includes malnutrition and other nutritional deficiencies. In ICD-10-CM, malnutrition is classified within a separate subchapter (E40–E46) and so has other nutritional deficiencies (E50–E64).

ICD-9-CM

Nutritional Deficiencies (260–269)

260	**Kwashiorkor**
261	**Nutritional marasmus**
262	**Other severe, protein-calorie malnutrition**
263	**Other and unspecified protein-calorie malnutrition**
264	**Vitamin A deficiency**
265	**Thiamin and niacin deficiency states**
266	**Deficiency of B-complex components**
267	**Ascorbic acid deficiency**
268	**Vitamin D deficiency**
269	**Other nutritional deficiencies**

ICD-10-CM

Malnutrition (E40–E46)

E40	**Kwashiorkor**
E41	**Nutritional marasmus**
E42	**Marasmic kwashiorkor**
E43	**Unspecified severe protein-calorie malnutrition**
E44	**Protein-calorie malnutrition of moderate and mild degree**

| E45 | Retarded development following protein-calorie malnutrition |
| E46 | Unspecified protein-calorie malnutrition |

Other Nutritional Deficiencies (E50–E64)

E50	Vitamin A deficiency
E51	Thiamine deficiency
E52	Niacin deficiency [pellagra]
E53	Deficiency of other B group vitamins
E54	Ascorbic acid deficiency
E55	Vitamin D deficiency
E56	Other vitamin deficiencies

Category Title Changes

A number of category title revisions were made in chapter 4. Titles were changed to better reflect the category's content, which was often necessary when specific types of diseases were given their own block, a new category was created, or an existing category was redefined.

ICD-9-CM

| 265 | Thiamin and niacin deficiency states |
| 266 | Deficiency of B-complex components |

ICD-10-CM

E51	Thiamine deficiency
E52	Niacin deficiency [pellagra]
E53	Deficiency of other B group vitamins

Organizational Adjustments

When comparing ICD-9-CM to ICD-10-CM, some codes have been added, deleted, combined, or moved. A code for certain types of adult osteomalacia was a subcategory code of vitamin D deficiency in ICD-9-CM. These conditions were relocated in ICD-10-CM to a separate three-character category for adult osteomalacia in the musculoskeletal and connective tissue disease chapter. For example:

ICD-9-CM

| 268 | Vitamin D deficiency |
| | 268.2 | Osteomalacia, unspecified |

ICD-10-CM

M83	Adult osteomalacia
	M83.0	Puerperal osteomalacia
	M83.1	Senile osteomalacia
	M83.2	Adult osteomalacia due to malabsorption
	M83.3	Adult osteomalacia due to malnutrition
	M83.4	Aluminum bone disease
	M83.5	Other drug-induced osteomalacia in adults
	M83.8	Other adult osteomalacia
	M83.9	Adult osteomalacia, unspecified

QUICK TIP

Although their alpha placement is purely coincidental, it may help in remembering code families to consider the following:

Most neoplasm codes begin with "C," as in cancer.

- Diabetes and other endocrine disorders begin with "E," as in endocrinology.
- Musculoskeletal codes begin with "M."
- Nephrology codes can be found under "N."
- Obstetrical codes begin with the letter "O."
- Perinatal codes begin with the letter "P."

KEY POINT

There are many reasons for changes to the contents of the chapters, including the need for increased clinical detail about a specific disorder, and the reclassification of diseases due to increased knowledge of their causes.

Complications

In ICD-10-CM, postoperative complications have been moved to procedure-specific body system chapters. Complications are split into two separate sections within chapter 4. Intraoperative complications of the endocrine system are classified to category E36, whereas postprocedural endocrine and metabolic complications and disorders, not elsewhere classified are assigned to category E89. Fourth- and fifth-character subcategory complications specify the type or nature of the complication, with the exception of those classified to other (.8) or (.89) and code E89.1 Postprocedural hypoinsulinemia, in which an additional code to specifically describe the nature of the complication is required. For example:

E36   **Intraoperative complications of endocrine system**

    E36.8   **Other intraoperative complications of endocrine system**
       Use additional code, if applicable to further specify disorder

E89   **Postprocedural endocrine and metabolic complications and disorders, not elsewhere classified**

    E89.1   **Postprocedural hypoinsulinemia**
       Use additional code, if applicable, to identify:
         acquired absence of pancreas (Z90.41-)
         diabetes mellitus (postpancreatectomy) (postprocedural) (E13.-)
         insulin use (Z79.4)

    E89.89   **Other postprocedural endocrine and metabolic complications and disorders**
         Use additional code, if applicable to further specify disorder

Drug-Induced Conditions

Combination codes that include both the causal drug (e.g., benzodiazepines), and external cause (e.g., therapeutic use), replace the need for a separate external cause code. Conditions due to the effects of drugs are coded with the nature of the adverse effect sequenced first. Instructional notes in the text direct the coder to assign the appropriate code from categories T36–65 in addition to the code for the specific manifestation or condition. Code section T36–T50 includes poisoning by, adverse effects of, and underdosing of drugs, medicaments, and biological substances. Conditions due to the adverse effects of drugs in therapeutic use are classified with fifth or sixth character 5. Code section T51–T65 describes toxic effects of substances chiefly nonmedicinal as to source. For example, category E09 classifies drug-induced diabetes mellitus:

ICD-10-CM

E09   **Drug or chemical induced diabetes mellitus**
       Code first poisoning due to drug or toxin, if applicable (T36–T65 with fifth or sixth character 1–4 or 6)
       Use additional code for adverse effect, if applicable, to identify drug (T36–T50 with fifth or sixth character 5)
       Use additional code to identify and insulin use (Z79.4)

Diagnosis: Initial encounter for corticosteroid-induced diabetes mellitus, requiring insulin

E09.9   **Drug or chemical induced diabetes mellitus without complications**

T38.0X5A   **Adverse effects of glucocorticoids and synthetic analogues, initial encounter**

Z79.4   **Long term (current) use of insulin**

Chapter 4 Coding Guidance

Diabetes Mellitus

Diabetes mellitus classification has been significantly revised in ICD-10-CM. Currently, ICD-9-CM includes diabetes code categories with other endocrine diseases classifiable to the same code grouping or code block (e.g., 252 Disorders of parathyroid gland, 254 Disorders of thymus gland). ICD-10-CM has designated a unique code block specifically for diabetes codes. Classification categories have been restructured as follows:

ICD-9-CM

Diseases of other endocrine glands (249–259)

249	Secondary diabetes mellitus
250	Diabetes mellitus

ICD-10-CM

Diabetes mellitus (E08–E13)

E08	Diabetes mellitus due to underlying condition
E09	Drug or chemical induced diabetes mellitus
E10	Type 1 diabetes mellitus
E11	Type 2 diabetes mellitus
E13	Other specified diabetes mellitus

Whereas ICD-9-CM incorporated the use of fifth-digit subclassifications to designate diabetes by type, ICD-10-CM classifies diabetes to separate categories by cause or type within a single code block (E08–E13), as noted above.

Additionally, ICD-10-CM no longer distinguishes between controlled and uncontrolled disease. The alphabetic index provides the following instruction:

Diabetes, diabetic
    inadequately controlled—code to Diabetes, by type, with hyperglycemia
    out of control—code to Diabetes, by type, with hyperglycemia
    poorly controlled—code to Diabetes, by type, with hyperglycemia

In ICD-10-CM, the diabetic manifestation is represented by the fourth-, fifth-, and sixth-code characters. The etiology/manifestation coding convention of ICD-9-CM has been replaced by combination codes. As such, certain manifestations of diabetes, formerly requiring mandatory dual coding, are reportable with a single code in ICD-10-CM. These combination codes classify diabetes by type, body system, and certain complications. For example:

Diagnosis: Type 2 diabetes mellitus with moderate nonproliferative diabetic retinopathy and macular edema

ICD-9-CM

250.50	Diabetes with ophthalmic manifestations
362.05	Moderate nonproliferative diabetic retinopathy
362.07	Diabetic macular edema

ICD-10-CM

E11.331   **Type 2 diabetes mellitus with moderate nonproliferative diabetic retinopathy with macular edema**

Furthermore, note how the following classifications specify the manifestation within the ICD-10-CM code. For example:

ICD-9-CM

250.60   **Diabetes with neurological manifestations**
Use additional code to identify manifestation

ICD-10-CM

E11.41   **Type 2 diabetes mellitus with diabetic mononeuropathy**
E11.42   **Type 2 diabetes mellitus with diabetic polyneuropathy**
E11.43   **Type 2 diabetes mellitus with diabetic autonomic (poly)neuropathy**
E11.44   **Type 2 diabetes mellitus with diabetic amyotrophy**

Although these combination codes streamline diabetes classification, multiple codes are often necessary to report a condition in its entirety. Instructional notes within the ICD-10-CM text prompt the coder when additional codes are necessary. For example:

Diagnosis: Type 2 diabetes mellitus with stage 3 chronic kidney disease

E11.22   **Diabetes mellitus with diabetic chronic kidney disease**
Type 2 diabetes mellitus with chronic kidney disease due to conditions classified to .21 and .22
Use additional code to identify stage of chronic kidney disease (N18.1–N18.6)

N18.3   **Chronic kidney disease, stage 3 (moderate)**
Code first any associated:
diabetic chronic kidney disease (E08.22, E09.22, E10.22, E11.22, E13.22)

Note that code subcategory E11.2 contains an inclusion note which states a hierarchy exists, in which diabetes with kidney complications (e.g., nephropathy) that result in chronic kidney disease are reported to a specific code (E11.22). In the alphabetic index, the main terms "Nephropathy" and "Nephritis" list subterms that reference diabetes codes E08–E13 with characters .21:

Nephropathy (*see also* Nephritis) N28.9
diabetic—*see* E09–E13 with .21

The inclusion note at code E11.22, however, states that diabetic renal complications classifiable to E11.21 are reported with E11.22 when the condition results in chronic kidney disease, which takes precedence in code assignment. This classification provides a severity mechanism to report disease progression. An additional code is required to report the specific stage of disease (N18.1–N18.6). Similar hierarchies exist within diabetes classifications E08–E13.

Instructions regarding the coding and reporting of diabetes mellitus in ICD-10-CM mirror those for ICD-9-CM. Although guideline content has been edited to apply to the classification changes inherent in ICD-10-CM, the underlying concepts and sequencing rules for diabetes remain largely unchanged. These key concepts include:

- Assign as many codes as necessary and appropriate to describe the complications of the disease.

- When multiple body system complications coexist (E08–E13), report all complications as documented. Sequencing is determined by the reason for the encounter.

- If the type of diabetes is not documented, assign type 2 (E11.-) by default.

- Report code Z79.4 for patients requiring long-term insulin therapy. Do not assign Z79.4 for temporary insulin to administered to bring a type 2 patient's blood sugar under control.

- Insulin pump malfunction resulting in either underdosing or overdosing of insulin is reported with the subcategory T85.6 mechanical complication code listed first, followed by the appropriate T38.3X6- code for the poisoning or adverse effect. Assign additional codes to report the type of diabetes mellitus and any associated complications.

- Secondary diabetes is always caused by another condition or event (e.g., malignant neoplasm, adverse effect of drug, poisoning, sequela of poisoning, disease). Instructional notes within the tabular list provide sequencing instruction. For example:

  E08   **Diabetes mellitus due to underlying condition**
  Code first the underlying condition

  E09   **Drug or chemical induced diabetes mellitus**
  Code first poisoning due to drug or toxin, if applicable (T36–T65 with fifth or sixth character 1–4 or 6)
  Use additional code for adverse effect, if applicable, to identify drug (T36–T50 with fifth or sixth character 5)

- Postpancreatectomy diabetes mellitus (due to surgical removal of all or part of the pancreas) is classified to code E89.1 Postprocedural hypoinsulinemia. The appropriate codes from categories E13 Other specified diabetes mellitus, and Z90.41.- Acquired absence of pancreas, are reported as additional diagnoses.

  Refer to the "ICD-10-CM Draft Official Guidelines for Coding and Reporting" in appendix A of this book for additional information.

Chapter 4 Coding Exercises

Assign the appropriate ICD-10-CM diagnosis codes for all reportable diagnoses, excluding external causes of morbidity (V00–Y99).

Answers to coding exercises are listed in the back of the book.

1. Congenital hypothyroidism without goiter _____

    _____

2. Type 2 diabetes mellitus with hyperosmolarity, without coma

    _____

    _____

3. Addison's disease _____

    _____

4. Vitamin B12 deficiency _____

    _____

5. Type 1 diabetes mellitus with ketoacidosis and coma

   _____

   _____

6. Graves' disease with thyrotoxic crisis _____

   _____

Chapter 4 Coding Scenarios

Assign the appropriate ICD-10-CM diagnosis codes for all reportable diagnoses, excluding external causes of morbidity (VØØ–Y99).

Answers to coding exercises are listed in the back of the book.

1. A 16-year-old female presents with her mother to the gynecologist's office for amenorrhea. Review of systems is within normal limits. Physical exam is normal with the exception of abnormal genitourinary findings. Upon pelvic exam, the patient is noted to have a short vaginal length and absent uterus. Intra-abdominal testicles are present on radiological exam. Surgical options and hormone replacement therapies were discussed with the patient and her mother. Referral was made to clinical psychologist and contact information for an Androgen Insensitivity Syndrome (AIS) support group was provided to assist in their decisions. Diagnosis is consistent with complete androgen insensitivity syndrome.

   _____

   _____

2. A 72-year old patient presents for evaluation and treatment of a stage 2 diabetic ulcer of the right heel due to systemic complications of his type 1 diabetes mellitus. Examination of the right foot reveals a 1cm ulcerative lesion with skin breakdown and exposed subcutaneous tissue, without necrosis or exposure of muscle. History is remarkable for peripheral vascular complications due to chronic, progressive diabetic peripheral angiopathy. Examination reveals lower extremity muscle weakness and marked decreased sensation in the feet and toes consistent with diabetic peripheral neuropathy.

   _____

   _____

3. A 34-year-old female presents post-assessment and treatment of associated glandular conditions by her endocrinologist. Family history is positive for multiple endocrine neoplasia (MEN) syndrome of similar type, with one ancestor's demise attributed to complications of thyroid cancer. Diagnostic workup and thyroid biopsy reveals bilateral medullary carcinoma of the upper central lobe of thyroid, with secondary hypertension and hyperparathyroidism due to underlying MEN syndrome, type IIA.

   _____

   _____

4. An 18-month-old toddler presents to the emergency department with a three-day history of watery diarrhea and decreased fluid intake. Fussy baby cries constantly, but lately has had "no tears." Mucous membranes appear dry and the child has become listless and fatigued. Parent has attempted to keep the child hydrated with apple juice and water. Attempts at oral rehydration with juice and water have replaced the patient's free water but not the sodium and other solutes. The patient is not dehydrated but has a metabolic solute deficit. The physician documents volume depletion secondary to viral gastroenteritis.

    _____

    _____

5. A 47-year-old male presents for his annual exam. History is significant for a 12-pound weight gain over the past year, and a total 22-pound weight gain during the past five years. The patient states that he injured his back last year and has had to limit his physical activity due to the injury. He has not made dietary modifications accordingly. Physical exam reveals no acute injury. BP is normal, cholesterol is slightly elevated at 272. Height 72 inches, weight 205 pounds; BMI 27.9. Diagnoses on exam are primary hypercholesterolemia and overweight.

    _____

    _____

6. An 18-year-old female ballet dancer presents for workup of fatigue and syncope. Her parents note a dramatic weight loss over the past seven months, with altered perception of appearance. The patient is underweight, with height 71 inches; weight 117 pounds; pediatric BMI 16.4; ECG shows prolonged QT interval. History and examination are consistent with anorexia nervosa with secondary amenorrhea and with moderate protein-calorie malnutrition. Follow-up includes psychiatric evaluation and dietary evaluation and nutrition/electrolyte support.

    _____

    _____

CHAPTER 5. MENTAL, BEHAVIORAL, AND NEURODEVELOPMENTAL DISORDERS (F01–F99)

Chapter 5 contains 11 code families with the first character "F." The coding families classified to chapter 5 are:

F01–F09	Mental disorders due to known physiological conditions
F10–F19	Mental and behavioral disorders due to psychoactive substance use
F20–F29	Schizophrenia, schizotypal and delusional, and other non-mood psychotic disorders
F30–F39	Mood [affective] disorders
F40–F48	Anxiety, dissociative, stress-related, somatoform and other nonpsychotic mental disorders
F50–F59	Behavioral syndromes associated with physiological disturbances and physical factors
F60–F69	Disorders of adult personality and behavior
F70–F79	Intellectual disabilities
F80–F89	Pervasive and specific developmental disorders
F90–F98	Behavioral and emotional disorders with onset usually occurring in childhood and adolescence
F99	Unspecified mental disorder

ICD-10-CM Subchapter Restructuring

Chapter 5 underwent a number of revisions, including expansion of the number of subchapters and code groupings (i.e., sections, blocks). Note how the ICD-10-CM code families in the list above contrasts with the previous ICD-9-CM classifications:

ICD-9-CM

Chapter 5. Mental Disorders (290–319)

290–299	Psychoses
290–294	Organic psychotic conditions
295–299	Other psychoses
300–316	Neurotic disorders, personality disorders, and other nonpsychotic mental disorders
317–319	Intellectual disabilities

With the expansion, ICD-10-CM now arranges specific disorders differently than in ICD-9-CM, and broadens the clinical detail. Based on the arrangement of chapter 5, ICD-10-CM has made further modifications to these expanded subchapter divisions and titles. Titles were changed to better reflect the content, which was often necessary when specific types of diseases were given their own block or defined differently.

Organizational Adjustments

When comparing ICD-9-CM to ICD-10-CM, some codes have been added, deleted, combined, or moved. The code for tension headache was found in ICD-9-CM chapter 5 under the subchapter "Neurotic Disorders, Personality Disorders, and Other Nonpsychotic Mental Disorders (300–316)." The code for this condition has been moved in ICD-10-CM and is now located in chapter 6, "Diseases of the Nervous System." These changes were made to maintain

 KEY POINT

Three chapters in ICD-10 underwent substantial review and revision: chapters 5, 19, and 20. The coder must understand the changes made to these chapters in order to code correctly from them.

consistency between ICD-9-CM and ICD-10-CM classification systems. Specific codes that classify tension headache by type and severity were added to ICD-9-CM effective October 1, 2009. For example:

ICD-9-CM

Chapter 5. Mental Disorders (290–319)

307   Special symptoms or syndromes, not elsewhere classified
    307.8   Pain disorders related to psychological factors
       307.81   Tension headache

ICD-10-CM

Chapter 6. Diseases of the Nervous System (G00–G99)

G44   Other headache syndromes
    G44.2   Tension-type headache
       G44.20   Tension-type headache, unspecified
          G44.201   Tension-type headache, unspecified, intractable
          G44.209   Tension-type headache, unspecified, nonintractable
             Tension headache NOS

Similarly, ICD-10-CM chapter 8, "Diseases of the Ear and Mastoid Process," includes central auditory processing disorder (ICD-9-CM code 315.32), which was formerly classified as a developmental delay in ICD-9-CM chapter 5, "Mental Disorders." ICD-10-CM reclassified the condition to category H93 as a disorder of the sense organs. This reclassification more appropriately identifies the underlying physiological factors associated with the manifestation of disease.

ICD-9-CM

Chapter 5. Mental Disorders (290–319)

315   Specific delays in development
    315.3   Developmental speech or language disorder
       315.32   Mixed receptive-expressive language disorder
          Central auditory processing disorder

ICD-10-CM

Chapter 8. Diseases of the Ear and Mastoid Process (H60–H95)

H93   Other disorders of ear, not elsewhere classified
       H93.25   Central auditory processing disorder
          Congenital auditory imperception
          Word deafness

Additionally, the specific code for psychogenic dysmenorrhea has been deleted in ICD-10-CM. This condition that is currently classified to code 306.52 will now be coded to the residual subcategory F45.8.

ICD-9-CM

       306.52   Psychogenic dysmenorrhea

ICD-10-CM

F45.8 **Other somatoform disorders**
Psychogenic dysmenorrhea
Psychogenic dysphagia, including "globus hystericus"
Psychogenic pruritus
Psychogenic torticollis
Somatoform autonomic dysfunction
Teeth-grinding

There were no codes in ICD-9-CM to distinguish between clinical subtypes of anorexia nervosa. As such, separate codes have been added to ICD-10-CM accordingly:

 DEFINITIONS

somatoform disorder. Chronic, but fluctuating, neurotic disorder that begins early in life, characterized by recurrent and multiple somatic complaints for which medical attention is sought, but are not due to any apparent physical illness.

ICD-10-CM

F50.0 **Anorexia nervosa**
F50.00 **Anorexia nervosa, unspecified**
F50.01 **Anorexia nervosa, restricting type**
F50.02 **Anorexia nervosa, binge eating/purging type**

Chapter 5 Coding Guidance

Pain Disorders Related to Psychological Factors
Subcategory F45.4 Pain disorders related to psychological factors, contains two fifth-character codes that differentiate between pain disorder exclusively related to psychological factors (F45.41) and pain disorder with related psychological factors (F45.42). For codes classified to subcategory F45.4, more than one code may be necessary to report these conditions in entirety. The following provides coding guidance for pain:

- Assign code F45.41 for pain that is exclusively psychological. For that reason, code F45.41 should not be assigned with category G89 Pain, not elsewhere classified. The Excludes 1 note at category G89 prohibits the reporting these codes together.

- An instructional note at code F45.42 states to code also any associated acute or chronic pain (G89.-) Report a code from category G89 with code F45.42 if documentation states a psychological component for the pain.

- An instructional note at category G89 Pain, not elsewhere classified states to also code related psychological factors associated with pain (F45.42).

Psychoactive Substance Use, Abuse, and Dependence
Many significant organizational and classification changes have been made to the code categories specific to alcohol and drug related-disorders. These changes include:

- Drug and alcohol abuse and dependence codes no longer identify continuous or episodic use. Instead, other data have been identified of greater value for reporting purposes.

- Combination codes for drug and alcohol use include associated conditions (e.g., withdrawal, sleep disorders and psychosis)

- Unique classification subcategories exist for specific status: use, abuse, and dependence.

- History of drug or alcohol dependence is classified as "in remission."

- An additional code is necessary to report blood alcohol level (Y9Ø.-), when documented.

Code block F1Ø–F19 Mental and behavioral disorders due to psychoactive substance use, includes the following code categories:

F1Ø	**Alcohol related disorders**
F11	**Opioid related disorders**
F12	**Cannabis related disorders**
F13	**Sedative, hypnotic or anxiolytic related disorders**
F14	**Cocaine related disorders**
F15	**Other stimulant related disorders**
F16	**Hallucinogen related disorders**
F17	**Nicotine dependence**
F18	**Inhalant related disorders**
F19	**Other psychoactive substance related disorders**

Within these code categories, fourth-character subcategories designate substance abuse (.1-), dependence (.2-), and use (.9-). Fifth characters designate status of condition, which, depending on the substance and status, such as those conditions presenting as uncomplicated, or may include:

- Intoxication
- Mood disorder
- Psychotic disorder
- Other disorder
- Unspecified disorder

Where applicable, sixth-place characters further specify the presence of certain complications, including:

- Delirium
- Delusions
- Hallucinations
- Perceptual disturbance

Certain codes with a fifth character "8" include sixth characters, which further classify the presence of specific complications as with:

Ø	**Anxiety disorder**
1	**Sexual dysfunction**
2	**Sleep disorder**
8	**Other psychoactive substance-induced disorder**

When provider documentation refers to use, abuse and dependence of the same psychoactive substance, report only one code as documented, per substance in accordance with the highest degree of clinical hierarchy. In those circumstances where the provider does not document abuse or dependence, the condition is classified to the "use" subcategory, as appropriate. Substance use may progress to substance abuse, which may result in dependence. Substance use status lies at the lowest severity end of the substance status scale, with dependence at the highest level of severity. Regarding psychoactive substance status of the same (one) substance, if both use and abuse of that substance are documented, report only the abuse. If abuse and dependence of that substance are both documented, report only the dependence. If both use and dependence of that substance are documented, report only the dependence. Excludes 1 notes are listed at each subcategory level, to indicate that use, abuse, and dependence of the same substance (classified within a subcategory) is not allowed. Note that an Excludes 1 note may be interpreted as "not coded here." As such, the subcategory codes, and those excluded by an Excludes 1 note, may not be reported together. For example:

> **Diagnosis:** Chronic alcohol abuse with dependence

F10.20   Alcohol dependence, uncomplicated

Since dependence represents a disease progression in severity from abuse to dependence, only the dependence is reported. In coding classification, dependence succeeds abuse in hierarchy. The Excludes 1 note at subcategory F10.2 states that alcohol abuse is not classified here, but more appropriately to subcategory F10.1-. For example:

> **Diagnosis:** Cannabis use with anxiety disorder due to cannabis abuse

F12.180   Cannabis abuse with cannabis-induced anxiety disorder.

Since abuse represents a disease progression in severity from use to abuse, only the abuse is reported. In coding classification, abuse succeeds use in hierarchy. The Excludes 1 note at category F12.1 states that cannabis use is not classified here, but more appropriately to subcategory F12.9-.

Mental and Behavioral Disorders Due to Psychoactive Substance Use

Codes for psychoactive substance use should only be assigned when supported by provider documentation, and when the substance use meets the definition of a reportable diagnosis. (See section III of the "ICD-10-CM Draft Official Guidelines for Coding and Reporting; Reporting Additional Diagnoses.") According to coding guidelines, codes F10.9-, F11.9-, F12.9-, F13.9-, F14.9-, F15.9- and F16.9- should only be reported when the physician documents an association between the psychoactive substance and a mental or behavioral disorder.

Remission status (-.21) for code categories F10–F19 Mental and behavior disorders due to psychoactive substance use, are assigned only on the basis of provider documentation of remission status.

Refer to the "ICD-10-CM Draft Official Guidelines for Coding and Reporting" in appendix A of this book for additional information.

Intellectual Disabilities

ICD-10-CM instructional notes state a change in sequencing of intellectual disability codes (F70–F79) from previous 1CD-9-CM instruction. In ICD-10-CM, the associated physical or developmental disorder is listed first, followed by the appropriate code from F70–F79, whereas in ICD-9-CM, the intellectual disability code (317–319) was sequenced first. Note that the terminology has been revised within the coding instruction from "psychiatric" disorders to "developmental" disorders.

ICD-9-CM

Intellectual Disabilities (317–319)
Use additional code(s) to identify any associated psychiatric or physical condition

ICD-10-CM

Intellectual Disabilities (F70–F79)
Code first any associated physical or developmental disorders

Level of Detail in Coding

As in ICD-9-CM, diagnosis codes are to be used and reported to the highest degree of specificity available. ICD-10-CM provides, in the majority of cases, an exponentially increased level of specificity than ICD-9-CM. In chapter 5, this code expansion is intended to facilitate identification of specific types or manifestations of disease that are now separately identifiable. Many of these changes are due to advances in our understanding of disease, or have been made in accordance with updates of currently applicable clinical terminology. For example:

ICD-9-CM		ICD-10-CM	
307.46	Sleep arousal disorder	F51.3	Sleepwalking [somnambulism]
		F51.4	Sleep terrors [night terrors]

New ICD-10-CM codes have been created for specific diseases or disorders not previously identifiable with unique codes in ICD-9-CM. For example:

ICD-9-CM		ICD-10-CM	
300.29	Other isolated or specific phobias	F40.210	Arachnophobia
		F40.218	Other animal type phobia
		F40.220	Fear of thunderstorms
		F40.228	Other natural environment type phobia
		F40.230	Fear of blood
		F40.231	Fear of infections and transfusions

Multiple Coding

Instructional notes appear throughout the text to provide sequencing instruction when more than one code is necessary to report the diagnosis in completion. Many codes classified to chapter 5 either necessitate or require the assignment of more than one code to report the condition in its entirety. For example, code block F01–F09, "Mental Disorders Due to Known Physiological Conditions," provides classification codes for mental disorders due to cerebral disease, injury, and other dysfunction and systemic diseases that adversely affect the brain, causing mental or behavioral disorders. This block lists an instructional note at the category level, and multiple notes at the category, subcategory, and additional character levels, which provide instruction regarding multiple coding and code sequencing. For example:

F01 **Vascular dementia**
Code first the underlying physiological condition or sequelae of cerebrovascular disease

F02 **Dementia in other diseases classified elsewhere**
Code first the underlying physiological condition, such as:
Alzheimer's (G30-)
cerebral lipidosis (E75.4)
Creutzfeldt-Jakob disease (A81.0-)

F04 **Amnestic disorder due to known physiological condition**
Code first the underlying physiological condition

Intellectual Disabilities (F70–F79)
Code first any associated physical or developmental disorders

F94.1 **Restrictive attachment disorder of childhood**
Use additional code to identify any associated failure to thrive or growth retardation

F98.1 **Encopresis not due to a substance or known physiological condition**
Use additional code to identify the cause of any coexisting constipation

Chapter 5 Coding Exercises
Assign the appropriate ICD-10-CM diagnosis codes for all reportable diagnoses, excluding external causes of morbidity (V00–Y99).

Answers to coding exercises are listed in the back of the book.

1. Alcohol dependence with intoxication _____

   _____

2. Caffeine use with stimulant-induced anxiety disorder _____

   _____

3. Mild major depressive disorder, recurrent episodes _____

   _____

4. Chronic post-traumatic stress disorder (PTSD) _____

   _____

5. Alcohol abuse with cannabis use _____

   _____

6. Attention deficit disorder (ADD) _____

   _____

7. Bipolar disorder, moderate manic episode _____

   _____

Chapter 5 Coding Scenarios

Assign the appropriate ICD-10-CM diagnosis codes for all reportable diagnoses, excluding external causes of morbidity (VØØ–Y99).

Answers to coding exercises are listed in the back of the book.

1. A 47-year-old female presents upon referral for evaluation of temporal lobe epilepsy and review of medications. History is remarkable for a marked increase in hypergraphia with compulsive writing and drawing and other impulsive behaviors. The patient's hypergraphia displays voluminous detailed artwork and writing consistent with predominately moral and religious themes. The patient's partner notes marked intensity in their relationship with increased religiosity and hyposexuality. Upon examination, the patient displays impaired memory, specifically in topic shifting with increased verbalization and reduced naming ability. As such, the patient's reactions to the awareness of her personality changes have resulted in significant frustration and emotional distress for the patient and her partner. Diagnosis is consistent with epilepsy personality syndrome secondary to temporal lobe epilepsy.

   _____

   _____

2. A 17-year-old male presents for adjustments of autism medications. He has comorbid mild intellectual disability and profound bilateral sensorineural hearing loss.

   _____

   _____

3. A 32-year-old female presents with nausea and vomiting, diaphoresis, and irregular heart beat following a 72-hour period of insomnia, increased irritability, restlessness, formication, and paranoid ideation. Exam reveals impaired judgment, multiple superficial abrasions to the face and lower arms and poor oral hygiene consistent with methamphetamine-associated behaviors. Drug toxicity screening is positive for methamphetamine. Blood alcohol level is 0.10 percent and is equal to 22 mg/l00 ml consistent with alcohol use with intoxication. The patient admits to a two-year crystal meth habit. She is transferred to the detoxification unit with the diagnosis of methamphetamine withdrawal and dependence.

   _____

   _____

4. A 74-year-old patient is seen for evaluation after being found wandering in his neighborhood, unable to find his home. History is consistent with progressive speech difficulties, inability to recall vocabulary and word dissociations. Examination reveals increasingly impaired motor coordination, urinary incontinence, progressive memory loss, and frustration consistent with progressive Alzheimer's dementia. The patient was referred to a partial hospitalization program for therapy.

   _____

   _____

CHAPTER 6. DISEASES OF THE NERVOUS SYSTEM (G00–G99)

This chapter contains 11 code families with the first character "G." The coding families classified to chapter 6 are:

G00–G09	Inflammatory diseases of the central nervous system
G10–G14	Systemic atrophies primarily affecting the central nervous system
G20–G26	Extrapyramidal and movement disorders
G30–G32	Other degenerative diseases of the nervous system
G35–G37	Demyelinating diseases of the central nervous system
G40–G47	Episodic and paroxysmal disorders
G50–G59	Nerve, nerve root and plexus disorders
G60–G65	Polyneuropathies and other disorders of the peripheral nervous system
G70–G73	Diseases of myoneural junction and muscle
G80–G83	Cerebral palsy and other paralytic syndromes
G89–G99	Other disorders of the nervous system

ICD-10-CM Category and Chapter Restructuring

ICD-10-CM contains many changes to the classification of diseases of the nervous system and special senses. In ICD-9-CM, diseases of the eye and ear were classified to the same chapter as nervous system disease. In ICD-10-CM, disorders of the eye and ear are now classified to separate chapters.

ICD-9-CM

Chapter 6. Disease of the Nervous System and Sense Organs (320–389)

ICD-10-CM

Chapter 6. Diseases of the Nervous System (G00–G99)

Chapter 7. Diseases of the Eye and Adnexa (H00–H59)

Chapter 8. Diseases of the Ear and Mastoid Process (H60–H95)

Throughout ICD-10-CM, certain disease categories have been restructured in such a way as to bring together related conditions into contiguous classifications. For example, toward the end of chapter 6, new categories for intraoperative complications and postprocedural disorders specific to the nervous system were created. In ICD-9-CM, these conditions were divided between two separate chapters. Complications that are specific to the nervous system are now classified together with diseases of the nervous system in ICD-10-CM. For example:

ICD-9-CM

349.0	Reaction to spinal or lumbar puncture
349.1	Nervous system complications from surgically implanted device
997.0	Nervous system complications
997.00	Nervous system complication, unspecified
997.01	Central nervous system complication
997.02	Iatrogenic cerebrovascular infarction or hemorrhage
997.09	Other nervous system complications

KEY POINT

Diseases of the eye and ear are no longer grouped with nervous system diseases. In ICD-10-CM, eye and ear diseases are found in two separate chapters, sharing the letter "H."

KEY POINT

No change was made to the classification of those situations where postprocedural conditions are *not* specific to a particular body system. They can be found in ICD-10-CM chapter 19, "Injury, Poisoning and Certain Other Consequences of External Causes," similarly to where they are located within ICD-9-CM.

998.1	Hemorrhage or hematoma or seroma complicating a procedure
998.11	Hemorrhage complicating a procedure
998.12	Hematoma complicating a procedure
998.13	Seroma complicating a procedure
998.2	Accidental puncture or laceration during a procedure

ICD-10-CM

G97 **Intraoperative and postprocedural complications and disorders of nervous system, not elsewhere classified**

G97.0 **Cerebrospinal fluid leak from spinal puncture**

G97.1 **Other reaction to spinal and lumbar puncture**

G97.2 **Intracranial hypotension following ventricular shunting**

G97.3 **Intraoperative hemorrhage and hematoma of a nervous system organ or structure complicating a procedure**

G97.31 **Intraoperative hemorrhage and hematoma of a nervous system organ or structure complicating a nervous system procedure**

G97.32 **Intraoperative hemorrhage and hematoma of a nervous system organ or structure complicating other procedure**

G97.4 **Accidental puncture and laceration of a nervous system organ or structure during a procedure**

G97.41 **Accidental puncture or laceration of dura during a procedure**

G97.48 **Accidental puncture and laceration of other nervous system organ or structure during a nervous system procedure**

G97.49 **Accidental puncture and laceration of other nervous system organ or structure during other procedure**

G97.5 **Postprocedural hemorrhage and hematoma of a nervous system organ or structure following a procedure**

G97.51 **Postprocedural hemorrhage and hematoma of a nervous system organ or structure following a nervous system procedure**

G97.52 **Postprocedural hemorrhage and hematoma of a nervous system organ or structure following other procedure**

G97.8 **Other intraoperative and postprocedural complications and disorders of nervous system**
Use additional code to further specify disorder

G97.81 **Other intraoperative complications of nervous system**

G97.82 **Other postprocedural complications and disorders of nervous system**

Category Title Changes

A number of category title revisions were made in chapter 6. Titles were changed to better reflect categorical content. This was often necessary when specific types of diseases were given unique classification blocks, a new category was created, or an existing category was redefined.

ICD-9-CM

354 **Mononeuritis of upper limb and mononeuritis multiplex**

ICD-10-CM

G56 **Mononeuropathies of upper limb**

Organizational Adjustments

After reviewing the different disease categories, the developers of ICD-10-CM restructured some of them to bring together those groups that are more closely related by underlying pathology. ICD-10-CM maintains separation of conditions primarily affecting the central nervous system from those affecting the peripheral nervous system; however, conditions representing symptoms (pain) and operative complications have been restructured toward the end of the chapter. For example, organic sleep disorders (327), previously sequenced after inflammatory diseases of the central nervous system (320–326) in ICD-9-CM have been reclassified in ICD-10-CM to code section G40–G47 Episodic and paroxysmal disorders. Similarly, certain hereditary, demyelinating and degenerative conditions once classified together have been reclassified between three separate sections in ICD-10-CM, which more clearly differentiate between causal pathologies. Close examination of the central nervous system disease code groupings illustrates the rationale of the restructuring. For example:

ICD-9-CM

320–326	**Inflammatory Diseases of the Central Nervous System**
327	**Organic Sleep Disorders**
330–337	**Hereditary and Degenerative Diseases of the Central Nervous System**
338	**Pain** (Restructured to section G89 Pain, not elsewhere classified, under category G89–G99, "Other Disorders of the Nervous System" in ICD-10-CM.)
339	**Other Headache Syndromes**
340–349	**Other Disorders of the Central Nervous System**

ICD-10-CM

G00–G09	**Inflammatory diseases of the central nervous system**
G10–G14	**Systemic atrophies primarily affecting the central nervous system**
G20–G26	**Extrapyramidal and movement disorders**
G30–G32	**Other degenerative diseases of the central nervous system**
G35–G37	**Demyelinating diseases of the central nervous system**
G40–G47	**Episodic and paroxysmal disorders**

A thorough understanding of the terminology and pathological disease processes inherent in ICD-10-CM coding is essential to clarify categorical content. As such, many codes have been added, deleted, combined, or moved. For example, the code for Tay-Sachs disease, which includes gangliosidosis, found in the nervous system and sense organs chapter in ICD-9-CM, has been moved in ICD-10-CM. Specific codes were created for Tay-Sachs and the different types of gangliosidosis in ICD-10-CM are found in chapter 4, "Endocrine, Nutritional and Metabolic Disorders." For example:

ICD-9-CM

330.1	**Cerebral lipidoses**
	Amaurotic (familial) idiocy
	Disease:
	Batten
	Jansky-Bielschowsky
	Kufs'
	Spielmeyer-Vogt
	Tay-Sachs
	Gangliosidosis

 DEFINITIONS

gangliosidosis. Abnormal harmful accumulation of certain lipids (gangliosides) due to enzyme deficiency; causing progressive destruction of nervous system tissues

ICD-10-CM

E75.0   **GM2 gangliosidosis**

    E75.00   **GM2 gangliosidosis, unspecified**

    E75.01   **Sandhoff disease**

    E75.02   **Tay-Sachs disease**

    E75.09   **Other GM2 gangliosidosis**

E75.1   **Other and unspecified gangliosidosis**

    E75.10   **Unspecified gangliosidosis**

    E75.11   **Mucolipidosis IV**

    E75.19   **Other gangliosidosis**

The code for eosinophilic meningitis has been reassigned in ICD-10-CM and is now classified in chapter 1, "Certain Infectious and Parasitic Diseases." For example:

ICD-9-CM

322.1   **Eosinophilic meningitis**

ICD-10-CM

Meningitis G03.9

  eosinophilic B83.2

    B83.2   **Angiostrongyliasis due to Parastrongylus cantonensis**

      Eosinophilic meningoencephalitis due to Parastrongylus cantonensis

While ICD-9-CM does have code 331.0 Alzheimer's disease, it provides no further detail about the disorder. Alzheimer's has been assigned its own category in ICD-10-CM, with four new valid four-character codes to classify this disorder based on onset. For example:

ICD-10-CM

G30   **Alzheimer's disease**

    INCLUDES   Alzheimer's dementia senile and presenile forms

    Use additional code to identify:

      delirium, if applicable (F05)

      dementia with behavioral disturbance (F02.81)

      dementia without behavioral disturbance (F02.80)

    EXCLUDES 1   *senile degeneration of brain NEC (G31.1)*

      senile dementia NOS (F03)

      senility NOS (R41.81)

G30.0   **Alzheimer's disease with early onset**

G30.1   **Alzheimer's disease with late onset**

G30.8   **Other Alzheimer's disease**

G30.9   **Alzheimer's disease, unspecified**

ICD-10-CM expanded certain disease classifications at the third- and fourth-character levels to provide additional codes. Fifth and sixth characters exist for each subcategory. This expansion is identifiable by an alpha character in the fourth-character position, previously populated by numbers. Category G43 Migraine, was expanded at the fourth-character subcategory level accordingly. For example:

G43 **Migraine**

    G43.7 **Chronic migraine without aura**

    G43.A **Cyclical vomiting**

    G43.B **Ophthalmoplegic migraine**

    G43.C **Periodic headache syndromes in child or adult**

    G43.D **Abdominal migraine**

    G43.8 **Other migraine**

    G43.9 **Migraine, unspecified**

Although the subcategory of disease status in epilepsy (e.g., intractable, not intractable, with or without status epilepticus) and migraine (e.g., intractable, not intractable, with or without status migrainosus) remains similar to that of ICD-9-CM, the hierarchy within code categories has been restructured. For example, localization-related epilepsy (G40.0–G40.2) has been sequenced before generalized epilepsy (G40.3–G40.4) in ICD-10-CM. Status epilepticus remains a severity indicator within the classification that indicates the presence of a severe, life-threatening state of persistent seizures with periods of coma.

ICD-10-CM restructuring has resulted in the movement of certain disorders once classified to chapter 7, "Diseases of the Circulatory System" in ICD-9-CM to chapter 6 in ICD-10-CM. These conditions include basilar and carotid artery syndromes, transient global amnesia and transient ischemic attack. These conditions, although vascular in origin, manifest neurological symptoms and sequelae due to the anatomy involved. Conversely, paralytic sequelae of cerebral infarct/stroke are classified to chapter 9, "Diseases of the Circulatory System" in ICD-10-CM.

Code categories G45 and G46 contain expanded subcategories that include specific types of vascular conditions with updated terminology. Certain conditions previously separately classified have either been combined, or else other conditions previously classified to an other specified (.8) code or "ill-defined" codes in ICD-9-CM have been assigned unique codes in ICD-10-CM. These reclassifications provide greater specificity by which to differentiate certain TIA syndromes by type or affected anatomic site. It is important to note a difference between G45 and G46 in whether the underlying cerebrovascular disease is coded. The instructional note under G46 states to "code first" the category I60–I69 code. In contrast, category G45 has no such instruction and is in fact excluded from I60–I69 by an "Excludes 1" indicating they are mutually exclusive. In ICD-10-CM, there will be circumstances in which the underlying cerebrovascular disease is coded and sequenced either first or in addition to other codes as documented or determined by the circumstances of the encounter.

ICD-9-CM		ICD-10-CM	
435.0	Basilar artery syndrome	G45.0	Vertebro-basilar artery syndrome
435.1	Vertebral artery syndrome	G45.0	Vertebro-basilar artery syndrome
435.3	Vertebrobasilar artery syndrome	G45.0	Vertebro-basilar artery syndrome
435.8	Other specified transient cerebral ischemias	G45.1	Carotid artery syndrome
		G45.2	Multiple and bilat precerebral artery syndromes
362.34	Amaurosis fugax	G45.3	Amaurosis fugax

ICD-9-CM		ICD-10-CM	
437.7	Transient global amnesia	G45.4	Transient global amnesia
435.2	Subclavian steal syndrome	G45.8	Othr transient cerebral ischemic attacks and related syndromes
435.8	Othr transient cerebral ischemias	G45.8	Othr transient cerebral ischemic attacks and related syndromes
435.9	Unspecified transient cerebral ischemia	G45.9	Transient cerebral ischemic attack, unspecified
435.8	Othr transient cerebral ischemias	G46.0	Middle cerebral artery syndrome
435.8	Othr transient cerebral ischemias	G46.1	Anterior cerebral artery syndrome
		G46.2	Posterior cerebral artery syndrome
437.8	Other ill-defined cerebrovascular disease	G46.3	Brain stem stroke syndrome
		G46.4	Cerebellar stroke syndrome
		G46.5	Pure motor lacunar syndrome
		G46.6	Pure sensory lacunar syndrome
		G46.7	Other lacunar syndromes
		G46.8	Othr vascular syndromes of brain in cerebrovascular diseases

DEFINITIONS

embolism. Circulating matter or particle (e.g., blood clot or plaque) which causes a circulatory obstruction and associated physiologic disruptions.

lacunar. Pertaining to discontinuity of space within an anatomical structure; pits, depressions or hollows.

motor. Of or relating to a motor nerve; one which causes or imparts motion.

sensory. Of or relating to the senses; including vision, hearing, tactile, or taste.

Chapter 6 Coding Guidance

Official Guidelines

The ICD-10-CM official guidelines for chapter 6 are similar to those in ICD-9-CM. Although the guidelines for reporting pain (category G89) have been reorganized, the concepts and sequencing rules remain the same. However, the addition of laterality to the reporting hemiparesis and monoplegia has resulted in some significant changes:

- The unspecified option (∅) should only be used when no documentation of laterality (right or left side affected) is available.

- Dominant and nondominant side designations remain in ICD-10-CM for the following categories and subcategories:

  G81   **Hemiplegia and hemiparesis**
  G83.1 Monoplegia of lower limb
  G83.2 Monoplegia of upper limb
  G83.3 Monoplegia, unspecified

- If the affected side is documented (right or left) but **not** further specified as dominant or nondominant, the following default code selections apply:

  – ambidextrous patients: default is dominant
  – left side affected: default is nondominant
  – right side affected: default is dominant

For example:

Diagnosis: Hemiplegia affecting right (dominant) side

G81.91   **Hemiplegia, unspecified affecting right dominant side**

Diagnosis: Spastic hemiplegia of right side

G81.11   **Spastic hemiplegia affecting right dominant side**

Diagnosis: Flaccid hemiplegia of left side

G81.04   Flaccid hemiplegia affecting left nondominant side

Multiple Coding

Similar to ICD-9-CM, certain codes within this chapter require either multiple codes or specific sequencing in order to properly report the condition. However, due to the increased data granularity (specificity) of the ICD-10 system, manifestation code edits have been reduced in number. For example, code section G00–G09 Inflammatory diseases of the central nervous system contains a reduction from 18 such codes in ICD-9-CM to five codes in ICD-10-CM.

A manifestation code is not allowed to be reported as a principal or first-listed diagnosis because each describes a manifestation of some other underlying disease, not the disease itself. This is important to understand when reporting CNS infections, since the causal infection or organism is often necessary to assign as additional codes. Certain CNS infections represent a primary infection; one which originates within the central nervous system. Alternately, other CNS infections present as secondary sites from an infection that originated elsewhere within the body. Therefore, it is important to understand the clinical terminology as it applies to many of the disease classifications included in this chapter. Generally, the ICD-10-CM code set describes conditions in a more clinically or anatomically specific manner than the ICD-9-CM system.

In following example, ICD-10-CM requires multiple coding, when ICD-9-CM classified the condition to a single, specific classification code. Similarly, certain conditions represented with unique classification codes in ICD-9-CM have been reclassified in ICD-10-CM. As such, manifestation/etiology edits indicate that the manifestation code must be sequenced secondary to the underlying disease or condition.

ICD-9-CM		ICD-10-CM	
321.1	Meningitis in other fungal diseases	G02	Meningitis in other infect & parasitic dz classified elsw
321.2	Meningitis due viruses NEC	G02	Meningitis in other infect & parasitic dz classified elsw
321.3	Meningitis due to trypanosomiasis	G02	Meningitis in other infect & parasitic dz classified elsw
321.4	Meningitis in sarcoidosis	G02	Meningitis in other infect & parasitic dz classified elsw

ICD-10-CM

G02   Meningitis in other infectious and parasitic diseases classified elsewhere
  Code first underlying disease, such as:
    Poliovirus infection (A80.-)

The above examples illustrate reclassification of infectious meningitis to the causal infectious disease code in chapter 1, thereby conserving space within the classification for future expansion and minimizing redundancies.

Unspecified Codes

Certain ICD-10-CM classifications differentiate specific conditions that were previously classified together. For example, 323.9 Unspecified causes of encephalitis, myelitis and encephalomyelitis, is equivalent to two possible codes in ICD-10-CM. For example:

ICD-9-CM

323.9   **Unspecified causes of encephalitis, myelitis and encephalomyelitis**

ICD-10-CM

G04.90   **Encephalitis and encephalomyelitis, unspecified**

G04.91   **Myelitis, unspecified**

When coding and reporting conditions classified to section G00-G09 Inflammatory diseases of the central nervous system, it is important to distinguish between the site and type of infection as specified in the diagnosis.

Drug-Induced Conditions

Unique codes have been established throughout this chapter to differentiate drug-induced nervous system disorders from those otherwise specified, including extrapyramidal and abnormal movement disorders:

G24.02   **Drug induced acute dystonia**

G24.09   **Other drug induced dystonia**

G25.1   **Drug-induced tremor**

G25.4   **Drug-induced chorea**

G25.61   **Drug induced tics**

G25.70   **Drug induced movement disorder, unspecified**

G25.71   **Drug induced akathisia**

G25.79   **Other drug induced movement disorders**

In ICD-10-CM, code sequencing practices have aligned with ICD-9-CM, utilizing chapter 19 poisoning and adverse effect codes, with specific identification of the causal agent (drug). Follow sequencing instruction in the ICD-10-CM text. Note that chapter 19 codes, which classify adverse effects of drugs in therapeutic use, are sequenced secondary to the nature of the condition, manifestation, or affect (e.g., Parkinsonism, dystonia, myoclonus), whereas in poisonings, overdoses, and other circumstances, the chapter 19 code is sequenced first.

Refer to the "ICD-10-CM Draft Official Guidelines for Coding and Reporting" in appendix A of this book for additional information.

As such, it is necessary for the coder to accurately identify the appropriate clinical code for the type of disease manifestation, accurately identify the causal substance and sequence the conditions in accordance with coding practices as directed by the ICD-10-CM classification. For example:

ICD-9-CM

333.92   **Neuroleptic malignant syndrome**
         Use additional E code to identify drug

            EXCLUDES *neuroleptic induced Parkinsonism (332.1)*

ICD-10-CM

G21.0   **Malignant neuroleptic syndrome**
         Use additional code for adverse effect, if applicable, to identify drug
         (T43.3X5, T43.4X5, T43.505, T43.595)

            EXCLUDES1 *neuroleptic induced parkinsonism (G21.11)*

Diagnosis: Initial encounter for neuroleptic malignant syndrome due to adverse effects in therapeutic use of haloperidol

G21.Ø   **Malignant neuroleptic syndrome**

T43.4X5A **Adverse effect of butyrophenone and thiothixene neuroleptics**

Epilepsy and Migraine

Classifications for epilepsy, migraine and headache are generally similar between systems. However, ICD-10-CM includes expanded characters, which differentiate headache as "intractable" or "not intractable," by type similar to existing classifications for epilepsy and migraine. A note at category G4Ø Epilepsy and recurrent seizures, and G43 Migraine, provides synonymous terms for the classification of "intractable," including:

- Pharmacoresistant (pharmacologically resistant)
- Treatment resistant
- Refractory (medically)
- Poorly controlled

Cluster Headache

ICD-10-CM classifications for headache syndromes are similar to their ICD-9-CM counterparts, with the exception of a sixth-character severity indicator that differentiates between intractable versus nonintractable presentations. However, there are many clinical variations of headache pain with distinct characteristics and treatments. Treatment is reliant upon accurate diagnosis; therefore, differentiation between headache syndromes is essential.

ICD-9-CM		ICD-10-CM	
339.ØØ	Cluster headache syndrome, intractable	G44.ØØ1	Cluster headache syndrome, unspecified, intractable
		G44.ØØ9	Cluster headache syndrome, unspecified, not intractable
339.Ø1	Episodic cluster headache	G44.Ø11	Episodic cluster headache, intractable
		G44.Ø19	Episodic cluster headache not intractable
339.Ø2	Chronic cluster headache	G44.Ø21	Chronic cluster headache, intractable
		G44.Ø29	Chronic cluster headache, not intractable

DEFINITIONS

neuroleptic (drug). Antipsychotic, tranquilizing medication.

DEFINITIONS

epilepsy. Brain disorder characterized by electrical-like disturbances; may include occasional impairment or loss of consciousness, abnormal motor phenomena and psychic or sensory disturbances.

intractable. Difficult to manage, change or resolve; strong-willed or resistant.

migraine. Benign vascular headache of extreme pain; commonly associated with irritability, nausea, vomiting and often photophobia; premonitory visual hallucination of a crescent in the visual field (scotoma).

Chapter 6 Coding Exercises

Assign the appropriate ICD-10-CM diagnosis codes for all reportable diagnoses, excluding external causes of morbidity (VØØ–Y99).

Answers to coding exercises are listed in the back of the book.

1. Recurrent seizures _____

   _____

2. Bacterial meningitis due to streptococcus B _____

   _____

3. Subsequent encounter for treatment of parkinsonism secondary to adverse effects of psychotropic phenothiazine in therapeutic use

   _____

   _____

4. Early onset Alzheimer's disease _____

   _____

5. Premenstrual migraine _____

   _____

6. Epilepsy with intractable complex partial seizures _____

   _____

7. Transient ischemic attack _____

   _____

Chapter 6 Coding Scenarios

Assign the appropriate ICD-10-CM diagnosis codes for all reportable diagnoses, excluding external causes of morbidity (VØØ–Y99).

Answers to coding exercises are listed in the back of the book.

1. A 30-year-old female presents with a recent history of progressive numbness and tingling of the lower extremities and increased difficulty walking, noting the tendency of her left foot to drag. She describes intense, shooting pains occurring intermittently in her lower extremities. There has been no known injury or precipitating factors. Physical examination reveals significantly impaired proprioception and vibration sense, lower extremity weakness and hyporeflexia and abnormality on MRI. The physician documents findings as consistent with a demyelinating process consistent with idiopathic transverse myelitis. Further workup will be undertaken to determine an underlying etiology and most appropriate course of treatment.

   _____

   _____

2. Patient presents for evaluation of persistent headache. Medication use is significant for overuse of Tylenol during the recovery and healing process from surgery two months prior. Upon exam, the patient states that she was taking Tylenol daily to prevent pain, as well as to alleviate pain when it occurs. She admits to some anxiety at the cessation of postoperative opiates in anticipation of pain, and has taken additional doses of Tylenol than is recommended. The physician documents diagnosis of drug-induced headache due to Tylenol overuse with chronic postoperative pain.

    _____

    _____

3. A 42-year-old left-handed male presents to the emergency department in distress. Chief complaints include severe headache, fever and chills, agitation, nausea and vomiting, photophobia, left arm paralysis, and stiff neck. Physical exam confirms the presence of tachycardia, fever, photophobia, fever, mental status changes, vomiting, and left extremity paralysis. History is negative for recent trauma or history of cardiovascular disease. Lumbar puncture was performed, which was negative for infectious pathogen. Diagnostic imaging was negative for cardiovascular pathology. The patient was admitted and placed in intravenous hydration. Admitting symptoms and findings on examination are documented as consistent with idiopathic aseptic meningitis with associated left extremity monoplegia.

    _____

    _____

4. A 36-year-old hospital employee presents with progressive numbness and tingling of the lower extremities and increasing difficulty walking. Onset of symptoms occurred approximately four weeks following administration of the first dose of hepatitis B vaccine, although she did not seek medical care for her symptoms at that time. One month later, following the second dose, the sensory disturbance ascended to the mid-trunk level, with progressive difficulty walking. Physical examination reveals significantly impaired sensation, lower extremity weakness and hyporeflexia and abnormality on MRI. Diagnosis was documented as acute disseminated postimmunization myelitis.

    _____

    _____

CHAPTER 7. DISEASES OF THE EYE AND ADNEXA (H00–H59)

Chapter 7 contains 12 code families with the first character "H," also shared with chapter 8, "Diseases of the Ear and Mastoid process." The coding families classified to chapter 7 are:

H00–H05	**Disorders of eyelid, lacrimal system and orbit**
H10–H11	**Disorders of conjunctiva**
H15–H22	**Disorders of sclera, cornea, iris and ciliary body**
H25–H28	**Disorders of lens**
H30–H36	**Disorders of choroid and retina**
H40–H42	**Glaucoma**
H43–H44	**Disorders of vitreous body and globe**
H46–H47	**Disorders of optic nerve and visual pathways**
H49–H52	**Disorders of ocular muscles, binocular movement, accommodation and refraction**
H53–H54	**Visual disturbances and blindness**
H55–H57	**Other disorders of eye and adnexa**
H59	**Intraoperative and postprocedural complications and disorders of eye and adnexa, not elsewhere classified**

ICD-10-CM Category Restructuring

The ICD-9-CM has only one subchapter for disorders of the eye and adnexa, which is included with the chapter for diseases of the nervous system. ICD-10-CM has reclassified these diseases into their own chapter, according to the blocks described above. For example, diseases of the eyelids fall into the middle in ICD-9-CM's subchapter. In ICD-10-CM, it is the first block.

As such, many codes have been added, deleted, combined, or moved. An excludes note has been added to the beginning of the chapter to clarify that certain conditions are more appropriately classified elsewhere, including:

- Certain conditions originating in the perinatal period (P04–P96)

- Certain infectious and parasitic diseases (A00–B99)

- Complications of pregnancy, childbirth and the puerperium (O00–O99)

- Congenital malformations, deformations, and chromosomal abnormalities (Q00–Q99)

- Diabetes mellitus related eye conditions (E09.3-, E10.3-, E11.3-, E13.3-)

- Endocrine, nutritional and metabolic diseases (E00–E88)

- Injury (trauma) of eye and orbit (S05.-)

ICD-10-CM restructuring reclassifies certain ophthalmic conditions to other chapters. Such is the case for ophthalmic manifestations of diabetes mellitus. ICD-10-CM effectively employs combination codes replacing etiology-manifestation coding for diabetic ophthalmic disease. For example:

👉 KEY POINT

Chapter 7, "Diseases of the Eye and Adnexa" is a separate ICD-10-CM chapter, as is chapter 8, "Diseases of the Ear and Mastoid Process." In ICD-9-CM, the codes for these diseases were included within chapter 6, Diseases of the Nervous System and Sense Organs.

ICD-9-CM		ICD-10-CM	
362.01	Background diabetic retinopathy	E10.311	Type 1DM w/uns diab retinop w/ME
		E10.319	Type 1DM w/uns diab retinop w/o ME
366.41	Diabetic cataract	E10.36	Type1 DM w/diabetic cataract
		E11.36	Type 2 DM w/diabetic cataract
		E13.36	Other spec diabetes mellitus w/diabetic cataract
362.07	Diabetic macular edema	E10.311	Type 1DM w/uns diab retinop w/ME
		E10.321	Type 1 DM w/mild non prolif diab retinpathy w/ME
		E10.331	Type 1 DM w/mod non prolif diab retinpathy w/ME
		E11.341	Type 1 DM w/sev nonprolif DR w/ME

In the example above, the ICD-10-CM chapter 4 codes (E00–E89) include the causal disease (diabetes mellitus), type of disease, specific ophthalmic manifestation, and associated conditions or complications. Conversely, ICD-10-CM classification of diabetes mellitus no longer includes an axis to indicate whether or not the disease is controlled. See the "ICD-10-CM Draft Official Guidelines for Coding and Reporting" for specific guidance regarding coding and reporting diabetes.

Category Title and Code Description Changes

A number of category title revisions were made in chapter 7. Titles were changed to better reflect categorical content, which was often necessary when specific types of diseases were given their own block, a new category was created, or an existing category was redefined. Note that the term "senile" has been replaced with the more appropriate term "age-related," where applicable.

ICD-9-CM

366.0	Infantile, juvenile, and presenile cataract
366.1	Senile cataract

ICD-10-CM

H25	Age-related cataract
H26	Other cataract
	H26.0	Infantile and juvenile cataract

Furthermore, ICD-10-CM contains code descriptions that have been updated to reflect current clinical terminology and to better represent conditions as they are understood by advancing medical technologies. For example, the diagnoses blind hypotensive eye and blind hypertensive eye have been revised to atrophy of the globe and absolute glaucoma, respectively.

ICD-9-CM		ICD-10-CM	
360.41	Blind hypotensive eye	H44.521	Atrophy of globe right eye
		H44.522	Atrophy of globe left eye
		H44.523	Atrophy of globe bilateral
		H44.529	Atrophy of globe unspecified eye

ICD-9-CM		ICD-10-CM	
360.42	Blind hypertensive eye	H44.511	Absolute glaucoma right eye
		H44.512	Absolute glaucoma left eye
		H44.513	Absolute glaucoma bilateral
		H44.519	Absolute glaucoma unspecified eye

ICD-10-CM includes unique codes for conditions not previously identified by ICD-9-CM. In the classification of retinoschisis and retinal cysts, new subcategory codes have been created to specifically identify cyst ora serrata; the junction between the retina and the ciliary body.

ICD-9-CM		ICD-10-CM	
361.19	Other retinoschisis and retinal cysts	H33.111	Cyst ora serrata right eye
		H33.112	Cyst ora serrata left eye
		H33.113	Cyst ora serrata bilateral
		H33.119	Cyst ora serrata unspecified eye

Although certain ICD-10-CM classifications that separate conditions according to severity of presentation are similar to those of ICD-9-CM, terminology has been updated to reflect current clinical language. For example, keratoconus was previously classified as unspecified (371.60), stable (371.61), or with acute hydrops (371.62). In ICD-10-CM, the term "unstable" replaces the less frequently documented "acute hydrops."

ICD-9-CM		ICD-10-CM	
371.62	Keratoconus, acute hydrops	H18.621	Keratoconus unstable, right eye
		H18.622	Keratoconus unstable, left eye
		H18.623	Keratoconus unstable, bilateral
		H18.629	Keratoconus unstable, unspecified eye

Organizational Adjustments

When comparing ICD-9-CM to ICD-10-CM, some codes have been added, deleted, combined, or moved. For example, in ICD-9-CM, the code for amaurosis fugax is an inclusion term under code 362.34. The code for this disease has been moved in ICD-10-CM. It now has its own code (G45.3) in chapter 6, "Diseases of the Nervous System," under category G45 Transient cerebral ischemic attacks and related syndromes.

ICD-9-CM

362.3 Retinal vascular occlusion
    362.34 Transient arterial occlusion
        Amaurosis fugax

ICD-10-CM

G45 Transient cerebral ischemic attacks and related syndromes
    G45.3 Amaurosis fugax

Laterality

The addition of laterality into ICD-10-CM classifications for diseases and disorders of paired organs and structures has resulted in some significant changes. Codes that specify bilateral conditions should always be reported when both eyes are affected. However, if no classification option for bilateral is available, and the condition affects both eyes, two codes may be assigned to report the condition in both the right and left eye. Many code categories within chapter 7 have been restructured, expanded, and new codes added to accommodate unique classifications. As such, the majority of diagnosis codes have been expanded to accommodate classifications for right, left, bilateral, or unspecified eye. Similarly, diagnoses specific to the eyelid are differentiated by laterality as well as upper or lower affected eyelid. ICD-10-CM classifications for aqueous misdirection (malignant glaucoma) have been expanded to designate laterality; the affected eye. For example:

ICD-9-CM

365.83	**Aqueous misdirection**
	Malignant glaucoma

ICD-10-CM

H40.83		**Aqueous misdirection**
		Malignant glaucoma
	H40.831	**Aqueous misdirection, right eye**
	H40.832	**Aqueous misdirection, left eye**
	H40.833	**Aqueous misdirection, bilateral**
	H40.839	**Aqueous misdirection, unspecified eye**

Paired Structures

ICD-10-CM classifications for hordeolum externum (stye) have been expanded to designate laterality and specific anatomic site, where paired structures (e.g., eyelids) exist:

H00.01		**Hordeolum externum**
	H00.011	**Hordeolum externum, right upper eyelid**
	H00.012	**Hordeolum externum, right lower eyelid**
	H00.013	**Hordeolum externum, right eye, unspecified eyelid**
	H00.014	**Hordeolum externum, left upper eyelid**
	H00.015	**Hordeolum externum, left lower eyelid**
	H00.016	**Hordeolum externum, left eye, unspecified eyelid**
	H00.019	**Hordeolum externum, unspecified eye, unspecified eyelid**

Anatomic Specificity

ICD-10-CM associates certain ophthalmic diseases with closely related manifestations separately. For example, parasitic endophthalmitis has been expanded to include separate classifications for parasitic cyst, by affected anatomic structure within the eye. Previously, ICD-10-CM classified parasitic endophthalmitis and parasitic cyst, regardless of affected site to a single code.

ICD-9-CM		ICD-10-CM	
360.13	Parasitic endophthalmitis, NOS	H21.331	Parasitic cyst iris, ciliary body or AC, right
		H33.121	Parasitic cyst of retina, right eye
		H44.121	Parasitic endophthalmitis, NOS right eye

Chapter 7 Coding Guidance

Official Guidelines

The *ICD-10-CM Draft Official Guidelines for Coding and Reporting* provide guidelines specific to glaucoma. These guidelines parallel ICD-9-CM in concept, with consideration to the structural classification changes inherent in ICD-10-CM. To ensure accurate code assignment throughout the remainder of this chapter, apply the ICD-10-CM conventions and instructions within the ICD-10-CM text.

Glaucoma

ICD-10-CM uses combination codes to classify glaucoma by type and stage to code section H40–H42. Category H40 classifies certain types of glaucoma by type, stage, and laterality. The absence of category H41 reserves space in the classification for future code expansion. Code H42 is a valid three-digit manifestation code that classifies glaucoma in diseases classified elsewhere. Instructional notes require the underlying disease or condition to be coded and sequenced first.

ICD-9-CM required multiple coding to report the type and stage of certain types of glaucoma. ICD-10-CM contains combination codes which classify the disease type, stage, and laterality in a single code in certain situations. For example, pigmentary glaucoma requires two codes in ICD-9-CM, whereas ICD-10-CM classifies pigmentary glaucoma by type, laterality, and stage in a single code.

ICD-9-CM

365.13   Pigmentary glaucoma
Use additional code to identify glaucoma stage (365.70–365.74)

ICD-9-CM		ICD-10-CM	
365.13	Pigmentary open-angle glaucoma	H40.1310	Pigmentary glaucoma, right eye, stage unspecified
		H40.1311	Pigmentary glaucoma, right eye, mild stage
		H40.1312	Pigmentary glaucoma, right eye, moderate stage
		H40.1313	Pigmentary glaucoma, right eye, severe stage
		H40.134	Pigmentary glaucoma, right eye, indeterminate stage

The *ICD-10-CM Draft Official Guidelines for Coding and Reporting* provide guidelines specific to glaucoma. Key concepts include:

- Assign as many as category H40 codes as necessary to identify glaucoma by type, laterality, and stage.

- Report bilateral glaucoma of the same type and stage in both eyes with a single bilateral classification code, if provided. The seventh character identifies the disease stage. If no bilateral classification exists, report only one code for the type of glaucoma with the appropriate seventh character.

- Bilateral glaucoma with different disease types or stages may require separate codes to identify each type and stage, as documented.

- If the stage of glaucoma progresses during the admission/encounter, assign the code for the highest stage documented.

- Do not assign the seventh character "4-Indeterminate stage" without documentation that the stage cannot be determined. If documentation does not specify disease stage, report seventh character "0-Unspecified stage."

Refer to the "ICD-10-CM Draft Official Guidelines for Coding and Reporting" in appendix A of this book for additional information.

The diagnosis of "glaucoma suspect" describes a patient with borderline signs and symptoms of glaucoma, such as a suspicious-looking optic nerve, a borderline high intraocular pressure (IOP), and associated visual field deficits. Ocular hypertension is an increase in the pressure inside the eye (IOP) and is higher than normal. Normal eye pressure ranges from 10 to 21 mm Hg. Eye pressure is measured in millimeters of mercury (mm Hg). The eye pressure for ocular hypertension is greater than 21 mm Hg. Code H40.0 describes high intraocular pressures, including those with no apparent cause, or other anatomic anomaly or pathology (e.g, anatomic narrow angle, ocular hypertension, borderline findings) that may create a minor block in aqueous outflow from the eye, but of which a definitive diagnosis of glaucoma is suspected, but has not yet been established.

Additionally, conditions once classified separately in ICD-9-CM have been moved to classification categories containing similar conditions or disease. For example, pseudoexfoliation glaucoma (365.52), has been reclassified as open angle, primary capsular glaucoma. The alphabetic index directs the coder accordingly. For example:

Glaucoma
    with
        pseudoexfoliation of lens—*see* Glaucoma, open angle, primary, capsular
        open angle H40.10-
            primary H40.11-
                capsular (with pseudoexfoliation of lens) H40.14-

Cataract

ICD-10-CM code descriptions for cataract classifications have been updated (similar to other ocular disorders) by replacing the term "senile" with "age-related," where appropriate. The term "senile" has been confused with an age-related dementia, cognitive decline, or other degenerative mental health condition beyond that associated with the normal aging process. Instead, the term "age-related" associates a stated condition occurring only with the natural aging process—without implying a change in mental or cognitive status. Otherwise, ICD-10-CM changes to terminology within the cataract classification categories include updated code descriptions for cataract revising "after-cataract" to "secondary cataract" and denoting hypermature senile cataract (366.18) as an age-related cataract, morgagnian type (H25.2-).

 DEFINITIONS

after-cataract. Cataract characterized by opacifications of the posterior capsule occurring subsequent to extracapsular cataract extraction *Syn. Secondary cataract.*

morgagnian-type cataract. A mature age-related cataract with lens opacification and a soft, liquefied or flattened fragile lens causing nuclear shifts to the bottom of the lens capsule.

ICD-9-CM		ICD-10-CM	
366.18	Hypermature senile cataract	H25.20	Age-related cataract morgagnian type, unspecified eye
		H25.21	Age-related cataract morgagnian type, right eye
		H25.22	Age-related cataract morgagnian type, left eye
		H25.23	Age-related cataract morgagnian type, bilateral

Code category H26.2 Complicated cataract, includes those associated with other systemic or ocular diseases. Instructional notes throughout this chapter prompt the coder to assign additional codes for associated cataract, where applicable. For example:

H20.1 **Chronic iridocyclitis**
Use additional code for any associated cataract (H26.21-)

H26.22 **Cataract secondary to ocular disorders (degenerative) (inflammatory)**
Code also associated ocular disorder

Infectious Disease Reclassifications

In ICD-10-CM many ophthalmic conditions of infectious origin have been reclassified to chapter 1, "Certain Infectious and Parasitic Diseases," including ocular manifestation of tuberculosis (A18.5-), and *Acanthamoeba* (B60.1-). ICD-9-CM required two codes in specific sequence to report ophthalmic infection with *Acanthamoeba*, whereas in ICD-10-CM, they are reported with a single code:

ICD-9-CM		ICD-10-CM	
136.21	Specific infection due to Acanthamoeba	B60.13	Keratoconjunctivitis due to Acanthamoeba
370.8	Other forms of keratitis		
136.21	Specific infection due to Acanthamoeba	B60.12	Conjunctivitis due to Acanthamoeba
372.15	Parasitic conjunctivitis		

Retained Foreign Body

Certain injuries involving retained or embedded fragments or splinters preclude removal due to technical difficulty, number of retained objects, or anatomically-sensitive locations in the body. Any embedded object (natural or synthetic) has the potential to cause infection, migrate, interfere with body functions, cause an immune response, or create other health problems. When an injury to the eye results in a retained foreign body, instructional notes within the text state to use an additional code to identify the foreign body by the type of embedded material. Subcategories Z18.0–Z18.1 and Z18.3–Z18.8 contain fifth characters that further specify the nature of the material (e.g., glass, stone, animal quills). For example:

H02.81 **Retained foreign body in eyelid**
Use additional code to identify the type of retained foreign body (Z18.-)

Z18 **Retained foreign body fragments**

Z18.0 **Retained radioactive fragments**

Z18.1 **Retained metal fragments**

Z18.2 **Retained plastic fragments**

Z18.3   **Retained organic fragments**

Z18.8   **Other specified retained foreign body**

Z18.9   **Retained foreign body fragments, unspecified material**

Codes from category Z18, however, are not applicable to, or overlap with, internal medical devices. These codes would be used as secondary status codes for cases such as injury codes that include the presence of a foreign body, or with toxic effect codes.

Drug- or Chemical-Induced Conditions

Combination codes, which include the causal drug or chemical and the external cause (e.g., therapeutic use), replace the need for a separate external cause code. Code section T36–T50 includes poisoning by, adverse effects of and underdosing of drugs, medicaments, and biological substances, whereas code section T51–T65 includes toxic effects of substances chiefly nonmedicinal as to source. When reporting a toxic-effect condition, use additional codes as necessary to report all associated manifestations of the toxic effect. Report adverse effects of drugs in therapeutic use with the appropriate chapter 19 code sequenced secondary to the nature of the complication or condition. Codes T36–T50 identify the causal drug. Adverse effects of drugs in therapeutic use are classified with fifth or sixth character 5. For example:

- Drug-induced condition in therapeutic use (T36–T50):

  H40.6 Glaucoma secondary to drugs
  > Use additional code for adverse effect, if applicable, to identify drug (T36–T50 with fifth or sixth character 5)

  Diagnosis: Secondary glaucoma due to adverse effects of ophthalmic corticosteroid therapy, subsequent encounter

  H40.6   **Glaucoma secondary to drugs**

  T49.5X5D   **Adverse effect of ophthalmological drugs and preparations**

- Chemical-induced condition (T51–T65):

  H46.3 Toxic optic neuropathy
  > Code first (T51–T65) to identify cause

  Diagnosis: Tobacco smoke-induced toxic optic neuropathy, accidental

  T65.221A   **Toxic effect of tobacco cigarettes, accidental (unintentional)**

  H46.3   **Toxic optic neuropathy**

When reporting from chapter 19 poisoning, adverse effect or toxicity diagnoses, additional codes may be required. Carefully consider instructional notes at the beginning of each code block (T36–T50, T51–T65) regarding the additional reporting of associated manifestations and intent.

Intraoperative and Postprocedural Complications of the Eye and Adnexa (H59)

In ICD-10-CM, postoperative complications have been moved to procedure-specific body system chapters. Postoperative eye and adnexal complication classifications contain certain unique diagnosis and surgery-specific complications. For example, category H59.4 specifically classifies inflammation (infection) of postprocedural bleb, by stage of severity. Code category H59 includes intraoperative complications (H59.1, H59.2), postprocedural complications (H59.3, H59.4) and those specifically associated with cataract surgery (H59.Ø), and other procedural complications (H59.8), including chorioretinal scars following retinal detachment surgery (H59.81). Code assignment is based on the provider's documentation of the relationship between the condition and the procedure. For example:

Diagnosis: Encounter for visual disturbance due to retina scar following retinal detachment surgery, right eye

H59.811   Chorioretinal scars after surgery for detachment, right eye

Chapter 7 Coding Exercises

Assign the appropriate ICD-10-CM diagnosis codes for all reportable diagnoses, excluding external causes of morbidity (VØØ–Y99).

Answers to coding exercises are listed in the back of the book.

1. Chalazion, left lower and upper eyelid _____

    _____

2. Dry eye syndrome, affecting both eyes _____

    _____

3. Accidental exposure with chlorine bleach conjunctivitis, right eye

    _____

    _____

4. Cornea edema due to contact lens, left eye _____

    _____

5. Senile cortical cataract, right eye _____

    _____

6. Retained magnetic foreign body in anterior chamber _____

    _____

Chapter 7 Coding Scenarios

Assign the appropriate ICD-10-CM diagnosis codes for all reportable diagnoses, excluding external causes of morbidity (V00–Y99).

Answers to coding exercises are listed in the back of the book.

1. A 6-year-old female presents for ophthalmologic evaluation. The mother reports squinting and avoidance of light, and has noticed at times the child seems unaware of people or objects in the periphery. Comprehensive eye examination reveals mild bilateral myopia at -1.75 right and -1.50 left. Direct examination reveals bilateral optic nerves to be underdeveloped. The ophthalmologist documents a diagnosis optic nerve hypoplasia. Further testing will be undertaken to determine the degree of impairment. Prescription for corrective lenses provided.

    _____

    _____

2. A 68-year-old patient presents in surgical consultation for treatment of complicated cataract with neovascularization of right eye and secondary noninfectious iridocyclitis.

    _____

    _____

3. A patient presents for an eye exam after spending years overseas in remote areas, without access to medical care. He presents today for assessment of persistent, worsening foggy vision, headaches, photophobia, and visual field disturbances. General eye examination with slit lamp and gonioscopy reveals glaucomatous findings. Ophthalmoscopy findings are consistent with chronic, bilateral primary angle closure glaucoma, mild disease in left eye with greater progression of disease in the right eye (moderate) and resultant ischemic neuropathy of the optic nerve.

    _____

    _____

CHAPTER 8. DISEASES OF THE EAR AND MASTOID PROCESS (H6Ø–H95)

Chapter 8 contains five code families with the first character "H," which is shared with chapter 7," Diseases of the Eye and Adnexa." The coding families classified to chapter 8 are:

H6Ø–H62	Diseases of external ear
H65–H75	Diseases of middle ear and mastoid
H8Ø–H83	Diseases of inner ear
H9Ø–H94	Other disorders of ear
H95	Intraoperative and postprocedural complications and disorders of ear and mastoid process, not elsewhere classified

ICD-10-CM classifies disorders of the ear and mastoid process by anatomic site, according to those conditions that affect the external (H6Ø–H62), middle (H65–H75), or inner (H8Ø–H83) ear. Additional classification sections follow that group together other disorders of ear (H9Ø–H94) and intraoperative or postprocedural disorders (H95).

ICD-10-CM Category Restructuring

Chapter 8, "Diseases of the Ear and Mastoid Process," is a separate chapter in ICD-10-CM, whereas in ICD-9-CM, the codes for these diseases were included within chapter 6, "Diseases of the Nervous System and Sense Organs." In addition, the ICD-9-CM has only one subchapter for disorders of the ear and mastoid process, whereas ICD-10-CM reclassified these diseases according to the blocks as described above.

ICD-10-CM separates the nervous system disease classifications from those of the sense organs (eye and ear), creating three separate chapters. Perhaps one of the most significant changes characteristic of the ICD-10-CM system is the incorporation of laterality into the classification, where paired organs and anatomic sites exist. Code classifications now exist to provide laterality options to report certain conditions as pertaining to a particular side (right or left), bilateral, or when not documented as to a specific side, unspecified. This is particularly evident in chapter 7, "Diseases of the Eye and Adnexa (HØØ–H59)," and chapter 8, "Diseases of the Ear and Mastoid Process. As such, many codes have been added, deleted, combined, or moved. An Excludes note has been added to the beginning of the chapter to clarify that certain conditions are more appropriately classified elsewhere, including:

- Certain conditions originating in the perinatal period (PØ4–P96)

- Certain infectious and parasitic diseases (AØØ–B99)

- Complications of pregnancy, childbirth and the puerperium (OØØ–O99)

- Congenital malformations, deformations and chromosomal abnormalities (QØØ–Q99)

- Endocrine, nutritional and metabolic diseases (EØØ–E88)

- Injury, poisoning and certain other consequences of external causes (S00–T88)

- Neoplasms (CØØ–D49)

- Symptoms, signs and abnormal clinical and laboratory findings, not elsewhere classified (R00–R94)

Category Title Changes

A number of category title revisions were made in chapter 8. Titles were changed to better reflect categorical content, which was often necessary when specific types of diseases were given their own block, a new category was created, or an existing category was redefined.

ICD-9-CM

381	Nonsuppurative otitis media and Eustachian tube disorders
382	Suppurative and unspecified otitis media

ICD-10-CM

H65	Nonsuppurative otitis media
H66	Suppurative and unspecified otitis media
H67	Otitis media in diseases classified elsewhere
H68	Eustchian salpingitis and obstruction
H69	Other and unspecified disorders of the Eustachian tube

Organizational Adjustments

When comparing ICD-9-CM to ICD-10-CM, some codes have been added, deleted, combined, or moved. For example, the code for cerebrospinal fluid otorrhea, found under the subchapter for diseases of the ear and mastoid process in the nervous system and sense organs chapter in ICD-9-CM, has not been included in the new chapter for diseases of the ear and mastoid process in ICD-10-CM, but is instead found in chapter 6, "Diseases of the Nervous System."

ICD-9-CM

388.61	Cerebrospinal fluid otorrhea

ICD-10-CM

G96.0	Cerebrospinal fluid leak

ICD-9-CM code 388.5 Disorders of acoustic nerve, has been expanded in ICD-10-CM to a subcategory level in which the fifth character is a placeholder "X"; reserving the character for future expansion.

ICD-9-CM

388.5	Disorders of acoustic nerve

ICD-10-CM

H93.3X	Disorders of acoustic nerve
	H93.3X1 Disorders of right acoustic nerve
	H93.3X2 Disorders of left acoustic nerve
	H93.3X3 Disorders of bilateral acoustic nerves
	H93.3X9 Disorders of unspecified acoustic nerve

Although there is no single specific code in ICD-9-CM for acute recurrent otitis media, ICD-10-CM provides several codes within three separate subcategories

KEY POINT

Some codes specific to certain disorders are being further subclassified in ICD-10-CM, to specify which side of the body is affected by that condition in a single code.

Example

380.31	Hematoma of auricle or pinna

This disorder is reported using one of four codes in ICD-10-CM:

H61.12	Hematoma of pinna Hematoma of auricle
H61.121	Hematoma of pinna, right ear
H61.122	Hematoma of pinna, left ear
H61.123	Hematoma of pinna, bilateral
H61.129	Hematoma of pinna, unspecified ear

DEFINITIONS

cerebrospinal fluid otorrhea. Discharge of cerebrospinal fluid escaping from the external ear canal as a result of fracture or disease of the temporal bone.

(H65.Ø, H65.1, H66.Ø) that classify acute otitis media by type (e.g., serous, nonsuppurative, suppurative) and laterality (unspecified, right, left bilateral). These codes also provide the option of classifying the condition as acute "recurrent." For example:

H65.Ø **Acute serous otitis media**
Acute and subacute secretory otitis

H65.ØØ	**Acute serous otitis media, unspecified ear**
H65.Ø1	**Acute serous otitis media, right ear**
H65.Ø2	**Acute serous otitis media, left ear**
H65.Ø3	**Acute serious otitis media, bilateral**
H65.Ø4	**Acute serous otitis media, recurrent, right ear**
H65.Ø5	**Acute serous otitis media, recurrent, left ear**
H65.Ø6	**Acute serous otitis media, recurrent, bilateral**
H65.Ø7	**Acute serous otitis media, recurrent, unspecified ear**

Chapter 8 Coding Guidance

Official Guidelines

At the time of this publication, no official coding guidelines have been published for chapter 8 classification codes. To ensure accurate code assignment, apply the ICD-10-CM conventions and instructions within the ICD-10-CM text. Many instructional notes have been added to this chapter. For example:

- Notes at the beginning of the chapter state to use an external cause code, if applicable, with chapter 8 codes, to identify causal factors.

- Multiple coding instructions "code also" or "use additional code, if applicable" are used to prompt that more than one code may be necessary to report a disease or condition in its entirety.

- Etiology/manifestation instruction (e.g., code first underlying disease/use additional code) is used for appropriate sequencing of otological disease manifestations secondary to causal condition classified elsewhere.

Ear Infections

The unique classification categories within chapter 8 of ICD-10-CM enable conditions to be reported with greater specificity, creating an increase in the granularity of data not available in the ICD-9-CM system. This is particularly evident in the ICD-10-CM classification of ear infections, in which code categories have been differentiated and expanded, not only to further specify site, laterality, and severity of presentation (i.e., acute, chronic, unspecified), but also to distinguish between specific types and characteristics of infection.

ICD-9-CM		ICD-1Ø-CM	
38Ø.1Ø	Unsp infective otitis externa	H6Ø.Ø1	Abscess of right external ear
		H6Ø.11	Cellulitis of right external ear
		H6Ø.311	Diffuse otitis externa, right ear
		H6Ø.321	Hemorrhagic otitis externa, right ear
38Ø.22	Other acute otitis externa	H6Ø.511	Acute actinic otitis externa, right ear
		H6Ø.521	Acute chemical otitis externa, right ear
		H6Ø.531	Acute contact otitis externa, right ear
		H6Ø.541	Acute eczematoid otitis externa, right ear
		H6Ø.551	Acute reactive otitis externa, right ear

As previously noted, ICD-10-CM includes separate classifications for *recurrent* acute otitis media. Such conditions were not specifically identifiable in ICD-9-CM. Furthermore, separate subcategories have been created in ICD-10-CM to differentiate specific nonsuppurative otitis media as acute serous otitis media (H65.0-) or other acute nonsuppurative otitis media (H65.1-). Within these subcategories, conditions are further identified by fourth, fifth and sixth characters that specify type (e.g., serous, allergic, other), laterality (e.g., right, left, bilateral), and presentation (recurrent or nonrecurrent).

ICD-9-CM

381   **Nonsuppurative otitis media and Eustachian tube disorders**

   381.0   **Acute nonsuppurative otitis media**

      381.01   **Acute serous otitis media**

ICD-10-CM

H65   **Nonsuppurative otitis media**

   H65.0   **Acute serous otitis media**

   H65.1   **Other acute nonsuppurative otitis media**

Code category H65 lists instructional notes that prompt the coder to use additional codes to identify associated perforated tympanic membrane (H72-) or certain significant exposures and environmental factors. An instructional note at category H72 Perforation of tympanic membrane, states to code first any associated otitis media. For example:

Diagnosis: Subacute allergic sanguinous otitis media, perforated tympanum, with chronic environmental exposure to tobacco smoke

H65.119   **Acute and subacute allergic otitis media (mucoid)(sanguinous)(serous), unspecified ear**

H72.90   **Unspecified perforation of tympanic membrane, unspecified ear**

Z77.22   **Contact with and (suspected) exposure to environmental tobacco smoke (acute)(chronic)**

Labyrinthitis

Although ICD-10-CM generally provides a far greater specificity than ICD-9-CM, certain classifications have been made less specific. For example, certain forms of vertigo, labyrinthitis, labyrinthine fistula and dysfunction once separately classified according to type, have been grouped together within revised subcategories, and are now identified by general diagnosis and laterality.

ICD-9-CM		ICD-10-CM	
386.19	Other and unspecified peripheral vertigo	H81.311	Aural vertigo right ear
386.31	Serous labyrinthitis	H83.01	Labyrinthitis right ear
386.32	Circumscribed labyrinthitis	H83.01	Labyrinthitis right ear
386.33	Suppurative labyrinthitis	H83.01	Labyrinthitis right ear
386.41	Round window fistula	H83.11	Labyrinthine fistula right ear
386.42	Oval window fistula	H83.11	Labyrinthine fistula right ear
386.43	Semicircular canal fistula	H83.11	Labyrinthine fistula right ear
386.51	Hyperactive labyrinth, unilateral	H83.2X1	Labyrinthine dysfunction, right ear

ICD-9-CM	ICD-10-CM
386.55 Loss of labyrinthine reactivity unilateral	H83.2X1 Labyrinthine dysfunction, right ear

Auditory Perception Disorders

Disorders of auditory perception may be congenital or acquired; however, the onset of either in early childhood can pose learning challenges. Individuals with impaired auditory perception may seem to either not respond well to auditory or verbal cues, not understand what they hear, or repetition of an auditory cue may be required to elicit a desired response. As such, these conditions are generally attributed to a disorder or dysfunction of the auditory nerve that more appropriately identifies the underlying physiological causal factors.

ICD-10-CM classifications for abnormal auditory perception disorders separately identify certain conditions (e.g., temporary auditory threshold shift), whereas other conditions (e.g., impairment of auditory discrimination) are grouped into general classification subcategories such as H93.29 Other abnormal auditory perceptions. Furthermore, central auditory processing disorder (ICD-9-CM code 315.32) was formerly classified as a developmental delay in chapter 5, "Mental Disorders," in ICD-9-CM. However, ICD-10-CM reclassified the condition to category H93 as a disorder of the sense organs. Auditory processing and perception disorders are not synonymous with deficits in general attention, language, or cognitive function, although such conditions may coexist or overlap.

ICD-9-CM		ICD-10-CM	
315.32	Central auditory processing disorder	H93.25	Central auditory processing disorder
388.40	Abnormal auditory perception, unspecified	H93.241	Temporary auditory threshold shift, right ear
		H93.291	Other abnormal auditory perceptions, right ear
388.43	Impairment of auditory discrimination	H93.299	Other abnormal auditory perceptions, unsp ear
388.45	Acquired auditory processing disorder	H93.299	Other abnormal auditory perceptions, unsp ear

Conductive Hearing Loss

Conductive hearing loss results from external or middle ear problems, which are often mechanical in nature. There are various causes for conductive hearing loss, including otitis media and otosclerosis. The most common cause of conductive hearing loss in children is otitis media infection in the middle ear cavity. The most common cause of conductive hearing loss in adults is otosclerosis. The loss results from fixation of the stapes (the third bone in the middle ear) so that sounds cannot be transported to the inner ear. Conductive hearing loss can be either temporary or permanent, and is treatable with medication and/or surgery.

ICD-10-CM has eliminated the classification of conductive hearing loss by site. The terms "external," "tympanic," and "middle ear" are no longer included. Instead, conductive hearing loss is included in subcategories H90.0–H90.2, regardless of site of origin. Although ICD-10-CM classifies types of hearing loss similarly to ICD-9-CM, the former describes laterality in a different manner, by stating the influence of the contralateral (other) side.

ICD-9-CM		ICD-10-CM	
389.03	Conductive hearing loss, middle ear	H90.0	Conductive hearing loss, bilateral
		H90.11	Conductive hearing loss, Rt ear, unilateral, unrestricted contralateral side
		H90.12	Conductive hearing loss, Lt ear, unilateral, unrestricted contralateral side
		H90.2	Conductive hearing loss, unspecified

Drug-Induced Conditions

Combination codes, which include both the causal drug (e.g., NSAIDs), and external cause (e.g., therapeutic use), replace the need for a separate external cause code. Effects of drugs are sequenced according to instruction in the ICD-10-CM text. Note that chapter 19 codes, which classify adverse effects of drugs in therapeutic use, are sequenced secondary to the nature of the condition, manifestation, or affect (e.g., hearing loss, labyrinthitis), whereas in poisonings, overdoses, and other circumstances, the chapter 19 code is sequenced first. Code section T36–T65 includes poisoning by, adverse effects of and underdosing of drugs, medicaments, and biological substances. Conditions due to the adverse effects of drugs in therapeutic use are classified with fifth or sixth character 5. For example:

Diagnosis: Hearing loss, left ear due to adverse effect of NSAIDs, initial encounter

H91.02 Ototoxic hearing loss, left ear

T39.315A Adverse effect of propionic acid derivatives, initial encounter

Refer to the "ICD-10-CM Draft Official Guidelines for Coding and Reporting" in appendix A of this book for additional information.

Intraoperative and Postprocedural Complications and Disorders of the Ear and Mastoid Process

In ICD-10-CM, postoperative complications have been moved to procedure-specific body system chapters. Postoperative ear complication classifications contain certain unique diagnosis and surgery-specific complications. For example, categories H95.0 and H95.1 specifically classify disorders of the ear following mastoidectomy. Code category H95.0 is diagnosis-specific; classifying recurrent postmastoidectomy cholesteatoma, whereas conditions within subcategory H95.1 classify specific postmastoidectomy complications such as inflammation, granulation, cysts, and other disorders. Subcategories H95.2- through H95.3- and H95.88 classify intraoperative complications, whereas subcategories H95.4- and H95.81- classify other postprocedural complications. Code assignment is based on the provider's documentation of the relationship between the condition and the procedure. For example:

Diagnosis: Stenosis of the left ear canal status post reconstructive surgery

H95.812 Postprocedural stenosis of left external ear canal

Chapter 8 Coding Exercises

Assign the appropriate ICD-10-CM diagnosis codes for all reportable diagnoses, excluding external causes of morbidity (V00–Y99).

Answers to coding exercises are listed in the back of the book.

1. Adhesive otitis, left ear _____

   _____

2. Impacted cerumen, left ear _____

   _____

3. Hemorrhagic otitis externa _____

   _____

4. Vertigo due to labyrinthine dysfunction, right ear _____

   _____

5. Otalgia with low frequency deafness, left ear _____

   _____

6. Recurrent postmastoidectomy granuloma, right ear _____

   _____

Chapter 8 Coding Scenarios

Assign the appropriate ICD-10-CM diagnosis codes for all reportable diagnoses, excluding external causes of morbidity (V00–Y99).

Answers to coding exercises are listed in the back of the book.

1. A 6-year-old child presents with fever and right ear pain. Examination reveals acute right serous otitis media with slight perforation of the central portion of the tympanic membrane. Of note, the patient's parents are smokers, and the patient is often exposed to cigarette smoke in the home and automobile.

    _____

    _____

2. A 48-year-old female presents with episodes of what she describes as a "spinning" dizziness of short duration, lasting approximately 20 seconds to two minutes at a time. She states that these episodes often occur upon rapidly standing from a sitting position or rising from a lying position, and interferes with certain daily activities, such as exercise. These episodes are often accompanied by nausea and visual disturbances in which she perceives that she "just cannot see straight." Examination reveals rotational nystagmus, but is negative for weakness or significant neurological findings. Diagnosis is documented as benign paroxysmal positional vertigo. The patient is referred to a specialist for further diagnosis and benign paroxysmal positional vertigo (BPPV) therapy.

    _____

    _____

3. A 15-year-old athlete on the local high school swim team presents for recurrent left swimmer's ear. Of note, a recent school screening exam was suspicious for hearing loss in left ear. History is significant for recurrent otitis media during early childhood, treated with repeat myringotomy procedures. Examination reveals inflammatory changes of the ear canal with drainage consistent with swimmer's ear. White, calcified deposits are noted on the tympanum characteristic of tympanosclerosis. The patient will be referred to an audiologist for evaluation and a treatment plan for conductive hearing loss due to tympanosclerosis; etiology undetermined in relation to past recurrent infections and procedures. The patient is prescribed antibiotics for swimmer's ear.

    _____

    _____

CHAPTER 9. DISEASES OF THE CIRCULATORY SYSTEM (I∅∅–I99)

This chapter contains 10 code families with the first character "I." The coding families classified to chapter 9 are:

I∅∅–I∅2	Acute rheumatic fever
I∅5–I∅9	Chronic rheumatic heart diseases
I1∅–I15	Hypertensive diseases
I2∅–I25	Ischemic heart diseases
I26–I28	Pulmonary heart disease and diseases of pulmonary circulation
I3∅–I52	Other forms of heart disease
I6∅–I69	Cerebrovascular diseases
I7∅–I79	Diseases of arteries, arterioles and capillaries
I8∅–I89	Diseases of veins, lymphatic vessels and lymph nodes, not elsewhere classified
I95–I99	Other and unspecified disorders of the circulatory system

ICD-10-CM Category Restructuring

Although ICD-10-CM chapter 9, "Diseases of the Circulatory System," is structured similarly to its counterpart in ICD-9-CM, intraoperative and postoperative complications unique to the circulatory system are included in the last code block of this chapter (I97). In ICD-10-CM, postoperative complications have been moved to procedure-specific body system chapters. In chapter 9, category I97 contains diagnoses and surgery-specific complications unique to the circulatory system, as illustrated by the following subcategory classifications:

I97.∅	Postcardiotomy syndrome
I97.1	Other postprocedural cardiac functional disturbances
I97.2	Postmastectomy lymphedema syndrome
I97.3	Postprocedural hypertension
I97.4	Intraoperative hemorrhage and hematoma of a circulatory system organ or structure complicating a procedure
I97.5	Accidental puncture and laceration of a circulatory system organ or structure during a procedure
I97.6	Postprocedural hemorrhage and hematoma of a circulatory system organ or structure following a procedure
I97.7	Intraoperative cardiac functional disturbances
I97.8	Other intraoperative and postprocedural complications and disorders of the circulatory system, not elsewhere classified

When reporting complications of cardiovascular surgery, code assignment is based on the provider's documentation of a cause-and-effect relationship between the condition and the procedure.

Category Title Changes

A number of category title revisions were made in chapter 9 such as changes to certain titles to better represent categorical content. This was often necessary when specific types of diseases were given their own separate block, a new category was created, or an existing category was redefined. For example, the terminology for "intermediate coronary syndrome" has been updated to the more common clinical diagnosis of "unstable angina." Additionally, although

KEY POINT

The codes in this chapter (I∅∅–I99) and those in the chapter on pregnancy, childbirth and the puerperium (O∅∅–O99) represent a challenge in accurate reporting as the alpha character I and O can be recorded incorrectly as numeral one (1) and zero (∅) if preventive measures are not taken.

code categories 394–396 are classified within the ICD-9-CM section titled, "Chronic Rheumatic Heart Disease (393–398)," the code category titles did not include the term "rheumatic." In ICD-10-CM, the titles of such categories have been revised to include essential terminology that more thoroughly defines the classification.

ICD-9-CM

394	Diseases of mitral valve
395	Diseases of aortic valve
396	Diseases of mitral and aortic valves
397	Diseases of other endocardial structures

ICD-10-CM

I05	Rheumatic mitral valve diseases
I06	Rheumatic aortic valve diseases
I07	Rheumatic tricuspid valve diseases
I08	Multiple valve diseases

Organizational Adjustments

When comparing ICD-9-CM to ICD-10-CM, some codes have been added, deleted, combined, or moved. Conditions such as unspecified lymphadenitis (I88.-) and gangrene, not elsewhere classified (I96) have been moved from other chapters in ICD-9-CM and appropriately reclassified as diseases of the circulatory system. Conversely, transient cerebral ischemia (TIA) codes, which were included in chapter 7, "Diseases of the Circulatory System," in ICD-9-CM, have been moved in ICD-10-CM to chapter 6, "Diseases of the Nervous System."

ICD-9-CM

Chapter 7. Diseases of the Circulatory System

435		Transient cerebral ischemia
	435.0	Basilar artery syndrome
	435.1	Vertebral artery syndrome
	435.2	Subclavian steal syndrome
	435.3	Vertebrobasilar artery syndrome
	435.8	Other specified transient cerebral ischemias
	435.9	Unspecified transient cerebral ischemia

ICD-10-CM

Chapter 6. Diseases of the Nervous System

G45		Transient cerebral ischemic attacks and related syndromes
	G45.0	Vertebro-basilar artery syndrome
	G45.1	Carotid artery syndrome (hemispheric)
	G45.2	Multiple and bilateral precerebral artery syndromes
	G45.3	Amaurosis fugax
	G45.4	Transient global amnesia
	G45.8	Other transient cerebral ischemic attacks and related syndromes
	G45.9	Transient cerebral ischemic attack, unspecified

 QUICK TIP

Documentation requirements for circulatory disorders are greater with ICD-10-CM than under ICD-9-CM. For instance, in subdural hemorrhage, ICD-10-CM codes available for this condition specify acute, subacute, or chronic.

The codes that specified the type of hypertension—malignant, benign, or unspecified—have been deleted in ICD-10-CM. Hypertension no longer uses type as an axis of classification. As such, the hypertension table is no longer necessary.

ICD-9-CM

401   Essential hypertension

    401.0   Malignant

    401.1   Benign

    401.9   Unspecified

ICD-10-CM

I10   Essential (primary) hypertension

    INCLUDES high blood pressure
             hypertension (arterial) (benign) (essential) (malignant) (primary) (systemic)

    EXCLUDES 1 *hypertensive disease complicating pregnancy, childbirth and the puerperium (O10–O11, O13–O16)*

    EXCLUDES 2 *essential (primary) hypertension involving vessels of brain (I60–I69)*
              essential (primary) hypertension involving vessels of eye (H35.0)

Combination Codes

Certain disease classifications have been expanded in ICD-10-CM to facilitate identification of secondary disease processes, specific manifestations, or associated complications. As such, code to the highest degree of specificity as documented in the record. For example, coronary artery disease with associated angina pectoris required two codes to report in ICD-9-CM, whereas in ICD-10-CM, both conditions are reportable by a single combination code. Angina pectoris due to arteriosclerotic coronary artery disease is reported using one combination code from subcategory I25.11 or I25.7. For example:

Diagnosis: Native coronary artery atherosclerosis with unstable angina pectoris

ICD-9-CM

414.01   Coronary atherosclerosis of native coronary artery

411.1   Intermediate coronary syndrome

ICD-10-CM

I25.110   Atherosclerotic heart disease of native coronary artery with unstable angina pectoris

    EXCLUDES 1 *unstable angina without atherosclerotic heart disease (I20.0)*

When reporting codes from subcategories I25.1, I25.7, or code I25.81, use additional codes to identify lipid rich plaque (I25.83) and calcified coronary artery lesion (I25.84), if documented.

Category I70 Atherosclerosis, classifies arteriosclerotic vascular disease by type, associated condition (severity), anatomic site, and laterality. Specific subcategories include the following information:

- **Major anatomic site:** aorta, renal artery, extremities, other arteries, generalized disease, unspecified site

 KEY POINT

ICD-10-CM combined common symptoms and complications of certain diagnosis codes, resulting in an increased number of combination code classifications. A combination code is a single code used to classify two diagnoses, or a diagnosis with an associated manifestation or complication.

- **Type of affected vessel:** native or bypass graft

  - ICD-10-CM assumes native vessel unless otherwise stated. For example:

  Arteriosclerosis, arteriosclerotic
      extremities (native arteries) I70.209
          bypass graft I70.309
              autologous vein graft I70.409

- **Type of bypass graft (if present and affected):** unspecified, autologous, nonautologous

- **Graft subtypes:** nonautologous: unspecified, biological, nonbiological

- **Associated complications and manifestations:** rest pain, intermittent claudication, ulceration, gangrene

  - Report code I70.92 to identify chronic total occlusion of the artery, if documented.

  - Subcategories are hierarchical in nature. Each subcategory includes conditions specified in the former category. As such, the subcategories progress in severity from atherosclerosis unspecified to that with intermittent claudication, rest pain, ulceration to finally, gangrene.

  - Atherosclerosis with ulceration requires an additional code to identify the severity of the ulcer

  - Anatomic codes of ulcer sites are thigh, calf, ankle, heel and midfoot, other part of foot, other part of leg, unspecified.

- **Laterality:** right, left, bilateral, other, unspecified. For example:

I70.221	**Atherosclerosis of native arteries of extremities with rest pain, right leg**
I70.332	**Atherosclerosis of unspecified type of bypass graft(s) of right leg with ulceration of calf** (Use additional code to identify severity of ulcer)
I70.423	**Atherosclerosis of autologous vein bypass graft(s) of the extremities with rest pain, bilateral legs**
I70.518	**Atherosclerosis of nonautologous biological bypass graft(s) of the extremities with intermittent claudication other extremity**
I70.662	**Atherosclerosis of nonbiological bypass graft(s) of the extremities with gangrene, left leg** (Use additional code to identify severity of ulcer, if applicable)
I70.721	**Atherosclerosis of other type of bypass graft(s) of the extremities with rest pain, right leg**

At the category level, inclusion terms clarify categorical content. An instructional note at category I70 prompts the coder to use an additional code to identify the presence of certain associated clinical health risks and comorbid conditions. Excludes 2 notes specify multiple conditions classifiable elsewhere. Excludes 2 notes indicate that the excluded condition is not part of the condition it is excluded from, however, a patient may have both conditions at the same time; therefore, both the code and the excluded codes may be reported together if supported by the documentation.

Disease that is bilateral in nature, and not classifiable to a single code may require multiple codes to report separate affected vessel types (e.g., native, bypass graft), manifestations (e.g., rest pain, ulceration), or levels of severity in the affected extremities, in order to accurately represent the status of disease in its entirety. For example:

Diagnosis: A patient presents with right lower extremity native atherosclerosis with intermittent claudication. He also has a left lower extremity atherosclerosis of an autologous bypass vein graft with rest pain and ulceration of the heel with the breakdown of skin.

I70.211	**Atherosclerosis of native arteries of the extremities with intermittent claudication, right leg**
I70.444	**Atherosclerosis of autologous vein bypass graft(s) of the left leg with ulceration of heel and midfoot**
L97.421	**Non-pressure chronic ulcer of left heel and midfoot limited to breakdown of skin**

In the above example, although both legs were affected by atherosclerotic disease, the native vessel on the right and grafted vessels on the left require separate classification codes. Both conditions are coded to represent the highest degree of severity available. Code I70.444 represents disease progression to ulceration status, which includes rest pain. Code also the severity of ulceration (L97.-).

Certain conditions, such as the presence of an ulcer or gangrene, require an additional code to identify the severity of ulceration. Category L97 Non-pressure chronic ulcer of lower limb, not elsewhere classified, specifies anatomic site, laterality, and severity. For example:

Diagnosis: Atherosclerosis of left lower extremity autologous bypass vein graft with rest pain and ulceration of the heel with breakdown of skin and exposure of fat layer

I70.444	**Atherosclerosis of autologous vein bypass graft(s) of the left leg with ulceration of heel and midfoot**
L97.422	**Non-pressure chronic ulcer of left heel and midfoot with fat layer exposed**

In the above example, code I70.444 requires an additional code L97.422, to identify the severity of the ulcer. Chronic ulcer codes are classified progressively by severity from least severe to most severe, with an unspecified option. Remember, always code to the highest degree of severity as supported by medical documentation and/or diagnostic statement.

Complications

In ICD-10-CM, postoperative complications have been moved to procedure-specific body system chapters. Complications are classified to category I97. Intraoperative complications are classified to categories I97.4 and I97.7. Postprocedural complications are classified to categories I97.1 and I97.6. Fourth- and fifth-character subcategory complications specify the type or nature of the complication, with the exception of those classified to other (.8) or (.89) codes. Subcategory I97.8 includes both intraoperative and postprocedural complications that are not classifiable elsewhere. An additional code, however, is necessary to specify the nature of the complication. Certain classification code subcategories in I97 contain codes that identify diagnosis-specific types of complications. For example:

I97.0	**Postcardiotomy syndrome**
I97.13	**Postprocedural heart failure** Use additional code to identify heart failure (I50.-)
I97.3	**Postprocedural hypertension**

Although category I97 contains many specific codes that describe the nature and type of complication, additional codes may be necessary to report the complication in its entirety. Many categories contain a sixth character to further define the complication as following cardiac surgery, a specific cardiac procedure (e.g., bypass, catheterization), or other surgery; performed on a different organ or body system. For example:

I97.0   **Postcardiotomy syndrome**

I97.1   **Other postprocedural cardiac functional disturbances**

    I97.11   **Postprocedural cardiac insufficiency**

        I97.110   **Postprocedural cardiac insufficiency following cardiac surgery**

        I97.111   **Postprocedural cardiac insufficiency following other surgery**

    I97.12   **Postprocedural cardiac arrest**

        I97.120   **Postprocedural cardiac arrest following cardiac surgery**

        I97.121   **Postprocedural cardiac arrest following other surgery**

    I97.13   **Postprocedural heart failure**
        Use additional code to identify the heart failure (I50.-)

        I97.130   **Postprocedural heart failure following cardiac surgery**

        I97.131   **Postprocedural heart failure following other surgery**

Chapter 9 Coding Guidance

ICD-10-CM chapter 9 contains a wide range of cardiovascular disease classifications, including diseases and disorders of the heart, cardiopulmonary circulation, cerebrovascular circulation and the arteries, veins and lymphatic circulatory system. Cardiovascular diagnostic coding can be complex in nature; often requiring multiple codes in a specific sequence. As such, chapter 9 contains multiple instructional notes that are essential to ensuring correct coding practices. Optum's *ICD-10-CM—The Complete Official Draft Code Set* highlights these crucial coding instructions in red font for ease of reference. These notes appear at the section, category, and subcategory levels throughout the tabular list. For example:

- **Etiology/manifestation coding.** Codes identified as manifestation codes cannot be sequenced first or reported alone. Manifestation codes may be identified by the phrase "in diseases classified elsewhere" in the code title. A "use additional code" note is listed at the etiology code and a "code first" note at the manifestation code. Follow the sequencing rules in the text. Sequence these conditions secondary to the underlying disease.

    I39   *Endocarditis and heart valve disorders in diseases classified elsewhere*
            Code first underlying disease

    Certain manifestation codes do not specify "in diseases classified elsewhere" in the code title, but may include a "code first underlying disease" notation:

    I68.0   *Cerebral amyloid angiopathy*
            Code first underlying amyloidosis (E85.-)

- **Multiple coding.** Instructional notes that state "code first" and "use additional code" provide sequencing rules. However, they may not be included in the etiology/manifestation combination, yet require multiple codes in specific sequence. "Code first" manifestation codes may be reported alone in certain circumstances.

I20.8	**Other forms of angina pectoris**
	Use additional code(s) for symptoms associated with angina equivalent

I47	**Paroxysmal tachycardia**
	Code first tachycardia complicating:
	obstetric surgery and procedures (O75.4)

I50	**Heart failure**
	Code first:
	heart failure due to hypertension (I11.0-)

Drug-Induced Conditions

Combination codes, which include both the causal drug (e.g., benzodiazepines) and external cause (e.g., therapeutic use), replace the need for a separate external cause code. Effects of drugs are sequenced according to instruction in the ICD-10-CM text. Note that chapter 19 codes, which classify adverse effects of drugs in therapeutic use, are sequenced secondary to the nature of the condition, manifestation, or affect (e.g., arrhythmia, angina), whereas in poisonings, overdoses, and other circumstances, the chapter 19 code is sequenced first. Code section T36–T50 includes poisoning by, adverse effects of and underdosing of drugs, medicaments, and biological substances. Conditions due to the adverse effects of drugs in therapeutic use are classified with fifth or sixth character 5. For example:

I42.7	**Cardiomyopathy due to drug and external agent**
	Code first (T36–T65) to identify cause

Refer to the "ICD-10-CM Draft Official Guidelines for Coding and Reporting" in appendix A of this book for additional information.

Guidelines

Although much of the coding advice published in the "ICD-10-CM Draft Official Guidelines for Coding and Reporting" for the classification of circulatory diseases in ICD-10-CM parallels that of ICD-9-CM, the guidelines for hypertension and acute myocardial infarction have been revised to coordinate with the changes inherent in the ICD-10-CM coding system.

Hypertension

The codes that specified the type of hypertension—malignant, benign, or unspecified—have been deleted in ICD-10-CM. Hypertension no longer uses type as an axis of classification. As such, the hypertension table is no longer necessary. ICD-10-CM code I10 Essential (primary) hypertension, includes hypertension described as:

- Arterial
- Benign
- Essential
- Malignant
- Primary
- Systemic

Hypertension complicating pregnancy, childbirth and the puerperium (O10–O11, O13–O16), hypertension involving vessels of brain (I60–I69), and hypertension involving vessels of eye (H35.0) are excluded from code I10 Essential (primary) hypertension.

In general, underlying concepts and sequencing rules for the coding of hypertension and hypertensive diseases have not changed. These key concepts include:

- A causal relationship between hypertension and heart disease must be stated or implied to report codes from category I11 Hypertensive heart disease. Code also the type of heart failure. For example:

Diagnosis: Hypertensive heart disease with left heart failure

I11.Ø **Hypertensive heart disease with heart failure**
      Use additional code to identify type of heart failure (I5Ø-)
I5Ø.1 **Left ventricular failure**

- Contrary to the above guideline, a causal relationship between hypertension and chronic kidney disease (CKD) is **assumed** between hypertension and chronic kidney disease unless otherwise documented. Code also the stage of chronic kidney disease. For example:

Diagnosis: Hypertension with stage IV chronic kidney disease (CKD)

I12.9 **Hypertensive chronic kidney disease with stage 1 through stage 4 chronic kidney disease, or unspecified chronic kidney disease**
      Use additional code to identify the stage of chronic kidney disease
N18.4 **Chronic kidney disease, stage 4 (severe)**

- Combination codes in category I13 are used to report conditions classifiable to *both* categories I11 and I12. Therefore, I11 codes + I12 codes = Report I13 codes only. Do not report conditions classifiable to I11 and I12 separately. Use additional codes to report type of heart failure and stage of CKD. For example:

Diagnosis: Hypertensive heart and kidney disease with congestive heart failure and stage 2 chronic kidney disease

I13.Ø **Hypertensive heart and chronic kidney disease with heart failure and stage 1 through stage 4 chronic kidney disease, or unspecified chronic kidney disease**
      Use additional code to identify type of heart failure
      Use additional code to identify the stage of chronic kidney disease
I5Ø.9 **Heart failure, unspecified**
N18.2 **Chronic kidney disease, stage 2 (mild)**

  - Note that the default code for congestive heart failure is I5Ø.9 Heart failure, unspecified. Code category I5Ø heart failure contains 14 subcategory codes to report heart failure by type (e.g., left, systolic, diastolic, combined) and severity (e.g., acute, chronic, acute on chronic). Do not report I5Ø.9 if the type of heart failure can be further specified.

- Hypertensive cerebrovascular disease requires two codes: the appropriate I6Ø–I69 code followed by the appropriate hypertension code.

- Hypertensive retinopathy requires two codes: the appropriate subcategory H35.Ø code and code I1Ø essential hypertension. Sequencing is determined by the circumstances of the encounter.

- Secondary hypertension requires two codes: a code to identify the etiology and the appropriate I15 code. Sequencing is determined by the circumstances of the encounter.

- Transient hypertension (RØ3.Ø) is not synonymous with systemic hypertension. Transient HTN of pregnancy is reported with O13.- or O14.-, as appropriate.

- Uncontrolled hypertension is not identified by a unique code in ICD-10-CM. Report with the appropriate I1Ø–I15 code.

  Refer to the "ICD-10-CM Draft Official Guidelines for Coding and Reporting" in appendix A of this book for additional information.

Acute Myocardial Infarction

Although significant changes in structure and parameters for coding AMI have changed, many of the underlying concepts and sequencing rules for the coding of acute myocardial infarction are parallel to those in ICD-9-CM.

Instructional notes have been added at the category level for I21 and I22, which state to use additional codes to identify certain health hazards, including tPA status and tobacco exposure, use, or dependence. Significant changes have been made to the classification of acute myocardial infarction (AMI) in ICD-10-CM, including:

- Time parameters for reporting AMI have been changed from eight weeks or less in ICD-9-CM to four weeks or less in ICD-10-CM. For example:

  I21   ST elevation (STEMI) and non-ST elevation (NSTEMI) myocardial infarction
  [INCLUDES]   myocardial infarction specified as acute or with a stated duration of 4 weeks (28 days) or less from onset

  I22   Subsequent ST elevation (STEMI) and non-ST elevation (NSTEMI) myocardial infarction
  [INCLUDES]   acute myocardial infarction occurring within four weeks (28 days) of a previous acute myocardial infarction, regardless of site

- The episode of care concept has been eliminated in ICD-10-CM. Instead, ICD-10-CM classifies AMI into two categories, initial AMI or subsequent AMI, regardless of the episode of care:

  - Initial AMI:

    I21   ST elevation (STEMI) and non-ST elevation (NSTEMI) myocardial infarction
  - Subsequent AMI:

    I22   Subsequent ST elevation (STEMI) and non-ST elevation (NSTEMI) myocardial infarction

ICD-9-CM		ICD-10-CM	
410.10	AMI anterior wall, unspec episode	I21.Ø9	STEMI involving other coronary artery, anterior wall
410.11	AMI anterior wall, initial episode	I21.Ø1	STEMI involving LMCA
		I21.Ø2	STEMI involving LAD
		I21.Ø9	STEMI involving other coronary artery anterior wall
		I22.Ø	Subsequent STEMI anterior wall
410.12	AMI anterior wall, subsequent episode	I21.Ø9	STEMI involving other coronary artery, anterior wall

Note: ICD-10-CM has revised the anatomic specificity of the myocardial infarction codes to specify the affected coronary vessel. In the example above, note that subcategory I21.Ø includes site-specific fifth characters for the left main coronary artery (I21.Ø1) and the left anterior descending artery (I21.Ø2).

- An AMI documented as subendocardial or nontransmural is coded as such (I21.4, I22.2), even if the site of infarction is specified. However, if the NSTEMI converts to a STEMI, report only the STEMI code. If the STEMI converts to a NSTEMI due to thrombolytic therapy, it is reported as a STEMI. For example:

Diagnosis: A patient is admitted with an acute inferior NSTEMI that converts to a STEMI during the hospitalization.

I21.19   **ST elevation (STEMI) myocardial infarction involving other coronary artery of inferior wall**

- A code from I22 must be used in conjunction with a code from I21, when a patient who has suffered an AMI has a new AMI within four weeks from the initial AMI. See the following example:

Diagnosis: A patient who suffers an acute NSTEMI is readmitted two weeks later with a subsequent inferior STEMI

I22.1   **Subsequent STE elevation (STEMI) myocardial infarction if inferior wall**

I21.4   **Non-ST elevation NSTEMI myocardial infarction**

- Sequencing of AMI is determined by the circumstances of the encounter.
  - If a patient is admitted for AMI, but has a subsequent AMI while in the hospital, the initial I21 code would be sequenced first as the reason for admission, followed by the I22 code.
  - If a patient is discharged from the hospital for treatment of an initial AMI, then has a subsequent AMI after discharge requiring readmission, the I22 subsequent AMI code is sequenced first as the reason for readmission, followed by the I21 code to identify the site of the initial AMI. The secondary I21 code for the initial AMI reports the status of the four-week healing phase for the initial AMI.

- Category I22 is never reported alone. The guidelines for assigning the correct I22 code are the same as those for reporting the initial MI (I21). Sequencing of I21 and I22 codes depends on the circumstances of the encounter.

- Continued care for an AMI may be reported with I21 codes, as appropriate within the four-week timeframe, regardless of the health care setting (i.e., facility transfer). Report category I21 codes for encounters occurring within the four week timeframe, regardless of the setting (acute or postacute), when the patient receives continued care for the myocardial infarction. For example:

Diagnosis: A patient is readmitted for postinfarction pericarditis 2 weeks after acute transmural anterior wall STEMI

I24.1   **Dressler's syndrome**

I21.Ø9   **ST elevation (STEMI) myocardial infarction involving other coronary artery of anterior wall**

- Continued care provided *after* the four-week initial care timeframe is reported with the appropriate aftercare code.

- Code I25.2 Old myocardial infarction, is reported only for healed (exceeding four weeks or 28 days) or old myocardial infarction status, not requiring further care.

- Unspecified site: report AMI to the affected site as documented, if no specified site is documented, code I21.3 ST elevation (STEMI) myocardial infarction of unspecified site, is reported by default. Confirm with the provider or query to ensure accuracy.

  Refer to the "ICD-10-CM Draft Official Guidelines for Coding and Reporting" in appendix A of this book for additional information.

Sequelae of Cerebrovascular Disease

ICD-10-CM classifies late effects of cerebrovascular disease as "sequelae" to category I69. Sequelae codes specify the residual effect that remains after the acute phase of a previous illness or injury (I60–I67). Subcategory codes have been expanded from their ICD-9-CM equivalents to include greater specificity regarding the type of stroke (e.g., hemorrhage, infarction), type of condition (e.g., speech and language deficits, cognitive deficits, hemiplegia, monoplegia), and affected side (laterality). Note that instructional notes prompt the coder to the use of additional codes that identify certain specific syndromes or conditions (e.g., paralytic syndromes, dysphagia, other sequelae) for reporting the condition in its entirety. For example:

> **I69.091** **Dysphagia following nontraumatic subarachnoid hemorrhage**
> Use additional code to identify the type of dysphagia, if known (R13.1-)

There is no time limit restricting the reporting of sequelae (late effect) codes. Residual conditions may occur months or years following the causal condition. Two codes are often required: the condition resulting from the sequela is sequenced first, followed by the appropriate late effect code. Sequelae codes from category I69 may be reported with codes from I60–I67 when current cerebrovascular disease and residual deficits from old cerebrovascular disease coexist. When the patient presents with a history of transient ischemic attack (TIA) or cerebral infarction with out residual deficits, report code Z86.73. For example:

> **Diagnosis:** A patient suffered a stroke four years ago with residual right dominant hemiparesis. Currently, he presents with a new cerebral infarction of the right anterior cerebral artery with resultant aphasia.

> **I63.521** **Cerebral infarction due to unspecified occlusion or stenosis of right anterior cerebral artery**

> **R47.01** **Aphasia**

> **I69.351** **Hemiplegia and hemiparesis following cerebral infarction affecting right dominant side**

Note: In the above example, the aphasia is not coded as sequelae (I69), since the aphasia is due to the current CVA.

Category I69 classification of default dominant or nondominant side is determined by the affected side (ambidextrous, right or left) as documented. This classification mirrors certain chapter 6 Diseases of the Nervous System classifications. In the absence of documentation of dominance, classify the default as:

- For ambidextrous patients, the default should be dominant

- If the left side is affected, the default is non-dominant

- If the right side is affected, the default is dominant

Do not assign category I69 codes in the absence of neurological deficits.

Example
A patient presents with flaccid hemiparesis of the right side due to old cerebral infarction.

I69.351   Hemiplegia and hemiparesis following cerebral infarction affecting right dominant side

In this example, only the laterality was documented. If the dominance is not stated (whether the patient was right- or left-handed), it is assumed that the right side is dominant.

Chapter 9 Coding Exercises

Assign the appropriate ICD-10-CM diagnosis codes for all reportable diagnoses, excluding external causes of morbidity (VØØ–Y99).

Answers to coding exercises are listed in the back of the book.

1. Mitral valve prolapse _____

   _____

2. Type II atrioventricular heart block _____

   _____

3. Acute on chronic diastolic congestive heart failure _____

   _____

4. Patient with a history of mild, controlled hypertension presents with an acute cerebellar stroke due to nontraumatic hemorrhage

   _____

   _____

5. Stage III chronic kidney disease, hypertension, mild chronic heart failure

   _____

   _____

6. Arteriosclerosis of bilateral lower extremities with rest pain, history positive for 30-year tobacco use, 10-year cessation _____

   _____

7. Spastic angina pectoris in a patient s/p CABG x2 with progressive coronary artery disease of native vessels, and a 60 percent lipid-rich plaque occlusion of one autologous bypass graft _____

   _____

Chapter 9 Coding Scenarios

Assign the appropriate ICD-10-CM diagnosis codes for all reportable diagnoses, excluding external causes of morbidity (VØØ–Y99).

Answers to coding exercises are listed in the back of the book.

1. A 47-year-old female with a past medical history remarkable for anxiety disorder presents with symptoms of anginal-type chest pain, dyspnea, and electrocardiographic (ECG) and enzyme changes mimicking acute myocardial infarction. Onset of symptoms is associated with onset of acute emotional distress. Lab results revealed abnormal cardiac enzyme levels. In the absence of coronary artery disease and with the patient's history of panic disorder, coronary angiography was postponed in lieu of serial echocardiography results, which was positive for findings of an apical wall motion abnormality. The second echocardiography showed a characteristic wall motion pattern of significant apical dysfunction. A third echocardiography revealed normalization of the LV dysfunction. Workup ruled out the presence of coronary artery disease. The patient responded well to treatment with beta-blockers, angiotensin-converting enzyme inhibitors, and intravenous diuresis. The diagnosis was documented as stress-induced cardiomyopathy due to acute stress (crisis) reaction in a patient with anxiety disorder.

    _____

    _____

2. A 15-year-old female passes out after running a track and field event. She goes into ventricular fibrillation, requiring emergent resuscitation. The patient had a similar episode of syncope at age 8 following a vigorous swimming lesson, with spontaneous resolution of normal rhythm. Upon admission to the hospital, EKG is positive for prolonged QT intervals. Genotype testing reveals mutations in potassium ion-channel genes. The physician documents the final diagnosis as Romano-Ward syndrome.

    _____

    _____

3. A 75-year-old male with a history of coronary artery disease presents to the hospital with unstable angina pectoris. Past medical history is significant for remote history of nontransmural AMI, approximately 10 years ago, and systemic hypertension. Serial enzyme changes are indicative of injury. Initial and subsequent ECG reveals deep Q-wave patterns and ST segment elevation in the anterolateral leads consistent with ST elevation transmural myocardial infarction. Imaging is evident for left anterior descending coronary artery occlusion. The patient is treated with thrombolytics and percutaneous coronary intervention.

    _____

    _____

CHAPTER 10. DISEASES OF THE RESPIRATORY SYSTEM (J00–J99)

Chapter 10 contains 11 coding families with the first character "J." The coding families classified to chapter 10 are:

J00–J06	**Acute upper respiratory infections**
J09–J18	**Influenza and pneumonia**
J20–J22	**Other acute lower respiratory infections**
J30–J39	**Other diseases of upper respiratory tract**
J40–J47	**Chronic lower respiratory diseases**
J60–J70	**Lung diseases due to external agents**
J80–J84	**Other respiratory diseases principally affecting the interstitium**
J85–J86	**Suppurative and necrotic conditions of the lower respiratory tract**
J90–J94	**Other diseases of the pleura**
J95	**Intraoperative and postprocedural complications and disorders of respiratory system, not elsewhere classified**
J96–J99	**Other diseases of the respiratory system**

ICD-10-CM Category Restructuring

Chapter 10 of ICD-10-CM has been restructured to group together related conditions in a different manner than ICD-9-CM. For example, the category structure in ICD-9-CM grouped conditions as acute, other, pneumonia, or chronic. ICD-10-CM groups conditions according to anatomic site of infection, severity, and cause; in a progression from acute to other, then chronic.

For example, in ICD-9-CM, the pneumonia and influenza section is sequenced after other diseases of the upper respiratory tract, whereas in ICD-10-CM, influenza and pneumonia are sequenced immediately following acute upper respiratory tract infections, and before other acute lower respiratory tract infections. In general, respiratory system infections precede other (including chronic) diseases and those due to external causes.

ICD-9-CM

460–466	**Acute respiratory infections**
470–478	**Other diseases of the upper respiratory tract**
480–488	**Pneumonia and influenza**
490–496	**Chronic obstructive pulmonary disease and allied conditions**

ICD-10-CM

J00–J06	**Acute upper respiratory infections**
J09–J18	**Influenza and pneumonia**
J20–J22	**Other acute lower respiratory infections**
J30–J39	**Other diseases of upper respiratory tract**
J40–J47	**Chronic lower respiratory diseases**
J60–J70	**Lung diseases due to external agents**

An instructional note has been added to the beginning of chapter 10 that states:

"When a respiratory condition is described as occurring in more than one site and is not specifically indexed, it should be classified to the lower anatomic site (e.g., tracheobronchitis to bronchitis in J40)."

Per ICD coding conventions, includes, excludes, and instructional notations at the beginning of a chapter, category or subcategory apply to all the codes classified within that chapter, category, or subcategory, as indicated.

Category Title Changes

A number of category title revisions were made in chapter 10. Titles were changed to better reflect categorical content, which was often necessary when specific types of diseases were given their own block, a new category was created, or an existing category was redefined. For example, conditions classified to the influenza and pneumonia code block (J09–J18) have been reorganized and titles revised to reflect those organizational changes. Note the change in the title of the code blocks between the two coding systems, and how the ICD-10-CM categories are more specifically defined. Certain valid three-character codes remain, allowing for future code expansion (e.g., J13, J14, J17).

ICD-9-CM

Pneumonia and Influenza (480–488)

480	Viral pneumonia
481	Pneumococcal [Streptococcus pneumoniae pneumonia]
482	Other bacterial pneumonia
483	Pneumonia due to other specified organism
484	Pneumonia in infectious diseases classified elsewhere
485	Bronchopneumonia, organism unspecified
486	Pneumonia, organism unspecified
487	Influenza
488	Influenza due to certain identified influenza viruses

ICD-10-CM

Influenza and Pneumonia (J09–J18)

J09	Influenza due to certain identified influenza viruses
J10	Influenza due to other identified influenza viruses
J11	Influenza due to unidentified influenza viruses
J12	Viral pneumonia, not elsewhere classified
J13	Pneumonia due to Streptococcus pneumoniae
J14	Pneumonia due to Hemophilus influenzae
J15	Bacterial pneumonia, not elsewhere classified
J16	Pneumonia due to other infectious organisms, not elsewhere classified
J17	Pneumonia in diseases classified elsewhere
J18	Pneumonia, unspecified organism

 KEY POINT

While many conditions have been assigned a specific classification code in ICD-10-CM, certain disorders are being reclassified to the residual subcategory. For example:

ICD-9-CM:

519.2   Mediastinitis

In ICD-10-CM, this disorder is reported as:

J98.5 Diseases of mediastinum, not elsewhere classified

Fibrosis of mediastinum
Hernia of mediastinum
Retraction of mediastinum
Mediastinitis

Organizational Adjustments

When comparing ICD-9-CM to ICD-10-CM, some codes have been added, deleted, combined, or moved.

Acute Recurrent Sinusitis

There is no specific code in ICD-9-CM for acute recurrent sinusitis. Seven codes have been added to category JØ1 accordingly:

ICD-10-CM

JØ1.Ø1	**Acute recurrent maxillary sinusitis**
JØ1.11	**Acute recurrent frontal sinusitis**
JØ1.21	**Acute recurrent ethmoidal sinusitis**
JØ1.31	**Acute recurrent sphenoidal sinusitis**
JØ1.41	**Acute recurrent pansinusitis**
JØ1.81	**Other acute recurrent sinusitis**
JØ1.91	**Acute recurrent sinusitis, unspecified**

Asthma

The asthma codes in ICD-9-CM are classified as extrinsic, intrinsic, chronic obstructive, other, and unspecified. In ICD-10-CM, this organizational method of classifying asthma has been significantly restructured. Category J45 Asthma, is organized based largely on severity instead of type (with the exception of certain types of asthma classifiable to subcategory J45.9). ICD-10-CM has refined severity with greater complexity as compared to the former structure in ICD-9-CM. Fourth-character subcategories progress in severity from mild (J45.2, J45.3) to severe (J45.5), with a residual subcategory for other and unspecified asthma (J45.9Ø). Subcategories J45.2 and J45.3 differentiate mild asthma as either intermittent (J45.2) or persistent (J45.3). Subcategories J45.4 and J45.5 assume a persistent state of asthmatic disease. Sixth-character codes in subcategories J45.2–J45.9Ø designate status as uncomplicated (Ø), with (acute) exacerbation (1) or status asthmaticus (2).

ICD-9-CM		ICD-10-CM	
493.ØØ	**Extrinsic asthma, unspecified**	J45.2Ø	**Mild intermittent asthma, uncomplicated**
		J45.3Ø	**Mild persistent asthma, uncomplicated**
		J45.4Ø	**Moderate persistent asthma, uncomplicated**
		J45.5Ø	**Severe persistent asthma, uncomplicated**
493.Ø1	**Extrinsic asthma with status asthmaticus**	J45.22	**Mild intermittent asthma with status asthmaticus**
		J45.32	**Mild persistent asthma with status asthmaticus**
		J45.42	**Moderate persistent asthma with status asthmaticus**
		J45.52	**Severe persistent asthma with status asthmaticus**

ICD-9-CM		ICD-10-CM	
493.02	Extrinsic asthma, with exacerbation	J45.21	Mild intermittent asthma, with (acute) exacerbation
		J45.31	Mild persistent asthma with (acute) exacerbation
		J45.41	Moderate persistent asthma with (acute) exacerbation
		J45.51	Severe persistent asthma with (acute) exacerbation

Respiratory Failure

Category J96 Respiratory failure, not elsewhere classified, has been expanded to include combination codes that designate not only severity, but the presence of associated symptoms of hypoxia and hypercapnia. This differentiation describes an additional severity indicator to address the presence of factors that require specific treatment interventions and carry potentially disparate clinical outcomes due to their effect on body systems, organs and degree of function. For example:

J96.00 Acute respiratory failure, unspecified whether with hypoxia or hypercapnia

J96.01 Acute respiratory failure with hypoxia

J96.02 Acute respiratory failure with hypercapnia

Certain conditions once classified within ICD-9-CM category 518.8 Other diseases of lung, have been moved elsewhere in the classification. For example, acute respiratory distress syndrome (ARDS) has been moved from the respiratory failure classification to a different code block in ICD-10-CM. This reclassification groups ARDS to a more anatomically specific code block.

ICD-9-CM

Other Diseases of Respiratory System (510–519)

518 Other diseases of lung

    518.82 Other pulmonary insufficiency, not elsewhere classified
        Acute respiratory distress
        Acute respiratory insufficiency
        Acute respiratory distress syndrome NEC

ICD-10-CM

Other Respiratory Diseases Principally Affecting the Interstitium (J80–J84)

J80 Acute respiratory distress syndrome
    Acute respiratory distress syndrome in adult or child
    Adult hyaline membrane disease

Additional organizational adjustments include:

- Streptococcal sore throat has been reclassified to chapter 10, having been formerly classified in chapter 1, "Infectious and Parasitic Diseases," in ICD-9-CM.

- Code J18.1 is a unique code for lobar pneumonia of unspecified organism. Previously, this code was included in the ICD-9-CM code for pneumococcal pneumonia.

 QUICK TIP

ICD-10-CM uses combination codes to create organism-specific classifications for acute bronchitis. For example, "acute bronchitis due to streptococcus" is reported with code J20.2.

 DEFINITIONS

interstitium. Tissue located between the air sacs of the lungs.

Similarly, the prevalence of combination codes in the ICD-10-CM classification facilitate identification of secondary disease processes, specific manifestations, or associated complications that have resulted in many additional organizational adjustments, including:

- Acute chest syndrome in sickle-cell disease has been reclassified to chapter 4, "Diseases of the Blood and Blood-forming Organs and Certain Disorders Involving the Immune Mechanism (D5Ø–D89)." Category D57 Sickle-cell disorders, no longer requires dual classification with etiology/manifestation reporting. For example:

ICD-9-CM

517.3 Acute chest syndrome
   Code first sickle-cell disease in crisis (282.42, 282.62, 282.64, 282.69)

ICD-10-CM

D57.Ø1 **Hb-SS disease with acute chest syndrome**

D57.211 **Sickle-cell/Hb-C disease with acute chest syndrome**

D57.411 **Sickle-cell thalassemia with acute chest syndrome**

D57.811 **Other sickle-cell disorders with acute chest syndrome**

- Lung involvement in certain systemic connective tissue disorders (M3Ø–M36), such as collagen vascular disease, lupus, and other autoimmune diseases, have been reclassified to chapter13, "Diseases of the Musculoskeletal System and Connective Tissue (MØØ–M99)." For example:

ICD-9-CM

517.8 Lung involvement in other diseases classified elsewhere
   Code first underlying disease

ICD-10-CM

M32.13 **Lung involvement in systemic lupus erythematosus**

M35.Ø2 **Sicca syndrome with lung involvement**

Intraoperative and Postprocedural Complications

In ICD-10-CM, many postoperative complications have been moved to complication-specific code categories at the end of the individual body system chapters. Intraoperative and postprocedural complications and disorders of the respiratory system, not elsewhere classified, are found in category J95. Certain subcategories and classification codes classify diagnosis or procedure-specific complications. For example:

J95.Ø **Tracheostomy complications**

J95.4 **Chemical pneumonitis due to anesthesia [Mendelson's syndrome]**

H95.5 **Postprocedural subglottic stenosis**

Codes J95.1–J95.3 differentiate pulmonary insufficiency by severity and type of surgery (thoracic vs. nonthoracic). For example:

J95.1 **Acute pulmonary insufficiency following thoracic surgery**

J95.2 **Acute pulmonary insufficiency following nonthoracic surgery**

J95.3 **Chronic pulmonary insufficiency following surgery**

Intraoperative complications are classified to category J95.6 and J95.7, whereas postprocedural complications are classified to categories J95.0–J95.5 and J95.81–J95.84. There may be some overlap depending on the circumstances of the procedure and complication. For example, subcategory J95.8 includes both intraoperative and postprocedural complications. These codes include complications specific to the condition (e.g., respiratory failure, pneumothorax) or device (e.g., respirator). Multiple codes, often in a specific sequence, are necessary to further specify the nature of certain complications and conditions classifiable to this category J95. For example:

J95.02	**Infection of tracheostomy stoma**	
	Use additional code to identify type of infection	
J95.4	**Chemical pneumonitis due to anesthesia [Mendelson's syndrome]**	
	Use additional code for adverse effect, if applicable, to identify drug (T41.- with fifth or sixth character 5)	
J95.851	**Ventilator associated pneumonia**	
	Use additional code to identify organism, if known (B95.-, B96.-, B97.-)	
J95.89	**Other postprocedural complications and disorders of respiratory system, not elsewhere classified**	
	Use additional code to identify disorder	

Level of Detail in Coding

As in ICD-9-CM, diagnosis codes are to be used and reported to the highest degree of specificity available. ICD-10-CM provides, in the majority of cases, an exponentially increased level of specificity than ICD-9-CM. In chapter 10, this code expansion is intended to facilitate identification of specific types or causes of respiratory diseases. Many of these changes are due to advances in our understanding of diseases, have been developed to provide necessary data to support epidemiology and research efforts, and have been made in accordance with updates of currently applicable clinical terminology. As such, new ICD-10-CM codes have been created for specific diseases or disorders not previously identifiable with unique codes in ICD-9-CM. For example:

ICD-9-CM		ICD-10-CM	
503	Pneumoconiosis due to inorganic dust	J63.0	Aluminosis (of lung)
		J63.1	Bauxite fibrosis (of lung)
		J63.2	Berylliosis
		J63.3	Graphite fibrosis (of lung)
		J63.4	Siderosis
		J63.5	Stannosis
		J63.6	Pneumoconiosis due to other inorganic dusts

Chapter 10 Coding Guidance

Official Guidelines

In general, coding advice as published in the "ICD-10-CM Draft Official Guidelines for Coding and Reporting" parallels that of ICD-9-CM, with one significant exception.

Other Chronic Obstructive Pulmonary Disease (J44)

Chronic obstructive pulmonary disease (COPD) classifications have been streamlined and simplified in ICD-10-CM. Category J44 Other chronic obstructive pulmonary disease, includes the following conditions formerly classified as either chronic obstructive asthma (493.2x) or as obstructive chronic bronchitis (491.2x):

- Asthma with chronic obstructive pulmonary disease
- Chronic asthmatic (obstructive) bronchitis
- Chronic bronchitis with airway obstruction
- Chronic bronchitis with emphysema
- Chronic emphysematous bronchitis
- Chronic obstructive asthma
- Chronic obstructive bronchitis
- Chronic obstructive tracheobronchitis

The expansion of includes and excludes notes within code block J40–J47 Chronic lower respiratory diseases, serve to clarify some of the issues that complicated the coding of bronchitis, asthma, emphysema, and COPD in ICD-9-CM. In accordance with ICD coding conventions, includes, excludes, and instructional notes at the beginning of the category apply to all the codes within that category. Certain conditions require more than one code to report it in its entirety. For example:

- Assign additional codes to identify the **type** of asthma, if applicable
- Assign additional codes to report tobacco history, use status or exposure

Category J44 excludes bronchiectasis, conditions without an obstructive component, and those due to external agents.

Note that category J44 codes include combination codes with severity components, which differentiate between COPD with acute lower respiratory infection, COPD with acute exacerbation, and COPD without mention of such complication (unspecified). For example:

J44.0 **Chronic obstructive pulmonary disease with acute lower respiratory infection**
Use additional code to identify the infection

J44.1 **Chronic obstructive pulmonary disease with (acute) exacerbation**
Decompensated COPD
Decompensated COPD with (acute) exacerbation
EXCLUDES 2 *chronic obstructive pulmonary disease [COPD] with acute bronchitis (J44.0)*

J44.9 **Chronic obstructive pulmonary disease, unspecified**
Chronic obstructive airway disease NOS
Chronic obstructive lung disease NOS

Note that code J44.1 contains an Excludes 2 note, which indicates that both conditions may be reported together when an infectious component and acute exacerbation coexist. For example:

Diagnosis: Acute bronchitis with acute exacerbation of COPD

J44.0	**Chronic obstructive pulmonary disease with acute lower respiratory infection**
J44.1	**Chronic obstructive pulmonary disease with (acute) exacerbation**

Refer to the "ICD-10-CM Draft Official Guidelines for Coding and Reporting" in appendix A of this book for additional information.

Drug-Resistant Organisms

Category Z16 Infection with drug resistant microorganisms, is to be reported as an additional code to identify the presence of drug-resistant infectious organisms in infectious conditions, which are classified elsewhere. This category is pharmaceutical-specific, which provides flexibility and specificity within the classification system to identify drug-resistance. Certain combination codes exist which specify methicillin-resistant infections. If a combination code exists that includes the causal organism, condition and drug-resistance status, do not assign separate, redundant codes. For example:

Diagnosis: Methicillin-resistant *Staphylococcus aureus* (MRSA) pneumonia

J15.212	**Pneumonia due to Methicillin resistant Staphylococcus aureus**

Diagnosis: ESBL β-Lactam–Resistant *Streptococcus pneumoniae* pneumonia; resistant to cephalosporin and penicillin

J13	**Pneumonia due to streptococcus pneumonia**
Z16.12	**Resistance to antimicrobial drugs; extended spectrum beta lactamase (ESBL) antibiotics**

Combination Codes

Certain disease classifications have been expanded in ICD-10-CM to facilitate identification of secondary disease processes, specific manifestations, or associated complications. As such, code to the highest degree of specificity as documented in the medical record. For example, certain respiratory infections codes have been revised from a multiple coding convention that required two codes to a combination code reportable with a single classification code. For example:

ICD-9-CM Multiple Coding

Chapter 8. Diseases of the Respiratory System (460–519)
Use additional code to identify infectious organism

466	**Acute bronchitis and bronchiolitis**
466.0	**Acute bronchitis**

Diagnosis: Acute bronchitis due to Streptococcus A

466.0	**Acute bronchitis**
041.01	**Streptococcus, Group A**

 KEY POINT

Some common symptoms and complications were added as fifth characters to certain diagnosis codes in ICD-10-CM, resulting in an increased number of combination codes. A combination code is a single code used to classify two diagnoses, or a diagnosis with an associated manifestation or complication.

ICD-10-CM Combination Codes

J20.0	Acute bronchitis due to Mycoplasma pneumoniae
J20.1	Acute bronchitis due to Hemophilus influenzae
J20.2	Acute bronchitis due to streptococcus
J20.3	Acute bronchitis due to coxsackievirus
J20.4	Acute bronchitis due to parainfluenza virus
J20.5	Acute bronchitis due to respiratory syncytial virus
J20.6	Acute bronchitis due to rhinovirus
J20.7	Acute bronchitis due to echovirus
J20.8	Acute bronchitis due to other specified organisms
J20.9	Acute bronchitis, unspecified

Drug- or Chemical-Induced Conditions

Combination codes, which include the causal drug, chemical, or external agent and the external cause (e.g., therapeutic use), replace the need for external cause codes, when reporting adverse effects of drugs in therapeutic use. Conditions due to radiation exposure require an additional code from categories W88–W9Ø or X39.Ø-, as appropriate, to identify the external cause.

Effects of drugs are sequenced according to instruction in the ICD-10-CM text. Note that chapter 19 codes, which classify adverse effects of drugs in therapeutic use, are sequenced secondary to the nature of the condition, manifestation, or affect (e.g., inflammation, fibrosis), whereas in poisonings, overdoses, and other circumstances, the chapter 19 code is sequenced first. Code section T36–T5Ø includes poisoning by, adverse effects of, and underdosing of drugs, medicaments, and biological substances; whereas, section T51–T65 includes toxic effects of substances chiefly nonmedicinal as the source. For example:

- Drug-induced condition (T36–T5Ø) due to adverse effects in therapeutic use:

J70.2	Acute drug-induced interstitial lung disorders
	Use additional code for adverse effect, if applicable, to identify drug (T36–T5Ø with fifth or sixth character 5)

Diagnosis: Acute interstitial fibrosis due to adverse effects of amiodarone therapy, subsequent encounter

J70.2	Acute drug-induced interstitial lung disorders
T45.1X5D	Adverse effect of antineoplastic and immunosuppressive drugs

- Toxic effects condition (T51–T65):

J69.1	Pneumonitis due to inhalation of oils and essences
	Code first (T51–T65) to identify substance

Diagnosis: Accidental inhalation pneumonitis, benzoin (tincture) oil, initial encounter

T52.8X1A	Toxic effect of other organic solvents, accidental (unintentional)
J69.1	Pneumonitis due to inhalation of oils and essences

Chapter 10 Coding Exercises

Assign the appropriate ICD-10-CM diagnoses codes for all reportable diagnoses, excluding external causes of morbidity (VØØ–Y99).

Answers to coding exercises are listed in the back of the book.

1. Acute maxillary sinusitis due to recurrent *Streptococcus pneumoniae* infection

   _____

   _____

2. Croup due to adenovirus _____

   _____

3. Otitis media due to influenza type B infection _____

   _____

4. Viral pneumonia due to influenza with a secondary methicillin-suseptible Staphylococcus aureus pneumonia infection _____

   _____

5. Large right vocal cord polyp with right-sided paralysis of vocal cord

   _____

   _____

6. Status asthmaticus _____

   _____

7. Acute exacerbation of COPD _____

   _____

8. Paratracheostomy infection with cellulitis _____

   _____

Chapter 10 Coding Scenarios

Assign the appropriate ICD-10-CM diagnoses codes for all reportable diagnoses, excluding external causes of morbidity (VØØ–Y99).

Answers to coding exercises are listed in the back of the book.

1. A patient presents with an exacerbation of chronic obstructive asthma. History is consistent with moderate persistent asthma. Symptoms upon admission include increased shortness of breath, wheezing, dyspnea, and chest tightness. Bronchodilator therapies failed to abate symptoms, which progressed to acute respiratory distress, consistent with status asthmaticus. The patient was placed on IV steroids, after which the patient returned to baseline.

    _____

    _____

2. A 65-year-old male presents with fatigue, fever, dyspnea, productive cough, and right-sided chest wall pain. Examination is positive for productive cough with thick, yellow sputum. The patient describes pleuritic-type chest pain that intensifies upon coughing. Past medical history is positive for chronic emphysematous obstructive bronchitis, due to his 40+ year history of tobacco dependence. Cessation attempts have been unsuccessful. Chest x-ray reveals infiltrate in the left lower lobe. Sputum cultures are positive for *Hemophilus influenzae*. The patient is placed on IV antibiotics, steroidal therapy, and supplemental oxygen.

    _____

    _____

3. A patient presents to the emergency department in respiratory distress due to acute exacerbation of chronic obstructive bronchitis. Upon examination, the patient was cyanotic around the mouth and tips of the extremities, with impaired motor function, severe dyspnea, and depressed consciousness. Arterial blood gasses were consistent with reduced alveolar ventilation decrease PaO2 (hypoxemia) and normal PaCO2. Clinical findings were documented as consistent with acute hypoxic respiratory failure. The patient was admitted and placed on a ventilator for treatment.

    _____

    _____

4. A 47-year-old female with recurrent nasopharyngeal cancer presents with nasal mucositis characterized by pain, inflammation, and irritation of the nasal mucosa. She has also experienced a decreases sense of smell since completing her most recent course of radiation therapy. Lab results are negative for secondary infection. The patient has responded well to nasal irrigation and topical pain management.

    _____

    _____

CHAPTER 11. DISEASES OF THE DIGESTIVE SYSTEM (KØØ–K95)

Chapter 11 contains 10 coding families with the first character "K." The coding families classified to chapter 11 are:

KØØ–K14	Diseases of oral cavity and salivary glands
K2Ø–K31	Diseases of esophagus, stomach and duodenum
K35–K38	Diseases of appendix
K4Ø–K46	Hernia
K5Ø–K52	Noninfective enteritis and colitis
K55–K64	Other diseases of intestines
K65–K68	Diseases of peritoneum and retroperitoneum
K7Ø–K77	Diseases of liver
K8Ø–K87	Disorders of gallbladder, biliary tract and pancreas
K9Ø–K95	Other diseases of the digestive system

ICD-10-CM Category Restructuring

ICD-10-CM restructures classifications of related conditions and specific anatomic sites in a different manner than ICD-9-CM. In chapter 11, separate blocks were created to distinguish diseases of the intestine from those of other digestive sites. Blocks K7Ø–K77 Diseases of liver, and K8Ø–K87 Disorders of gallbladder, biliary tract and pancreas, differentiate between conditions affecting separate organs and their related structures into distinct coding families. In ICD-9-CM, diseases of the intestines are grouped together with diseases of the peritoneum. Likewise, ICD-9-CM groups together diseases and disorders of the liver, biliary tract, and pancreas into the "other diseases" classification. For example:

ICD-9-CM

56Ø–569	Other diseases of intestines and peritoneum
57Ø–579	Other diseases of the digestive system

ICD-10-CM

K55–K64	Other diseases of intestines
K65–K68	Diseases of peritoneum and retroperitoneum
K7Ø–K77	Diseases of liver
K8Ø–K87	Disorders of gallbladder, biliary tract and pancreas
K9Ø–K95	Other diseases of the digestive system

Category Title Changes

A number of category title revisions were made in chapter 11. Titles were changed to better reflect categorical content, which was often necessary when specific types of diseases were given their own block, a new category was created, or an existing category was redefined. For example:

ICD-9-CM

565	Anal fissure and fistula

ICD-10-CM

K6Ø	Fissure and fistula of anal and rectal regions

Organizational Adjustments

When comparing ICD-9-CM to ICD-10-CM, some codes have been added, deleted, combined, or moved. For example, certain diseases and disorders of the jaws that are classified to ICD-9-CM chapter 9, "Diseases of the Digestive System (570–579)," have been moved to ICD-10-CM chapter 13, "Diseases of the Musculoskeletal System and Connective Tissue (M00–M99)." ICD-9-CM codes reclassified in ICD-10-CM to chapter 13 include those conditions classified to categories 524 Dentofacial anomalies, including malocclusion, 525.7 Endosseous dental implant failure, and 526 Diseases of the jaws. For example:

ICD-9-CM

Chapter 9. Diseases of the Digestive System (520–579)

Diseases of Oral Cavity, Salivary Glands, and Jaws (520–529)

524	Dentofacial anomalies, including malocclusion
525	Other diseases and conditions of the teeth and supporting structures
525.7	Endosseous dental implant failure
526	Diseases of the jaws

ICD-10-CM

Chapter 13. Diseases of the Musculoskeletal System and Connective Tissue (M00–M99)

Dentofacial Anomalies [Including Malocclusion] and Other Disorders of Jaw (M26–M27)

M26	Dentofacial anomalies [including malocclusion]
M27	Other diseases of jaws
M27.6	Endosseous dental implant failure

The codes that specified whether obstruction was mentioned in conjunction with a gastric, duodenal, peptic, or gastrojejunal ulcer have been deleted in ICD-10-CM. Obstruction is no longer an axis of classification for ulcers. For example:

ICD-9-CM

531.00	Acute gastric ulcer with hemorrhage without mention of obstruction
531.01	Acute gastric ulcer with hemorrhage with obstruction

ICD-10-CM

K25.0	Acute gastric ulcer with hemorrhage

There was no single code in ICD-9-CM for alcoholic hepatitis with ascites. A new combination code has been added to ICD-10-CM to classify this type of hepatitis with an associated manifestation.

ICD-10-CM

K70.10	Alcoholic hepatitis without ascites
K70.11	Alcoholic hepatitis with ascites

Complications

In ICD-10-CM, many postoperative complication codes have been moved to complication-specific code categories at the end of the individual body system chapters. Depending on the nature of the condition, digestive system complications are classified to code block K90–K94. Intraoperative and postprocedural complications and disorders of the digestive system, not elsewhere classified, are assigned to category K91, whereas category K94 includes complications of artificial openings of the digestive system (i.e., colostomy, enterostomy).

Codes K91.0–K91.5 identify specific postoperative diagnoses or surgery-associated syndromes. For example:

K91.0	**Vomiting following gastrointestinal surgery**
K91.1	**Postgastric surgery syndromes**
K91.2	**Postsurgical malabsorption, not elsewhere classified**
K91.3	**Postprocedural intestinal obstruction**
K91.5	**Postcholecystectomy syndrome**

Code K91.89 Other postprocedural complications and disorders of digestive system is used to report digestive system complications that are not specifically classifiable elsewhere. An additional code, however, is necessary to specify the nature of the complication. For example:

Diagnosis: Functional diarrhea following gastrointestinal surgery

ICD-9-CM

997.4	**Digestive system complications**
564.5	**Functional diarrhea**

ICD-10-CM

K91.89	**Other postprocedural complications and disorders of digestive system**
K59.1	**Functional diarrhea**

Category K92 Other diseases of digestive system, is a nonspecific category that includes fourth- and fifth-character codes for conditions not elsewhere classified. This category includes mucositis, which requires the use of an additional code if associated with the effects of drug or radiation therapy. For example:

K92.81	**Gastrointestinal mucositis (ulcerative)**
	Code also type of associated therapy, such as:
	antineoplastic and immunosuppressive drugs (T45.1X-)
	radiological procedure and radiotherapy (Y84.2)

Category K92 also includes unspecified gastrointestinal hemorrhages (hematemesis, melena, and GI hemorrhage NOS) that are not complications of a procedure, nor associated with disease processes classifiable elsewhere by combination code. An Excludes 1 note indicates that the conditions listed, are more appropriately classified elsewhere. For example:

K92.2 **Gastrointestinal hemorrhage, unspecified**

> **EXCLUDES 1** *acute hemorrhagic gastritis (K29.Ø1)*
> *hemorrhage of anus and rectum (K62.5)*
> *angiodysplasia of stomach with hemorrhage (K31.811)*
> *diverticular disease with hemorrhage (K57-)*
> *gastritis and duodenitis with hemorrhage (K29-)*
> *peptic ulcer with hemorrhage (K25–K28)*

Category K94 Complications of artificial openings of the digestive system, contains four subcategories that specify the anatomic site and type of artificial opening. For example:

K94.Ø **Colostomy complications**

K94.1 **Enterostomy complications**

K94.2 **Gastrostomy complications**

K94.3 **Esophagostomy complications**

The fifth character specifies the nature of the complication. Infections of artificial openings require the use of an additional code to specify the type of infection. For example:

K94.ØØ **Colostomy complication, unspecified**

K94.Ø1 **Colostomy hemorrhage**

K94.Ø2 **Colostomy infection**
> Use additional code to specify type of infection, such as:
> cellulitis of abdominal wall (LØ3.311)
> sepsis (A4Ø.-, A41-)

K94.Ø3 **Colostomy malfunction**

K94.Ø9 **Other complications of colostomy**

Chapter 11 Coding Guidance

Official Guidelines

At the time of this publication, no official coding guidelines have been published for chapter 11 classification codes. To ensure accurate code assignment, apply the ICD-10-CM conventions and instructions within the ICD-10-CM text.

Level of Detail in Coding

As in ICD-9-CM, diagnosis codes are to be used and reported at the highest degree of specificity available. ICD-10-CM provides, in the majority of cases, an exponentially increased level of specificity than ICD-9-CM. In chapter 11, this code expansion is often used to facilitate the reporting of severity by classification of the condition to the extent of disease progression. For example:

ICD-9-CM		ICD-1Ø-CM	
521.Ø6	Dental caries pit and fissure	KØ2.51	Dental caries on pit and fissure surface, limited to enamel
		KØ2.52	Dental caries on pit and fissure surface, penetrating to dentin
		KØ2.53	Dental caries on pit and fissure surface, penetrating into pulp

ICD-9-CM		ICD-10-CM	
525.12	Loss of teeth due to periodontal disease	K08.121	Complete loss of teeth d/t PD, Class I
		K08.122	Complete loss of teeth d/t PD, Class II
		K08.123	Complete loss of teeth d/t PD, Class III
		K08.124	Complete loss of teeth d/t PD, Class IV
		K08.129	Complete loss of teeth d/t PD, Unsp class
		K08.421	Partial loss of teeth d/t PD, Class I
		K08.422	Partial loss of teeth d/t PD, Class II
		K08.423	Partial loss of teeth d/t PD, Class III
		K08.424	Partial loss of teeth d/t PD, Class IV
		K08.429	Partial loss of teeth d/t PD, Unsp class

Combination Codes

Certain disease classifications have been expanded in ICD-10-CM to facilitate identification of secondary disease processes, specific manifestations or associated complications. As such, code to the highest degree of specificity as documented in the medical record. For example, to report Crohn's disease with associated bowel obstruction, fistula, or abscess, two codes were required in ICD-9-CM; however, in ICD-10-CM, these conditions are reportable by a single combination code. For example:

Diagnosis: Crohn's disease of the large intestine with rectal abscess

ICD-9-CM

555.1   **Regional enteritis of large intestine**

566   **Abscess of anal and rectal regions**

ICD-10-CM

K50.114   **Crohn's disease of large intestine with abscess**

Diagnosis: Crohn's disease of the large intestine with colonic fistula

ICD-9-CM

555.1   **Regional enteritis of the large intestine**

569.81   **Fistula of intestine, excluding rectum and anus**

ICD-10-CM

K50.113   **Crohn's disease of large intestine with fistula**

Diagnosis: Crohn's disease of large intestine with bowel obstruction

ICD-9-CM

555.1   **Regional enteritis of large intestine**

560.89   **Other specified intestinal obstruction**

ICD-10-CM

K50.112   **Crohn's disease of large intestine with intestinal obstruction**

Similarly, ICD-10-CM classifications for diverticular disease of the intestine have been expanded with combination codes with revised specifications of anatomic bowel sites (e.g., small, large, small and large bowel) and associated complications (e.g., perforation and abscess). For example:

 KEY POINT

ICD-10-CM combines common symptoms and complications of certain diagnosis codes, resulting in an increased number of combination code classifications. A combination code is a single code used to classify two diagnoses, or a diagnosis with an associated manifestation or complication.

ICD-9-CM

562   Diverticula of intestine
Use additional code to identify any associated:
peritonitis (567.0–567.9)

562.1   Colon

562.10   Diverticulosis of colon (without mention of hemorrhage)

562.11   Diverticulitis of colon (without mention of hemorrhage)

562.12   Diverticulosis of colon with hemorrhage

562.13   Diverticulitis of colon with hemorrhage

ICD-10-CM

K57.20   Diverticulitis of large intestine with perforation and abscess without bleeding

K57.21   Diverticulitis of large intestine with perforation and abscess with bleeding

K57.30   Diverticulosis of large intestine without perforation or abscess without bleeding

K57.31   Diverticulosis of large intestine without perforation or abscess with bleeding

K57.32   Diverticulitis of large intestine without perforation or abscess without bleeding

K57.33   Diverticulitis of large intestine without perforation or abscess with bleeding

Drug-Induced Conditions

Combination codes, which include the causal drug (e.g., benzodiazepines), and external cause (e.g., therapeutic use), replace the need for a separate external cause code. Sequencing instructions may vary, depending on the notes in the text.

Effects of drugs are sequenced according to instruction in the ICD-10-CM text. Note that chapter 19 codes, which classify adverse effects of drugs in therapeutic use, are sequenced secondary to the nature of the condition, manifestation, or affect (e.g., inflammation, ulcer), whereas in poisonings, overdoses, and other circumstances, the chapter 19 code is sequenced first. Code section T36–T50 includes poisoning by, adverse effects of, and underdosing of drugs, medicaments, and biological substances. For example:

K22.1   Ulcer of esophagus
Code first poisoning due to drug or toxin, if applicable (T36–T65 with fifth
Use additional code for adverse effect, if applicable, to identify drug (T36–T50 with fifth or sixth character 5)

Diagnosis: Doxycycline-induced esophageal ulcer, adverse effect in therapeutic use, initial encounter

K22.10   Ulcer of esophagus without bleeding

T36.4X5A   Adverse effect of tetracyclines, initial encounter

Other conditions due to the effects of certain chemotherapeutic or radiation therapies require multiple codes, but the chapter 19 code may be sequenced in accordance with the circumstances of the encounter. As such, the notes in the text may direct the coder to sequence the causal therapeutic substance as an additional diagnosis, by stating to "code also drug," "code also type of therapy," or "use an additional external cause code." For example:

K92.81   **Gastrointestinal mucositis (ulcerative)**
Code also type of associated therapy, such as:
     antineoplastic and immunosuppressive drugs (T45.1X-)
     radiological procedure and radiotherapy (Y84.2)

Multiple Coding

Instructional notes appear throughout the text to provide sequencing instruction when more than one code is necessary to report a diagnosis in its entirety. Digestive system diseases or disorders associated with alcohol or tobacco substance abuse or exposures require the reporting of more than one code in a specific sequence. For example, category KØ5 Gingivitis and periodontal diseases, lists an instructional note at the beginning of the category:

KØ5   **Gingivitis and periodontal diseases**
Use additional code to identify:
     alcohol abuse and dependence (F1Ø-)
     exposure to environmental tobacco smoke (Z77.22)
     exposure to tobacco smoke in the perinatal period (P96.81)
     history of tobacco use (Z87.891)
     occupational exposure to environmental tobacco smoke (Z57.31)
     tobacco dependence (F17-)
     tobacco use (Z72.Ø)

Code First/Use Additional Code

These notes tell the coder that although certain conditions may occur independently of each other, multiple codes may be necessary to report associated conditions or designate underlying cause, as appropriate. For example:

K62.89   **Other specified diseases of anus and rectum**
Use additional code for any associated fecal incontinence (R15-)

K52.1   **Toxic gastroenteritis and colitis**
Code first (T51–T65) to identify toxic agent
Use additional code for adverse effect, if applicable, to identify drug
     (T36–T5Ø with fifth or sixth character 5)

Etiology/Manifestation Coding

The etiology/manifestation convention in ICD-10-CM *requires* the underlying condition to be sequenced first followed by the manifestation. Codes that may not be reported alone or sequenced as a first-listed diagnosis may be identified by the phrase "in diseases classified elsewhere" in the code title. Not all manifestation codes are identified by the phrase "in diseases classified elsewhere." When the conventions "code first underlying disease" and "use additional code" are noted in the text, the sequencing rules apply. For example:

K87   **Disorders of gallbladder, biliary tract and pancreas in diseases classified elsewhere**
     Code first underlying disease

Code Also

This note alerts the coder that more than one code may be necessary to report the condition in its entirety. Code sequencing is discretionary. Factors that may determine sequencing include severity and reason for the encounter. For example:

K08.0 Exfoliation of teeth due to systemic causes
Code also underyling systemic condition

Diagnosis Premature exfoliation of teeth due to disseminated Langerhans-cell histiocytosis

K08.0	**Exfoliation of teeth due to systemic causes**
C96.0	**Multifocal and multisystemic (disseminated) Langerhans-cell histiocytosis**

Chapter 11 Coding Exercises

Assign the appropriate ICD-10-CM diagnoses codes for all reportable diagnoses, excluding external causes of morbidity (V00–Y99).

Answers to coding exercises are listed in the back of the book.

1. Periodontal abscess _____

2. Recurrent acute parotitis _____

3. Reflux esophagitis _____

4. Chronic bleeding duodenal ulcer _____

5. Chronic superficial gastritis _____

6. Hepatic encephalopathy with coma, chronic hepatic failure
_____
_____

Chapter 11 Coding Scenarios

Assign the appropriate ICD-10-CM diagnoses codes for all reportable diagnoses, excluding external causes of morbidity (VØØ–Y99).

Answers to coding exercises are listed in the back of the book.

1. A 62-year-old woman presents with a two-day history of abdominal pain. The abdomen is tender to palpation, no peritoneal signs, with reactive Murphy's sign. WBCs are elevated at 15.7. Diagnostic imaging of the abdomen is positive for a nonobstructive gas pattern with multiple calcifications in the right upper quadrant. Enhanced CT of the abdomen is positive for elongated gallbladder, thickened gallbladder wall, pericholecystic inflammation, and multiple stones in the gallbladder and gallbladder neck. The patient was taken to surgery where the gallbladder was removed without incident. Diagnosis is documented as acute cholecystitis with cholelithiasis.

   _____

   _____

2. A 57-year-old male presents with increased back pain, chills, and vomiting. The patient took Tylenol and a Compazine suppository without relief. Physical examination of the abdomen was positive for RUQ tenderness with no rebound. Rectal exam was negative for occult blood. Labs were positive for leukocytosis, elevated bilirubin and a markedly elevated Amylase. Chest x-ray and KUB were unremarkable. Abdominal CT was positive for acute inflammatory changes of the pancreas and bile ducts. The patient was admitted for acute pancreatitis with cholangitis, kept NPO and started on Cefoxitin. An endoscopic retrograde cholangiopancreatography (ERCP) was performed with removal of an obstructing common bile duct stone. Blood cultures remained negative. The patient's amylase returned to normal. He was discharged in improved condition.

   _____

   _____

3. A 45-year-old female patient who is currently undergoing chemotherapy for breast cancer presents with oral mucosal inflammation that has worsened over the past week to the point where eating and drinking are painful. She has intermittent nausea and vomiting as a result of the chemotherapy, and this has exacerbated her oral symptoms. Examination reveals ulcerative mucosa of the oral cavity. Diagnosis is documented as ulcerative mucositis due to antineoplastic therapy. She was prescribed an anesthetic gel and acetaminophen for pain control.

   _____

   _____

CHAPTER 12. DISEASES OF THE SKIN AND SUBCUTANEOUS TISSUE (LØØ–L99)

Chapter 12 contains nine coding families, with the first character "L." The coding families classified to chapter 12 are:

LØØ–LØ8	**Infections of the skin and subcutaneous tissue**
L1Ø–L14	**Bullous disorders**
L2Ø–L3Ø	**Dermatitis and eczema**
L4Ø–L45	**Papulosquamous disorders**
L49–L54	**Urticaria and erythema**
L55–L59	**Radiation-related disorders of the skin and subcutaneous tissue**
L6Ø–L75	**Disorders of skin appendages**
L76	**Intraoperative and postprocedural complications of skin and subcutaneous tissue**
L8Ø–L99	**Other disorders of the skin and subcutaneous tissue**

Note that ICD-10-CM chapter 12, "Diseases of the Skin and Subcutaneous Tissue (LØØ–L99), follows chapter 11, "Diseases of the Digestive System (KØØ–K94)." The body system chapters have been restructured to place both the skin and musculoskeletal disease chapters before the genitourinary chapter.

ICD-9-CM Chapter Sequence

Chapter 9. Diseases of the Digestive System (52Ø–579)

Chapter 1Ø. Diseases of the Genitourinary System (58Ø–629)

Chapter 11. Complications of Pregnancy, Childbirth and the Puerperium (63Ø–679)

Chapter 12. Diseases of the Skin and Subcutaneous Tissue (68Ø–7Ø9)

Chapter 13. Diseases of the Musculoskeletal System and Connective Tissue (71Ø–739)

ICD-10-CM Chapter Sequence

Chapter 11. Diseases of the Digestive System (KØØ–K95)

Chapter 12. Diseases of the Skin and Subcutaneous Tissue (LØØ–L99)

Chapter 13. Diseases of the Musculoskeletal System and Connective Tissue (MØØ–M99)

Chapter 14. Diseases of the Genitourinary System (NØØ–N99)

ICD-10-CM Subchapter and Category Restructuring

Chapter 12 of ICD-10-CM has been restructured to group together related conditions differently than in the current coding system. ICD-9-CM groups conditions into three subchapters, whereas ICD-10-CM has nine code blocks containing related types of dermatological disorders as listed above.

ICD-9-CM

68Ø–686	**Infections of Skin and Subcutaneous Tissue**
69Ø–698	**Other Inflammatory Conditions of Skin and Subcutaneous Tissue**
7ØØ–7Ø9	**Other Diseases of Skin and Subcutaneous Tissue**

Category and Code Title Changes

A number of category title revisions were made in chapter 12. Titles were changed to better reflect categorical content, which were often necessary when specific types of diseases were given unique blocks, a new category was created, or an existing category was redefined. For example:

ICD-9-CM

68Ø	**Carbuncle and furuncle**
681	**Cellulitis and abscess of finger and toe**
682	**Other cellulitis and abscess**
683	**Acute lymphadenitis**

ICD-10-CM

LØ2	**Cutaneous abscess, furuncle and carbuncle**
LØ3	**Cellulitis and acute lymphangitis**
LØ4	**Acute lymphadenitis**

Title changes within categories LØ2–LØ4 reflect the system expansion. This expansion includes fifth and sixth characters, which specify severity (acute), anatomic site (e.g., trunk, buttock, limb), type of lesion (e.g., abscess, carbuncle, furuncle), and laterality (e.g., right, left, unspecified), where applicable.

Code title changes reflect the expansion of carbuncle and furuncle codes, which contain codes that specify anatomic site and laterality. For example:

LØ2.42	**Furuncle of limb**	
	LØ2.421	**Furuncle of right axilla**
	LØ2.422	**Furuncle of left axilla**
	LØ2.423	**Furuncle of right upper limb**
LØ2.43	**Carbuncle of limb**	
	LØ2.431	**Carbuncle of right axilla**
	LØ2.432	**Carbuncle of left axilla**
	LØ2.433	**Carbuncle of right upper limb**

The ICD-10-CM category titles and code descriptions have been revised to more accurately reflect current clinical terminology. These revisions parallel the changes to the classification system. For example, cellulitis and acute lymphangitis have been separated by condition (cellulitis vs. lymphangitis), and further classified by site (e.g., finger, toe, axilla) and laterality (e.g., right, left, unspecified) where applicable. For example:

ICD-9-CM

681	**Cellulitis and abscess of finger and toe**	
	INCLUDES that with lymphangitis	
681.Ø	**Finger**	
	681.ØØ	**Cellulitis and abscess, unspecified**
	681.Ø1	**Felon**
	681.Ø2	**Onychia and paronychia of finger**

ICD-10-CM

L03.0	**Cellulitis and acute lymphangitis of finger and toe**		
	L03.01	**Cellulitis of finger**	
		L03.011	**Cellulitis of right finger**
		L03.012	**Cellulitis of left finger**
		L03.019	**Cellulitis of unspecified finger**
	L03.02	**Acute lymphangitis of finger**	
		L03.021	**Acute lymphangitis of right finger**
		L03.022	**Acute lymphangitis of left finger**
		L03.029	**Acute lymphangitis of unspecified finger**

Organizational Adjustments

When comparing ICD-9-CM to ICD-10-CM, some codes have been added, deleted, combined, or moved. For example, carbuncle and furuncle of the breast is listed as an inclusion site under code 680.2 in ICD-9-CM; however, ICD-10-CM has reclassified this condition to chapter 13, "Diseases of the Genitourinary System (NØØ–N99)." For example:

ICD-9-CM

Chapter 12. Diseases of the Skin and Subcutaneous Tissue (LØØ–L99)

680.2 **Carbuncle and furuncle, trunk**

ICD-10-CM

Chapter 14. Diseases of the Genitourinary System (NØØ–N99)

N61 **Inflammatory disorders of breast**

Similarly, dermatological infections due to infectious and parasitic disease may be more appropriately classified to chapter 1, "Certain Infectious and Parasitic Diseases." For example, there is no specific classification code in ICD-9-CM to classify cutaneous strongyloidiasis. The default code listed in the alphabetic index is specifically for intestinal infection (127.2). ICD-10-CM, however, lists a unique code for this infection in chapter 1, category B78 Strongyloidiasis. For example:

ICD-9-CM

127 **Other intestinal helminthiasis**

 127.2 **Strongyloidiasis**

The general equivalence mappings (GEM) link code B78.1 to code 686.8 in ICD-9-CM:

ICD-9-CM

686.8 **Other specified local infections of the skin and subcutaneous tissue**

ICD-10-CM

B78.1 **Cutaneous strongyloidiasis**

Furthermore, dermatological manifestations of diabetes mellitus require etiology/manifestation reporting, whereby the appropriate code for the diabetes with skin complications (EØ8.62-, EØ9.62-, E1Ø.62-, E11.62-, E13.62-) is listed

---

KEY POINT

Many chapter 12 conditions have been assigned unique codes in ICD-10-CM, with specific codes that report the type of skin condition or lesion as well as anatomic site and laterality.

first, followed by the specific chapter 12 code that further describes the dermatological manifestation. For example:

Diagnosis: Type 1 diabetes mellitus with diabetic foot ulcer, right heel

E10.621   Type 1 diabetes mellitus with foot ulcer
Use additional code to identify the site of ulcer (L97.4-, L97.5-)

L97.419   Non-pressure chronic ulcer of right heel and midfoot with unspecified severity

Level of Detail in Coding

Chapter 12 of ICD-10-CM provides greater classification detail by condition, severity, anatomic site and laterality. For example:

Condition (e.g., furuncle, carbuncle) and anatomic site:

ICD-9-CM		ICD-10-CM	
680.2	Carbuncle and furuncle of trunk	L02.221	Furuncle of abdominal wall
		L02.222	Furuncle of back [any part, except buttock]
		L02.223	Furuncle of chest wall
		L02.224	Furuncle of groin
		L02.225	Furuncle of perineum
		L02.226	Furuncle of umbilicus
		L02.229	Furuncle of trunk, unspecified
		L02.231	Carbuncle of abdominal wall
		L02.232	Carbuncle of back [any part, except buttock]
		L02.233	Carbuncle of chest wall
		L02.234	Carbuncle of groin
		L02.235	Carbuncle of perineum
		L02.236	Carbuncle of umbilicus
		L02.239	Carbuncle of trunk, unspecified

In ICD-9-CM, subcategory 707.0 reports pressure ulcer by anatomic site, whereas subcategory 707.2 specifies the stage of the pressure ulcer. Two codes are required to report pressure ulcers in ICD-9-CM. For example:

ICD-9-CM

707.0   Pressure ulcer
Use additional code to identify pressure ulcer stage (707.20–707.25)

707.02   Upper back
Shoulder blades

707.03   Lower back
Coccyx
Sacrum

In ICD-10-CM, separate classifications for pressure ulcers identify the severity of the ulcers by stage (e.g., unstageable, stages 1 to 4, and unspecified), and further refine the specification of anatomic site. For example, in subcategory L89.1 these sites include:

- Unspecified part of back
- Right upper back
- Left upper back

 DEFINITIONS

abscess. Circumscribed collection of pus resulting from bacteria, frequently associated with swelling and other signs of inflammation.

carbuncle. Necrotic infection of the skin and subcutaneous tissues, occurring mainly in the neck and back, that produces pus and forms drainage cavities.

furuncle. Inflamed, painful cyst or nodule on the skin caused by bacteria, often staphylococcus, entering along the hair follicle.

- Right lower back
- Left lower back
- Sacral region

Thirty-five codes are currently listed in ICD-10-CM subcategory L89.1 Pressure ulcer of back (excluding the sacral region), including the following. For example:

L89.14 Pressure ulcer of left lower back

L89.140 Pressure ulcer of left lower back, unstageable

L89.141 Pressure ulcer of left lower back, stage 1
Healing pressure ulcer of left lower back,
stage 1
Pressure pre-ulcer skin changes limited to persistent focal edema, left lower back

L89.142 Pressure ulcer of left lower back, stage 2
Healing pressure ulcer of left lower back,
stage 2
Pressure ulcer with abrasion, blister, partial thickness skin loss involving epidermis and/or dermis, left lower back

L89.143 Pressure ulcer of left lower back, stage 3
Healing pressure ulcer of left lower back,
stage 3
Pressure ulcer with full thickness skin loss involving damage or necrosis of subcutaneous tissue, left lower back

L89.144 Pressure ulcer of left lower back, stage 4
Healing pressure ulcer of left lower back,
stage 4
Pressure ulcer with necrosis of soft tissues through to underlying muscle, tendon, or bone, left lower back

L89.149 Pressure ulcer of left lower back, unspecified stage
Healing pressure ulcer of left lower back NOS
Healing pressure ulcer of left lower back, unspecified stage

In ICD-9-CM, subcategory 707.1 reports nonpressure ulcers of lower limbs by site. ICD-10-CM has expanded these classifications to include site, laterality and severity, as measured by the degree of erosion through the tissues; from the skin to bone. The staging system that applies to pressure ulcerations of the skin, does not apply to nonpressure ulcers. For example:

ICD-9-CM

707.13   Ulcer of ankle

ICD-10-CM

L97.301   Non-pressure chronic ulcer of unspecified ankle limited to breakdown of skin

L97.302   Non-pressure chronic ulcer of unspecified ankle with fat layer exposed

L97.303   Non-pressure chronic ulcer of unspecified ankle with necrosis of muscle

L97.304   Non-pressure chronic ulcer of unspecified ankle with necrosis of bone

L97.309   Non-pressure chronic ulcer of unspecified ankle with unspecified severity

L97.311   Non-pressure chronic ulcer of right ankle limited to breakdown of skin

L97.312   Non-pressure chronic ulcer of right ankle with fat layer exposed

L97.313   Non-pressure chronic ulcer of right ankle with necrosis of muscle

L97.314   Non-pressure chronic ulcer of right ankle with necrosis of bone

L97.319	**Non-pressure chronic ulcer of right ankle with unspecified severity**
L97.321	**Non-pressure chronic ulcer of left ankle limited to breakdown of skin**
L97.322	**Non-pressure chronic ulcer of left ankle with fat layer exposed**
L97.323	**Non-pressure chronic ulcer of left ankle with necrosis of muscle**
L97.324	**Non-pressure chronic ulcer of left ankle with necrosis of bone**
L97.329	**Non-pressure chronic ulcer of left ankle with unspecified severity**

Category L97 contains extensive includes, excludes, and instructional notes in the ICD-10-CM tabular list to facilitate accurate coding and reporting. Category L97 codes may be sequenced as first listed diagnoses if no underlying condition is documented as the cause of the ulcer. However, if one of the following underlying conditions is documented with a lower extremity ulcer, sequence the underlying associated condition first, such as:

- Atherosclerosis of the lower extremities (I70.23-, I70.24-, I70.33-, I70.34-, I70.43-, I70.44-, I70.53-, I 70.54-, I70.63-, I70.64-, I70.73-, I70.74-)

- Chronic venous hypertension (I87.31-, I87.33-)

- Diabetic ulcers (E08.621, E08.622, E09.621, E09.622, E10.621, E10.622, E11.621, E11.622, E13.621, E13.622)

- Gangrene (I96)

- Postphlebitic syndrome (I87.01-, I87.03-)

- Postthrombotic syndrome (I87.01-, I87.03-)

- Varicose ulcer (I83.0-, I83.2-)

    For example:

    Diagnosis: Atherosclerotic vascular disease right leg with chronic superficial plantar skin ulceration

I70.234	**Atherosclerosis of native arteries of right leg with ulceration of heel and midfoot**
	Use additional code to identify severity of ulcer (L97.- with fifth character 1)
L97.411	**Non-pressure chronic ulcer of right heel and midfoot limited to breakdown of skin**

Chapter 12 Coding Guidance

Official Guidelines

Pressure Ulcer
In general, coding advice as published in the "ICD-10-CM Draft Official Guidelines for Coding and Reporting" parallels that of ICD-9-CM, except where the changes in pressure ulcer classification have resulted in revision of the guidelines. The underlying concepts, however, remain the same. These key concepts include:

- Assign as many codes as necessary from category L89 to identify multiple pressure ulcers, by anatomic site and stage. For example:

    Diagnosis: Pressure ulcers of the sacrum, stage 2 and right lower back, stage 1

L89.152   **Pressure ulcer of sacral region, stage 2**

L89.131   **Pressure ulcer of right lower back, stage 1**

- Any associated gangrene (I96) should be sequenced first.

- Unstageable pressure ulcers (L89.--Ø) are those for which the stage cannot be determined based upon the documentation. These codes may be assigned to report deep tissue injury not due to trauma and ulcers covered by eschar or treated with a skin or muscle graft. Unstageable ulcers are not synonymous with unspecified ulcers (L89.--9)

- Assign the ulcer stage based on the clinical documentation and guidance in the alphabetic index list of terms and subterms and verification of code assignment in the tabular list.

- Query the physician, as appropriate if the documentation is insufficient to assign an appropriate code.

- No code is assigned for a pressure ulcer described as "healed."

- Pressure ulcers described as "healing" should be reported with the appropriate code based upon the clinical documentation. When the documentation is unclear at to whether the patient has a current ulcer or if the patient is being treated for a healing pressure ulcer, query the provider. For example:

Diagnosis: Healing pressure ulcer of left heel, stage 2

L89.622   **Pressure ulcer of left heel, stage 2**

- A pressure ulcer that evolves from one stage to the next during the course of treatment is reported only at the highest level of severity as supported by the documentation. For example:

Diagnosis: A stage I pressure ulcer of the right buttock worsens to stage II during the hospital stay

L89.312   **Pressure ulcer of right buttock, stage 2**

Chapter 12 Coding Exercises

Assign the appropriate ICD-10-CM diagnoses codes for all reportable diagnoses, excluding external causes of morbidity (VØØ–Y99).

Answers to coding exercises are listed in the back of the book.

1. Staphylococcal boil, left groin _____

   _____

2. Pilonidal fistula with abscess _____

   _____

3. Seborrheic dermatitis of the scalp _____

   _____

4. Drug rash due to adverse effects of erythromycin, initial encounter

   _____

   _____

5. Localized subacute cutaneous lupus erythematous _____

   _____

6. Healing pressure ulcer of the left ankle _____

   _____

7. Foreign body granuloma of left palm _____

   _____

Chapter 12 Coding Scenarios

Assign the appropriate ICD-10-CM diagnoses codes for all reportable diagnoses, excluding external causes of morbidity (VØØ–Y99).

Answers to coding exercises are listed in the back of the book.

1. A 6-year-old patient presents with erythema multiforme minor due to amoxicillin prescribed for otitis media. The patient has approximately 13 percent body surface exfoliation, primarily on his limbs.

   _____

   _____

2. A type 1 diabetic patient with progressive diabetic peripheral vascular disease presents for treatment of a nonhealing chronic right foot ulcer. Examination reveals significant breakdown of the overlying skin at plantar surface of the foot at the base of the calcaneus with erosion in the subcutaneous tissue and a central, focal necrosis of the underlying muscle.

   _____

   _____

3. An elderly patient presents for treatment of a gangrenous stage 3 sacral pressure ulcer, a stage 2 healing decubitus ulcer of the left buttock, and preulcer skin changes of the right hip.

   _____

   _____

CHAPTER 13. DISEASES OF THE MUSCULOSKELETAL SYSTEM AND CONNECTIVE TISSUE (MØØ–M99)

Chapter 13 contains 18 coding families, with the first character "M." The coding families classified to chapter 13 are:

MØØ–MØ2   Infectious arthropathies

MØ5–M14   Inflammatory polyarthropathies

M15–M19   Osteoarthritis

M2Ø–M25   Other joint disorders

M26–M27   Dentofacial anomalies [including malocclusion] and other disorders of jaw

M3Ø–M36   Systemic connective tissue disorders

M4Ø–M43   Deforming dorsopathies

M45–M49   Spondylopathies

M5Ø–M54   Other dorsopathies

M6Ø–M63   Disorders of muscles

M65–M67   Disorders of synovium and tendon

M7Ø–M79   Other soft tissue disorders

M8Ø–M85   Disorders of bone density and structure

M86–M9Ø   Other osteopathies

M91–M94   Chondropathies

M95   Other disorders of the musculoskeletal system and connective tissue

M96   Intraoperative and postprocedural complications and disorders of musculoskeletal system, not elsewhere classified

M99   Biomechanical lesions, not elsewhere classified

ICD-10-CM Category Restructuring

Chapter 13 of ICD-10-CM has been restructured to bring together related conditions. ICD-9-CM groups conditions into the four subchapters listed below, whereas ICD-10-CM separates the classification into 18 distinct code blocks as listed above, each containing related categories of musculoskeletal and connective tissue disorders.

ICD-9-CM

71Ø–719   Arthropathies and Related Disorders

72Ø–724   Dorsopathies

725–729   Rheumatism, Excluding the Back

73Ø–739   Osteopathies, Chondropathies and Acquired Musculoskeletal Deformities

In ICD-9-CM, category 711 Arthropathy associated with infections, is included in the first subchapter, "Arthropathies and Related Disorders (71Ø–719)." However, ICD-10-CM contains, a specific block with code categories that classify arthropathies associated with infection by etiology, type, and the nature of the infection.

Category Title Changes

A number of category title revisions were made in chapter 10. Titles were changed to better reflect categorical content, which was often necessary when specific types of diseases were given their own block, a new category was created, or an existing category was redefined. For example, rheumatoid arthritis classification has been refined from one general code category to four distinct code categories.

ICD-9-CM

714   Rheumatoid arthritis and other inflammatory polyarthropathies

ICD-10-CM

M05   Rheumatoid arthritis with rheumatoid factor
M06   Other rheumatoid arthritis
M07   Enteropathic arthropathies
M08   Juvenile arthritis

Organizational Adjustments

When comparing ICD-9-CM to ICD-10-CM, many codes have been added, deleted, combined, or moved. ICD-10-CM, chapter 13, contains significant revisions and expansions when compared with ICD-9-CM by means of classification refinement regarding type, etiology, severity, and laterality of condition. For example, in ICD-9-CM, gout is classified to chapter 3, "Endocrine, Nutritional and Metabolic Diseases, and Immunity Disorders (240–279)," whereas in ICD-10-CM, it is classified to chapter 13, "Diseases of the Musculoskeletal System and Connective Tissue (M00–M99)." Furthermore, gout classification was extensively expanded to differentiate between severity (third character), etiology or type (fourth character), anatomic site (fifth character), and laterality (sixth character). A seventh character represents tophi status—an additional severity indicator that represents disease progression. The three-character code categories reflect this expansion by the use of an alphabetic character in the third-character position.

ICD-9-CM

Chapter 3. Endocrine, Nutritional and Metabolic Diseases, and Immunity Disorders (240–279)

Other Metabolic and Immunity Disorders (270–279)

274   Gout
    274.0   Gouty arthropathy
    274.1   Gouty nephropathy
    274.8   Gout with other specified manifestations
    274.9   Gout, unspecified

ICD-10-CM

Chapter 13. Diseases of the Musculoskeletal System and Connective Tissue (MØØ–M99)

Inflammatory polyarthropathies (MØ5–M14)

The appropriate 7th character is to be added to each code from category M1A.

    Ø   **without tophus (tophi)**
    1   **with tophus (tophi)**

M1A   **Chronic gout**

    M1A.Ø   **Idiopathic chronic gout**

    M1A.1   **Lead-induced chronic gout**

    M1A.2   **Drug-induced chronic gout**

    M1A.3   **Chronic gout due to renal impairment**

    M1A.4   **Other secondary chronic gout**

    M1A.9   **Chronic gout, unspecified**

M1Ø   **Gout**

    M1Ø.Ø   **Idiopathic gout**

    M1Ø.1   **Lead-induced gout**

    M1Ø.2   **Drug-induced gout**

    M1Ø.3   **Gout due to renal impairment**

    M1Ø.4   **Other secondary gout**

    M1Ø.9   **Gout, unspecified**

ICD-10-CM combination codes classify the combination of osteoporosis and pathological fracture and facilitate reporting of certain specific types of osteoporosis, anatomic site of fracture, and laterality. Seventh characters identify the circumstances of the encounter. These seventh characters also apply to pathological fractures classified to categories M84.3–M84.6. For example:

ICD-10-CM

M8Ø   **Osteoporosis with current pathological fracture**

The appropriate 7th character is to be added to each code from category M8Ø.

    A   **initial encounter for fracture**
    D   **subsequent encounter for fracture with routine healing**
    G   **subsequent encounter for fracture with delayed healing**
    K   **subsequent encounter for fracture with nonunion**
    P   **subsequent encounter for fracture with malunion**
    S   **sequela**

    M8Ø.Ø   **Age-related osteoporosis with current pathological fracture**
        Involutional osteoporosis with current pathological fracture
        Osteoporosis NOS with current pathological fracture
        Postmenopausal osteoporosis with current pathological fracture
        Senile osteoporosis with current pathological fracture

        M8Ø.ØØ   **Age-related osteoporosis with current pathological fracture, unspecified site**

        M8Ø.Ø1   **Age-related osteoporosis with current pathological fracture, shoulder**

            M8Ø.Ø11   **Age-related osteoporosis with current pathological fracture, right shoulder**

M80.012   Age-related osteoporosis with current pathological fracture, left shoulder

M80.019   Age-related osteoporosis with current pathological fracture, unspecified shoulder

Certain diseases and disorders of the jaws which are classified to ICD-9-CM chapter 9, "Diseases of the Digestive System (520–579)," have been moved to ICD-10-CM chapter 13, "Diseases of the Musculoskeletal System and Connective Tissue (M00–M99)." ICD-9-CM codes reclassified in ICD-10-CM to chapter 13 include those condition complications classified to category 524 Dentofacial anomalies, including malocclusion, 525.7 Endosseous dental implant failure, and category 526 Diseases of the jaws. For example:

ICD-9-CM

Chapter 9. Diseases of the Digestive System (520–579)

Diseases of Oral Cavity, Salivary Glands and Jaws (520–529)

524   Dentofacial anomalies, including malocclusion

525   Other diseases and conditions of the teeth and supporting structures

     525.7   Endosseous dental implant failure

526   Diseases of the jaws

ICD-10-CM

Chapter 13. Diseases of the Musculoskeletal System and Connective Tissue (M00–M99)

Dentofacial Anomalies [including malocclusion] and other Disorders of Jaw (M26–M27)

M26   Dentofacial anomalies [including malocclusion]

M27   Other diseases of jaws

     M27.6   Endosseous dental implant failure

Complications

In ICD-10-CM, many postoperative complication codes have been moved to complication-specific code categories at the end of the individual body system chapters. Musculoskeletal system complications are classified to category M96. Intraoperative complications and certain postprocedural complications, including accidental punctures, hemorrhage, and hematoma, are classified to subcategory M96.8. Code M96.89 includes both intraoperative and postprocedural complications that are not classifiable elsewhere. An additional code, however, is necessary to specify the nature of the complication. Subcategories M96.0–M96.6 contain codes that identify diagnosis or surgery-specific types of complications. For example:

M96.0   Pseudarthrosis after fusion or arthrodesis

M96.1   Postlaminectomy syndrome, not elsewhere classified

M96.2   Postradiation kyphosis

M96.3   Postlaminectomy kyphosis

M96.4   Postsurgical lordosis

M96.5   Postradiation scoliosis

M96.6   Fracture of bone following insertion of orthopedic implant, joint prosthesis, or bone plate

Biomechanical Lesions

Category M99 Biomechanical lesions, not elsewhere classified, is used to report conditions that cannot better be classified to a more specific code. Subcategories include terminology commonly used in osteopathic and chiropractic medicine, and may be used interchangeably, or with a certain degree of clinical overlap. Structural deviation, misalignment, or stenosis can often be readily identified upon diagnostic imaging; however, the mechanical nature of the associated dysfunction and manifestations in the body often require further assessment or diagnosis.

For example, subcategory M99.0 Segmental and somatic dysfunction, may be used to classify conditions in which an anatomical state of altered function occurs in the musculoskeletal system. The bones, muscles, fascia, ligaments, discs, and related nerves and vessels may be affected, resulting in impaired function. Associated symptoms may include pain, inflammation, tenderness, muscle spasms, rigidity, and tension. Conditions classified to ICD-10-CM subcategory M99.0 are classified to category 739 in ICD-9-CM, and include both segmental and somatic dysfunction of specified anatomic sites.

As such, conditions classified to M99.0 are not new to the ICD system. The World Health Organization's (WHO) ICD-10 includes these classifications, which have been modified for use in the United States in ICD-10-CM. These codes comprise a unique category with specific codes for distinct conditions formerly classified as spinal stenosis, or to other nonspecific codes, in ICD-9-CM.

ICD-9-CM		ICD-10-CM	
723.0	Spinal stenosis in cervical region	M99.2	Subluxation of neural canal
		M99.3	Subluxation complex (vertebral)
		M99.4	Connective tissue stenosis of neural canal
		M99.5	Intervertebral disc stenosis of neural canal
		M99.6	Osseous stenosis of neural canal
		M99.7	Connective tissue and disc stenosis of intervertebral foramina
724	Spinal stenosis, other than cervical	M99.2	Subluxation of neural canal
		M99.3	Subluxation complex (vertebral)
		M99.4	Connective tissue stenosis of neural canal
		M99.5	Intervertebral disc stenosis of neural canal
		M99.6	Osseous stenosis of neural canal
		M99.7	Connective tissue and disc stenosis of intervertebral foramina

Chapter 13 Coding Guidance

Official Guidelines

The "ICD-10-CM Draft Official Guidelines for Coding and Reporting," section C.13 provides the following essential instructions:

- Codes with site and laterality designations represent the affected bone, joint or muscle involved.

- Report the "multiple sites" designation when the condition affects more than one site within a classification category.

- If no "multiple site" designation is available, and multiple sites are involved, report multiple codes, as appropriate.

- For codes that specify a bone site near a joint structure, the site designation should be classified as affecting the bone, not the joint. For example:

  Diagnosis: Idiopathic aseptic osteonecrosis of the shoulder; avascular necrosis proximal greater tuberosity of the right humerus

  Assign: **M87.021 Idiopathic aseptic necrosis of right humerus**

  Do not assign: **M87.011 Idiopathic osteonecrosis of the shoulder**

- In general, most acute, traumatic musculoskeletal injuries are classified to chapter 19. Chapter 13 lists classification codes, which represent conditions due to healed, chronic, or recurrent injury.

- For pathological fractures, report the seventh character "A" for encounters during the active treatment phase (e.g., surgery, emergency medicine, evaluation, and treatment by new physician). Report the seventh character "D" for encounters following the completion of active treatment. Seventh characters G, K, P, and S represent complications of healing and treatment.

- Osteoporosis (M80, M81) is a systemic condition. The site-specific codes in category M81 represent the site of fracture, not the site of disease.

  - Report category M81 codes when a patient with osteoporosis does not have a *current* pathological fracture. History of osteoporosis fracture is reported with status code Z87.310.

  - Category M80 includes osteoporosis with current "fragility fracture;" a traumatic fracture in a patient with osteoporosis occurring due to a minor fall or trauma, in which the causal event would not normally cause fracture in healthy bone.

Refer to the "ICD-10-CM Draft Official Guidelines for Coding and Reporting" in appendix A of this book for additional information.

Multiple Coding

ICD-10-CM chapter 13 contains a wide range of musculoskeletal and connective tissue classifications, including diseases and disorders of the bones, joints, and accessory structures (e.g., tendons, bursae, ligaments, synovium), cartilage, muscles, and connective tissues. Chapter 13 includes many combination codes that associate the condition and certain secondary diseases processes, specific manifestation, and associated complications or infections. Such diagnostic coding can be complex in nature; often requiring multiple codes in a specific sequence. As such, chapter 13 contains multiple instructional notes that are essential to ensuring correct coding practices. Optum's *ICD-10-CM—The Complete Official Draft Code Set* highlights these crucial

CODING AXIOM

Category M80 includes fragility fracture sustained as the result of a minor fall or trauma occurring under circumstances which would not usually cause a normal, healthy bone to fracture.

coding instructions in red font for ease of reference. These notes appear at the section, category, subcategory, and individual code levels throughout the tabular list.

Etiology/Manifestation Coding

The etiology/manifestation convention in ICD-10-CM *requires* the underlying condition to be sequenced first, followed by the manifestation. These codes may be identified by the phrase "in diseases classified elsewhere" appearing in italicized type in the code title. Sequence these conditions secondary to the underlying disease. Not all manifestation codes are identified by the phrase "in diseases classified elsewhere." When the conventions "code first underlying disease" and "use additional code" are noted in the text, the sequencing rules apply. For example:

> **M14.851** **Arthropathies in other specified disease classified elsewhere, right hip**
> Code first underlying disease

> **M36.0** **Dermato(poly)myositis in neoplastic disease**
> Code first underlying neoplasm (C00–D49)

Code First/Use Additional Code

These notes tell the coder that although certain conditions may occur independently of each other, multiple codes may be necessary to report associated conditions or designate underlying cause, as appropriate. For example:

> **M02** **Postinfective and reactive arthropathies**
> Code first underlying disease, such as:
> congenital syphilis [Clutton's joints] (A50.5)
> enteritis due to Yersinia enterocolitica (A04.6)
> infective endocarditis (I33.0)
> viral hepatitis (B15–B19)

> **M34.2** **Systemic sclerosis induced by drug and chemical**
> Code first poisoning due to drug or toxin, if applicable (T36–T65 with fifth or sixth character 1–4 or 6)
> Use additional code for adverse effect, if applicable, to identify drug (T36–T50 with fifth or sixth character 5)

> **M60.0** **Infective myositis**
> Use additional code (B95–B97) to identify infectious agent

> **M93.0** **Slipped upper femoral epiphysis (nontraumatic)**
> Use additional code for associated chondrolysis (M94.3)

Code Also

This note alerts the coder that more than one code may be necessary to report the condition in its entirety. Code sequencing is discretionary. Factors that may determine sequencing include severity and reason for the encounter. For example:

> **M08** **Juvenile arthritis**
> Code also any associated underlying condition such as:
> regional enteritis [Crohn's disease] (K50-)
> ulcerative colitis (K51)

> **M84.5** **Pathological fracture in neoplastic disease**
> Code also underlying neoplasm

CODING AXIOM

ICD-10-CM includes specific classifications for pathological fracture by type or cause, including due to osteoporosis (M80), neoplastic disease (M84.5), or other specified disease (M84.6).

Combination Codes

Certain chapter 13 disease classifications have been expanded in ICD-10-CM to facilitate identification of secondary disease processes, specific manifestations, or associated complications. As such, code to the highest degree of specificity as documented in the record. Consult the instructions in the text to determine whether additional codes are necessary to report the associated conditions or manifestations. For example, ICD-10-CM category M32 Systemic lupus erythematosus (SLE), lists subcategories that specify type or cause (drug-induced) and disease with organ or disease-specific manifestations.

ICD-9-CM		ICD-10-CM	
710.0	Systemic lupus erythematosus	M32.0	Drug-induced systemic lupus erythematosus
		M32.10	Systemic lupus erythematosus, organ or system involvement unspecified
		M32.11	Endocarditis in systemic lupus erythematosus
		M32.12	Pericarditis in systemic lupus erythematosus
		M32.13	Lung involvement in systemic lupus erythematosus
		M32.14	Glomerular disease in systemic lupus erythematosus
		M32.15	Tubulo-interstitial nephropathy in systemic lupus erythematosus
		M32.19	Other organ or system involvement in systemic lupus erythematosus
		M32.8	Other forms of systemic lupus erythematosus
		M32.9	Systemic lupus erythematosus, unspecified

Drug- or Chemical-Induced Conditions

Combination codes, which include the causal drug, chemical, or external agent and the external cause (e.g., therapeutic use), replace the need for external cause codes. Yet, conditions due to radiation exposure require an additional code from categories W88–W90 or X39.0-, as appropriate, to identify the external cause.

Effects of drugs are sequenced according to instruction in the ICD-10-CM text. Note that chapter 19 codes, which classify adverse effects of drugs in therapeutic use, are sequenced secondary to the nature of the condition, manifestation, or affect (e.g., inflammation, ulcer), whereas in poisonings, overdoses, and other circumstances, the chapter 19 code is sequenced first.

Code section T36–T50 includes poisoning by, adverse effects of, and underdosing of drugs, medicaments, and biological substances, whereas section T51–T65 includes toxic effects of substances chiefly nonmedicinal as to source. For example:

- Drug-induced condition (T36–T50):

  M83.5   **Other drug-induced osteomalacia in adults**
  Use additional code for adverse effect, if applicable, to identify drug (T36–T50 with fifth or sixth character 5)

  Diagnosis: Phenobarbital induced osteomalacia in therapeutic use, subsequent encounter

M83.5   **Other drug-induced osteomalacia in adults**

M42.3X5D **Adverse effect of barbiturates, subsequent encounter**

- Toxic effects of nonmedicinal substance (T56.Ø-):

M1A.1   **Lead-induced chronic gout**
        Code first toxic effects of lead and its compounds (T56.Ø-)

Diagnosis: Accidental lead poisoning-induced chronic gouty arthropathy, right shoulder, subsequent encounter

T56.ØX1D **Toxic effect of lead and its compounds, accidental (unintentional), subsequent encounter**

M1A.111 **Lead-induced chronic gout, right shoulder**

Chapter 13 Coding Exercises

Assign the appropriate ICD-10-CM diagnoses codes for all reportable diagnoses, excluding external causes of morbidity (VØØ–Y99).

Answers to coding exercises are listed in the back of the book.

1. Charcot's joint, right shoulder, left ankle and left right foot _____

    _____

2. Primary gout flare, left foot _____

    _____

3. Sickle-cell arthropathy of the left knee in Hb-C disease _____

    _____

4. Osteoarthritis of the right hip _____

    _____

5. Displacement of intervertebral disc L2–L3, with radiculopathy

    _____

    _____

6. Old tear of the posterior horn of the medial meniscus, right knee

    _____

    _____

7. Myopathy due to juvenile polymyositis _____

    _____

Chapter 13 Coding Scenarios

Assign the appropriate ICD-10-CM diagnoses codes for all reportable diagnoses, excluding external causes of morbidity (VØØ–Y99).

Answers to coding exercises are listed in the back of the book.

1. A 20-year-old soccer league player with no previous injury or history of leg pain, presents with recent onset of a dull, persistent ache in the right anterolateral thigh. The pain has gradually increased since the last tournament game, and has become progressively worse. Chief complaint upon presentation was of severe right lateral leg pain. Upon examination, he was non-weight bearing, with strong pulses and good capillary return. Passive motion produced severe pain. Compartmental pressure was measured at 55 mm Hg, consistent with nontraumatic compartment syndrome.

   _____

   _____

2. A 68-year-old female presents with a history of breast cancer, for which she completed treatment three years ago. She was recently diagnosed with thoracic spine bone metastasis from the primary breast neoplasm. She now presents with acute pain of the dorsal spine after attempting to move a platter from the kitchen cupboard. Diagnostic imaging reveals an acute fracture of the sixth and seventh thoracic vertebrae with evidence of neoplastic lesion.

   _____

   _____

3. A 78-year-old male who is 15 years status post left total hip arthroplasty presents with increased pain and difficulty walking. He has had an unsteady gait for several years and has fallen on numerous occasions but refused evaluation prior to this visit. X-ray of the left femur reveals periprosthetic osteolysis with resulting major osseous defect. Arrangements will be made for revision hip replacement.

   _____

   _____

CHAPTER 14. DISEASES OF THE GENITOURINARY SYSTEM (NØØ–N99)

Chapter 14 contains 11 coding families, with the first character "N." The 11 coding families classified to chapter 14 are:

NØØ–NØ8	**Glomerular diseases**
N1Ø–N16	**Renal tubulo-interstitial diseases**
N17–N19	**Acute renal failure and chronic kidney disease**
N2Ø–N23	**Urolithiasis**
N25–N29	**Other disorders of kidney and ureter**
N3Ø–N39	**Other diseases of the urinary system**
N4Ø–N53	**Diseases of male genital organs**
N6Ø–N65	**Disorders of breast**
N7Ø–N77	**Inflammatory diseases of female pelvic organs**
N8Ø–N98	**Noninflammatory disorders of female genital tract**
N99	**Intraoperative and postprocedural complications and disorders of genitourinary system, not elsewhere classified**

ICD-10-CM Category Restructuring

Chapter 10 of ICD-10-CM has been restructured to group together related conditions in a different manner than ICD-9-CM. For example, ICD-9-CM contains only the two subchapter sections for renal disease classifications as listed below, compared to the six separate ICD-10-CM blocks as shown above.

ICD-9-CM

58Ø–589	**Nephritis, Nephritic Syndrome and Nephrosis**
59Ø–599	**Other Diseases of Urinary System**

For example, in ICD-9-CM, there is no separate subchapter for urolithiasis, and the various sites where a calculus may occur are not grouped together. A calculus affecting the upper urinary tract (kidney and ureter) is classified to category 592, whereas a calculus of the lower urinary tract is classified to category 593. In ICD-10-CM, this condition is classified to a unique code block, with affected anatomic sites classified to the three sequential code categories as listed below:

ICD-9-CM

Other Diseases of Urinary System (59Ø–599)

592	**Calculus of kidney and ureter**
593	**Other disorders of kidney and ureter**
594	**Calculus of lower urinary tract**

ICD-10-CM

Urolithiasis (N2Ø–N23)

N2Ø	**Calculus of kidney and ureter**
N21	**Calculus of lower urinary tract**
N22	**Calculus of urinary tract in diseases classified elsewhere**

Category Title Changes

A number of category title revisions were made to chapter 14. Titles were changed to better reflect categorical content, which was often necessary when specific types of diseases were classified to separate or unique code blocks, a new category was created, or an existing category was redefined. For example, those conditions classified to category 580 Acute glomerulonephritis, in ICD-9-CM are now redefined as glomerular diseases. They include expanded code classifications, which specify severity to differentiate between clinical subtypes. The term "acute glomerulonephritis" has been replaced with "acute nephritic syndrome." Note the specification of clinical subtypes in the code descriptions for the expanded acute glomerulonephritis codes.

ICD-9-CM

580.0	Acute glomerulonephritis with lesion of proliferative glomerulonephritis

ICD-10-CM

N00.0	Acute nephritic syndrome with minor glomerular abnormality
N00.1	Acute nephritic syndrome with focal and segmental glomerular lesions
N00.2	Acute nephritic syndrome with diffuse membranous glomerulonephritis
N00.3	Acute nephritic syndrome with diffuse mesangial proliferative glomerulonephritis
N00.4	Acute nephritic syndrome with diffuse endocapillary proliferative glomerulonephritis
N00.5	Acute nephritic syndrome with diffuse mesangiocapillary glomerulonephritis
N00.6	Acute nephritic syndrome with dense deposit disease
N00.7	Acute nephritic syndrome with diffuse crescentic glomerulonephritis

The ICD-10-CM category titles and code descriptions have been extensively revised to more accurately reflect current clinical terminology. For example, it should be noted that the term "pathological" in ICD-9-CM has been replaced with "morphological" in ICD-10-CM.

ICD-9-CM

580.9	Acute glomerulonephritis with unspecified pathological lesion in kidney

ICD-10-CM

N00.9	Acute nephritic syndrome with unspecified morphological changes

Organizational Adjustments

When comparing ICD-9-CM to ICD-10-CM, some codes have been added, deleted, combined, or moved. For example, the unique code used to report galactocele has been deleted in ICD-10-CM. Instead, this condition is coded in the residual three-character category for other disorders of breast.

ICD-9-CM

611.5	Galactocele

 DEFINITIONS

morphological. Pertaining to structure and function.

pathological. Pertaining to, or relating to disease.

ICD-10-CM

N64.89   **Other specified disorders of breast**
Galactocele
Subinvolution of breast (postlactational)

In some cases, renal manifestations of systemic diseases classified elsewhere have been moved to other body system chapters. In ICD-10-CM, combination codes associate diseases with secondary disease processes, specific manifestations, or associated complications. For example, certain nephrotic syndromes, nephritis, and nephropathies associated with diabetes mellitus have been reclassified to chapter 4, "Endocrine Nutritional and Metabolic Diseases (E00–E89)."

ICD-9-CM

Two codes are required in specific sequence (etiology/manifestation). For example:

250.40   **Diabetes with renal manifestations**

581.81   **Nephrotic syndrome with other specified pathological lesion in kidney**

ICD-10-CM

One combination code reports the underlying disease and renal manifestation. For example:

E10.21   **Type I diabetes mellitus with diabetic nephropathy**

E10.22   **Type 1 diabetes mellitus with diabetic chronic kidney disease**

E10.29   **Type 1 diabetes mellitus with other diabetic kidney complication**

Similarly, the following renal conditions due to systemic connective tissue disorders have been reclassified as:

M32.14   **Glomerular disease in systemic lupus erythematosus**

M32.15   **Tubulo-interstitial nephropathy in systemic lupus erythematosus**

M35.04   **Sicca syndrome with tubulo-interstitial nephropathy**

This classification change can be observed at code N08. This valid three-character code is used to report secondary renal manifestation of diseases classified elsewhere. In etiology/manifestation coding, the manifestation code cannot be a first-listed diagnosis, or reported alone. Note that code N08 lists the diagnosis due to both diabetes and lupus as Excludes 1 conditions. This indicates that the listed excluded conditions cannot be reported with N08, and are instead, more appropriately reported elsewhere. For example:

NØ8　**Glomerular disorders in diseases classified elsewhere**
>　　　Glomerulonephritis
>　　　Nephritis
>　　　Nephropathy
>　　　*Code first underlying disease, such as:*
>>　　　*amyloidosis (E85-)*
>>　　　*congenital syphilis (A5Ø.5)*
>>　　　*cryoglobulinemia (D89.1)*
>>　　　*disseminated intravascular coagulation (D65)*
>>　　　*gout (M1A-, M1Ø.-)*
>>　　　*microscopic polyangiitis (M31.7)*
>>　　　*multiple myeloma (C9Ø.Ø-)*
>>　　　*sepsis (A4Ø.Ø–A41.9)*
>>　　　*sickle-cell disease (D57.Ø–D57.8)*
>
>　EXCLUDES 1　*glomerulonephritis, nephritis and nephropathy (in):*
>>　　　*antiglomerular basement membrane disease (M31.Ø)*
>>　　　*diabetes (EØ8–E13 with .21)*
>>　　　*gonococcal (A54.21)*
>>　　　*Goodpasture's syndrome (M31.Ø)*
>>　　　*hemolytic-uremic syndrome (D59.3)*
>>　　　*lupus (M32.14)*
>>　　　*mumps (B26.83)*
>>　　　*syphilis (A52.75)*
>>　　　*systemic lupus erythematosus (M32.14)*
>>　　　*Wegener's granulomatosis (M31.31)*
>>　　*pyelonephritis in diseases classified elsewhere (N16)*
>>　　*renal tubulo-interstitial disorders classified elsewhere (N16)*

Intraoperative and Postprocedural Complications

In ICD-10-CM, many postoperative complication codes have been moved to complication-specific code categories at the end of the individual body system chapters. Intraoperative and postprocedural complications and disorders of the genitourinary system are classified to category N99. Certain subcategories and codes describe diagnosis or procedure-specific complications. Many subcategories include fifth and sixth characters that further specify the type of complication, type of procedure or anatomic site. Chapter 14 subcategories include:

N99.Ø　**Postprocedural (acute) (chronic) kidney failure**

N99.1　**Postprocedural urethral stricture**

N99.2　**Postprocedural adhesions of vagina**

N99.3　**Prolapse of vaginal vault after hysterectomy**

N99.4　**Postprocedural pelvic peritoneal adhesions**

N99.5　**Complications of stoma of urinary tract**

N99.6　**Intraoperative hemorrhage and hematoma of a genitourinary system organ or structure complicating a procedure**

N99.7　**Accidental puncture and laceration of a genitourinary system organ or structure during a procedure**

N99.8　**Other intraoperative and postprocedural complications and disorders of genitourinary system**

Level of Detail in Coding

As in ICD-9-CM, diagnosis codes are to be used and reported to the highest level of specificity available. ICD-10-CM provides, in the majority of cases, an exponentially increased level of specificity than ICD-9-CM. In chapter 14, this code expansion is intended to facilitate identification of specific types or causes of renal and other genitourinary diseases. Many of these changes are due to advances in our understanding of diseases, have been developed to provide necessary data to support epidemiology and research efforts, and have been made in accordance with updates of currently applicable clinical terminology. As such, new ICD-10-CM codes have been created for specific diseases or disorders not previously identifiable with unique codes in ICD-9-CM. For example:

ICD-9-CM		ICD-10-CM	
593.89	Other specified disorders of kidney and ureter	N28.82	Megaloureter
		N28.84	Pyelitis cystica

Certain classifications have been expanded, creating specific codes to the associated condition and underlying cause.

ICD-9-CM		ICD-10-CM	
606.1	Oligospermia	N46.11	Organic oligospermia
		N46.121	Oligospermia due to drug therapy
		N46.122	Oligospermia due to infection
		N46.123	Oligospermia due to obstruction of efferent ducts
		N46.124	Oligospermia due to radiation
		N46.125	Oligospermia due to systemic disease
		N46.129	Oligospermia due to other extratesticular causes

Chapter 14 Coding Guidance

Official Guidelines

Coding advice as published in the "ICD-10-CM Draft Official Guidelines for Coding and Reporting" parallels that of ICD-9-CM. Key concepts include:

- Chronic kidney disease classifications are based on severity as documented by the provider.

- If both a stage of chronic kidney disease (N18.-) and end stage renal disease (N18.6) are documented, assign only N18.6 to report the highest degree of severity.

- Assign both the appropriate N18 Chronic kidney disease (CKD), code and Z94.0 Kidney transplant status, to report CKD in a transplant patient.

- CKD in a transplant patient is not synonymous with a transplant complication. See the complications section of the guidelines (1.c.19.g) for clarification.

- The sequencing of CKD in relationship to other associated conditions is determined by the conventions and instructions in the ICD-10-CM text.

Refer to the "ICD-10-CM Draft Official Guidelines for Coding and Reporting" in appendix A of this book for additional information.

Multiple Coding

Instructional notes appear throughout the text to provide sequencing instructions when more than one code is necessary to report a diagnosis in its entirety. Genitourinary system diseases or disorders associated with other urinary tract conditions or symptoms may require the reporting of more than one code, often in a specific sequence. Please see the following instructional note in code N40.1. For example:

> **N40.1   Enlarged prostate with lower urinary tract symptoms [LUTS]**
> Use additional code for associated symptoms, when specified:
> incomplete bladder emptying (R39.14)
> nocturia (R35.1)
> straining on urination (R39.16)
> urinary frequency (R35.0)
> urinary hesitancy (R39.11)
> urinary incontinence (N39.4-)
> urinary obstruction (N13.8)
> urinary retention (R33.8)
> urinary urgency (R39.15)
> weak urinary stream (R39.12)

Code First/Use Additional Code

These notes tell the coder that although certain conditions may occur independently of each other, multiple codes may be necessary to report associated conditions or designate underlying cause, as appropriate. In chapter 14, many of these notations prompt the assignment of a causal underlying disease process first, or to assign additional codes to identify an infectious agent.

These notations may appear at the beginning of a code block, three-character category, or at the subcategory level, and in accordance with ICD coding conventions, will apply to all codes and subsequent codes therein. Instructional notations listed with a single code within a subcategory, apply only to that code. For example:

Notation at the beginning of code blocks that applies to code categories N00–N08:

> **Glomerular Diseases (N00–N08)**
> Code also any associated kidney failure (N17–N19)

Notation at the beginning of a three-character category that applies to all codes listed in category N30:

> **N30   Cystitis**
> Use additional code to identify infectious agent (B95–B97)

Notation at the subcategory level that applies to codes N48.30–N48.39:

> **N48.3   Priapism**
> Code first underlying cause

Notation at the individual code level that applies only to code N76.81:

> **N76.81   Mucositis (ulcerative) of vagina and vulva**
> Code also type of associated therapy, such as:
> antineoplastic and immunosuppressive drugs (T45.1X-)
> radiological procedure and radiotherapy (Y84.2)

Etiology/Manifestation Coding

The etiology/manifestation convention in ICD-10-CM *requires* the underlying condition to be sequenced first followed by the manifestation. Codes that may not be reported alone, or sequenced as a first-listed diagnosis may be identified by the phrase "In diseases classified elsewhere" in the code title. A "use additional code" note is listed at the etiology code and a "code first" note at the manifestation code. Follow the sequencing rules in the text. For example:

> **N37** **Urethral disorders in diseases classified elsewhere**
> *Code first underlying disease.*

Diagnosis: Reiter's urethritis

> **M02.30** **Reiter's disease, unspecified site**
>
> **N37** **Urethral disorders in diseases classified elsewhere**

Code Also

This note alerts the coder that more than one code may be necessary to report the condition in its entirety. Code sequencing is discretionary. Factors that may determine sequencing include severity and reason for the encounter. For example:

> **N39.3** **Stress incontinence (female) (male)**
> *Code also any associated overactive bladder (N32.81)*

Chapter 14 Coding Exercises

Assign the appropriate ICD-10-CM diagnoses codes for all reportable diagnoses, excluding external causes of morbidity (V00–Y99).

Answers to coding exercises are listed in the back of the book.

1. Atonic neuropathic bladder with urinary urge incontinence _____

   _____

2. Ureteral calculus with hydronephrosis _____

   _____

3. Chronic membranoproliferative glomerulonephritis with stage 3 chronic kidney disease _____

   _____

4. Benign prostatic hypertrophy (BPH) with urinary retention _____

   _____

5. Organic erectile dysfunction following radical prostatectomy _____

   _____

6. Tubo-ovarian endometriosis _____

   _____

Chapter 14 Coding Scenarios

Assign the appropriate ICD-10-CM diagnoses codes for all reportable diagnoses, excluding external causes of morbidity (VØØ–Y99).

Answers to coding exercises are listed in the back of the book.

1. A 13-year-old male presents to the emergency department with an acute onset of sharp, unilateral scrotal pain, nausea, and vomiting following soccer practice. Clinical signs of tenderness and swelling upon exam are consistent with the diagnosis of intravaginal (internal tunica vaginalis) spermatic cord torsion of the left testicle. Upon surgical exploration via midline scrotal incision, the left testicle was deemed salvageable with expedient intervention. A torsion of the spermatic cord within the tunica vaginalis on the left side was isolated and corrected with detorsion and fixation of the proximal spermatic cord and testicle to the scrotal wall. An incidental cystic lesion was excised from the left testicle. Tissue analysis confirmed benign cyst. Contralateral fixation of the viable testicle to the scrotal wall was performed with nonabsorbable sutures.

    _____

    _____

2. A 62-year-old female presents with prolapse of the cervical stump through the vaginal introitus. She had been experiencing progressive pelvic symptoms for approximately 18 months, including stress incontinence and overactive bladder. She now presents for correction of complete detachment of the cervical stump through the vaginal vault, occurring within the last 48 hours.

    _____

    _____

3. A 57-year-old patient was admitted to the hospital for a lengthy surgical repair of a dissecting thoracoabdominal aortic aneurysm. Postoperative course was complicated by a marked increase in serum creatinine with subsequent acute renal failure. The patient's renal function returned to baseline with hemodialysis.

    _____

    _____

CHAPTER 15. PREGNANCY, CHILDBIRTH, AND THE PUERPERIUM (OØØ–OØ9A)

Chapter 15 contains nine coding families, with the first character "O." The coding families classified to chapter 15 are:

OØØ–OØ8	**Pregnancy with abortive outcome**
OØ9	**Supervision of high risk pregnancy**
O1Ø–O16	**Edema, proteinuria and hypertensive disorders in pregnancy, childbirth and the puerperium**
O2Ø–O29	**Other maternal disorders predominantly related to pregnancy**
O3Ø–O48	**Maternal care related to the fetus and amniotic cavity and possible delivery problems**
O6Ø–O77	**Complications of labor and delivery**
O8Ø–O82	**Encounter for delivery**
O85–O92	**Complications predominantly related to the puerperium**
O94–O9A	**Other obstetric conditions, not elsewhere classified**

The code blocks in chapter 15 of ICD-10-CM differ significantly in sequence, structure, and title from their ICD-9-CM counterparts below. For example, notice the separation of hypertensive and related disorders from other complications of pregnancy. Similarly, a unique code block was created for otherwise uncomplicated deliveries; separating those classifications from code sections that include complications and other indications for care.

ICD-9-CM

Chapter 11. Complications of Pregnancy, Childbirth and the Puerperium (63Ø–679)

63Ø–633	**Ectopic and Molar Pregnancy**
634–639	**Other Pregnancy with Abortive Outcome**
64Ø–649	**Complications Mainly Related to Pregnancy)**
65Ø–659	**Normal Delivery, and Other Indications for Care in Pregnancy, Labor, and Delivery**
66Ø–669	**Complications Occurring Mainly in the Course of Labor and Delivery**
67Ø–677	**Complications of the Puerperium**
678–679	**Other Maternal and Fetal Complications**

ICD-10-CM Category Restructuring

Chapter 15 of ICD-10-CM has been restructured to group together certain related conditions in a different manner than in the current coding system. ICD-9-CM groups conditions into seven subchapters, whereas ICD-10-CM has the nine previously mentioned code blocks. For example, in ICD-9-CM, the codes representing encounter for supervision of high-risk pregnancy are found in the supplementary V code chapter. Yet, in ICD-10-CM, these codes have been moved to chapter 15, in a unique category, OØ9 Supervision of high risk pregnancy. Code classifications have been expanded to include the etiology of the high risk status and (current) trimester of pregnancy. For example:

ICD-9-CM

Supplementary Classification of Factors Influencing Health Status and Contact with Health Services (VØ1–V91)

Persons Encountering Health Services in Circumstances Related to Reproduction and Development (V2Ø–V29)

V23   Supervision of high risk pregnancy

ICD-10-CM

Chapter 15. Pregnancy, Childbirth and the Puerperium (OØØ–O9A)

Supervision of High Risk Pregnancy (OØ9)

OØ9   Supervision of high risk pregnancy

Category Title Changes

Many category title revisions were made in chapter 15. Titles were changed to better reflect categorical content, which was often necessary when specific types of diseases were given their own block, a new category was created, or an existing category was redefined.

Example 1

ICD-9-CM

652   Malposition and malpresentation of fetus

ICD-10-CM

O32   Maternal care for malpresentation of fetus

Example 2

ICD-9-CM

635   Legally induced abortion

ICD-10-CM

OØ4   Complications following (induced) termination of pregnancy

Organizational Adjustments

When comparing ICD-9-CM to ICD-10-CM, some codes have been added, deleted, combined, or moved.

The codes for complete legally and illegally induced abortions without complications are classified with all other abortion codes in ICD-9-CM. However, these codes have been reclassified in ICD-10-CM to the chapter 21 code, Z33.2 Encounter for elective termination of pregnancy. For example:

ICD-9-CM

635.92   Legally induced abortion without mention of complication, complete

636.92   Illegally induced abortion without mention of complication, complete

ICD-10-CM

Z33.2   Encounter for elective termination of pregnancy

The code for breech or other malpresentation successfully converted to cephalic presentation has been deleted in ICD-10-CM. This condition is now classified to the residual category under three-character code grouping O32. For example:

ICD-9-CM

652.1 **Breech or other malpresentation successfully converted to cephalic presentation**

ICD-10-CM

O32 **Maternal care for malpresentation of fetus**

There is no specific code in ICD-9-CM for a malignant neoplasm complicating pregnancy, childbirth, and the puerperium. A new category has been added to the ICD-10-CM to classify maternal malignant neoplasms and other harm or injury, confirmed or suspected, that affects any trimester, delivery, or the puerperium.

ICD-10-CM

O9A **Maternal malignant neoplasms, traumatic injuries and abuse classifiable elsewhere but complicating pregnancy, childbirth and the puerperium**

Combination Codes

Certain chapter 15 classifications have been expanded to facilitate identification of associated complications. As such, always code to the highest level of specificity as documented in the medical record. Consult instructions in the text to determine whether additional codes are necessary. For example, obstructed labor includes combination codes that specify the nature or reason for the obstruction. When reporting code O65.5, an additional code is necessary to identify the specific pelvic organ abnormality. For example:

O65.0	**Obstructed labor due to deformed pelvis**
O65.1	**Obstructed labor due to generally contracted pelvis**
O65.2	**Obstructed labor due to pelvic inlet contraction**
O65.3	**Obstructed labor due to pelvic outlet and mid-cavity contraction**
O65.4	**Obstructed labor due to fetopelvic disproportion, unspecified**
O65.5	**Obstructed labor due to abnormality of maternal pelvic organs** Use additional code to identify abnormality of pelvic organs (O34.-)
O65.8	**Obstructed labor due to other maternal pelvic abnormalities**
O65.9	**Obstructed labor due to maternal pelvic abnormality, unspecified**

Chapter 15 Coding Guidance

Official Guidelines and Conventions

In general, coding advice as published in the "ICD-10-CM Draft Official Guidelines for Coding and Reporting" parallels that of ICD-9-CM, except where the structure and classification have resulted in a revision of the guidelines. The underlying concepts, however, remain similar. Key concepts include:

- Chapter 15 codes are to be used only on the maternal record, never on the newborn record.

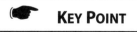 **KEY POINT**

The codes in chapter 15 should only be used on the mother's record and never on the newborn's record.

- Chapter 14 codes are used to report maternal or obstetric conditions related to, or aggravated by, the pregnancy, childbirth, or puerperium.

- Codes from chapter 15 take sequencing priority over codes from other chapters. For example:

  Retroversion, retroverted
  > uterus (acquired) (acute) (any degree) (asymptomatic) (cervix) (postinfectional) (postpartal, old) in pregnancy—*see* Pregnancy, complicated by, abnormal, uterus

- Notes at the beginning of the chapter apply to all codes within the chapter. Notes at the beginning of the code block apply to conditions within that block. Likewise, notes at the category level apply to the codes within the three-character category, and notes at the subcategory level apply to all codes within the subcategory. Notes listed at individual codes apply only to that code. For example, the note at the beginning of chapter 15 applies to all chapter 15 codes:

  Chapter 15. Pregnancy, Childbirth and the Puerperium (O00–O09A)
  > **NOTE** Codes from this chapter are for use only on maternal records—never on newborn records.

- The provider must document that a condition being treated is *not* affecting an existing pregnancy, otherwise the condition is classified to the appropriate chapter 15 code.

- Codes from other chapters may be assigned in addition to chapter 15 codes, when appropriate, to provide further specificity. For example:

  O22.3 Deep phlebothrombosis in pregnancy
  > Use additional code to identify the deep vein thrombosis (I82.4-, I82.5-, I82.62-, I82.72-)
  > Use additional code, if applicable, for associated long-term (current) use of anticoagulants (Z79.01)

- Selection of OB principal or first-listed diagnosis:

  - Routine outpatient prenatal visits without complications (Z34.-) cannot be reported in conjunction with chapter 15 codes.

  - Prenatal outpatient visits for high-risk patients (O09.-) may be reported with additional chapter 15 codes, as appropriate. For example:

    O09.291 Supervision of pregnancy with other poor reproductive or obstetric history, first trimester

    O26.21 Pregnancy care for patient with recurrent pregnancy loss, first trimester

  - The principal diagnosis should correspond to the reason for the encounter when an admission for delivery does not result in a delivery. In the event of multiple complications requiring treatment, any appropriate complication code may be sequenced first.

- The principal diagnosis in a patient with cesarean delivery should be the condition responsible for the patient's admission. If the patient was admitted with a condition that necessitated cesarean section, that condition should be listed first. If the reason for the admission was unrelated to the condition necessitating cesarean section, the condition that was the reason for the admission or encounter should be listed first.

- Assign an outcome of delivery (Z37.-) code on every maternal record during which a delivery occurs. Do not re-assign for subsequent admissions or on the newborn record.

- Assign codes from categories O35 and O36 only when the fetal condition is actually responsible for affecting or otherwise modifying the management of the mother's pregnancy.

- In utero surgery is reported with the appropriate code from category O35 on the mother's record. Do not assign chapter 16 codes on the mother's record. In utero surgery on a fetus is classified and reported as an obstetric encounter.

- Report an obstetric patient admitted with an HIV-related illness with the appropriate subcategory O98.7- code, followed by the specific code to report the illness. For example:

  O98.711   Human immunodeficiency virus [HIV] diseases complicating pregnancy, first trimester

  B2Ø   Human immunodeficiency virus [HIV] disease

  – Asymptomatic HIV infection status during pregnancy, childbirth, or the puerperium should be reported with the appropriate O98.7- code and code Z21 for the asymptomatic HIV status.

- Diabetes mellitus in pregnancy requires multiple coding; the appropriate O24 category code, followed by the appropriate diabetes code (E08–E13).

  – Report also any long-term use of insulin (Z79.4). For example:

    O24.Ø11 Pre-existing diabetes mellitus, type 1, in pregnancy, first trimester

    E1Ø.9   Type 1 diabetes mellitus without complications

    Z79.4   Long term (current) use of insulin

- Report gestational (pregnancy-induced) diabetes with the appropriate subcategory O24.4- code. Abnormal glucose tolerance is reported with the appropriate O99.81 subcategory code.

  – Gestational diabetes is classified into three subcategories: affecting the pregnancy, childbirth, or puerperium. The sixth character indicates the method of control: diet controlled, insulin controlled, or unspecified control.

- Assign the appropriate chapter 15 code for sepsis complicating abortion, pregnancy, childbirth, or the puerperium. Report also code R65.2- for severe sepsis, if documented.

  – Report the causal organism, when specified in the documentation. For example:

    O85   Puerperal sepsis

    R65.2Ø   Severe sepsis without septic shock

    B95.61   Methicillin susceptible Staphylococcus aureus as the cause of diseases classified elsewhere

- The postpartum period extends from delivery through the subsequent six weeks. The peripartum period extends from the last month of pregnancy to five months postpartum. Chapter 15 codes may be used to report peripartum or postpartum complications, if documented as such, by the provider.

- Routine postpartum care is reported with code Z39.Ø.

- See code O94 for instruction regarding sequelae (late effects) of complications of pregnancy, childbirth, and the puerperium.

- Attempted termination of pregnancy with live fetus is reported with code Z33.2 and Z37.- outcome codes. For example:

Z33.2   **Encounter for elective termination of pregnancy**

Z37.0   **Single live birth**

- Assign additional chapter 15 codes, as appropriate, to report any documented complications of pregnancy associated with conditions reported to categories O07 Failed attempted termination of pregnancy, and O08 Complications following ectopic and molar pregnancy.

- Subsequent encounters for retained products of conception following a spontaneous abortion or elective termination of pregnancy requires multiple codes to appropriately report the circumstances in their entirety:

  - The appropriate code from category O03 Spontaneous abortion

    or

  - Code O07.4 Failed attempted termination of pregnancy without complication, followed by code Z33.2 Encounter for elective termination of pregnancy

- The final character is designated for the trimester of pregnancy and should be based on the provider's documentation of the trimester for the current encounter.

  - If the trimester is not a component of a code, the condition is either classified to a specific trimester, or is not applicable to the condition.

  - During the delivery encounter, the "in childbirth" option should be reported for coexisting conditions.

- Select the appropriate code from category Z3A to report the weeks of gestation of pregnancy on the maternal record.

- Preterm labor (O60) is defined as before 37 completed weeks of gestation.

- Categories that do not distinguish between pre-existing conditions and pregnancy-related conditions may be used for either.

- When reporting an O10 hypertension code that includes hypertensive heart or chronic kidney disease, assign the appropriate code from the hypertension category as a secondary diagnosis. For example:

O10.211   **Pre-existing hypertensive chronic kidney disease complicating pregnancy, first trimester**

I12.9   **Hypertensive chronic kidney disease with stage 1 through stage 4 chronic kidney disease, or unspecified chronic kidney disease**
         Use an additional code to identify the stage of chronic kidney disease (N18.1–N18.4, N18.9)

N18.2   **Chronic kidney disease, stage 2 (mild)**

- Report substance abuse in pregnancy, childbirth, and the puerperium with a subcategory O99.31- code sequenced first. Assign an additional chapter 5 code to specify the substance abuse and dependence by type and severity. Report also any secondary diagnoses for manifestations or other status as prompted by coding conventions and notations within the ICD-10-CM text. For example:

O99.32   **Drug use complicating pregnancy, childbirth, and puerperium**
         Use additional codes from F11–F16 and F18–F19 to identify manifestations of the drug use

Diagnosis: Methamphetamine-induced mood disorder, first trimester pregnancy

O99.321	**Drug use complicating pregnancy, first trimester**
F15.14	**Other stimulant abuse with stimulant-induced mood disorder**

- Poisoning, toxic, adverse effects and underdosing in a pregnant patient is reported with the appropriate subcategory O9A.2- code sequence first, followed by the appropriate chapter 19 code.

O9A.211	**Injury, poisoning and certain other consequences of external causes complicating pregnancy, first trimester**
T58.11XA	**Toxic effect of carbon monoxide from utility gas, accidental (unintentional)**

- See code O8Ø for notations regarding the appropriate coding and reporting of an uncomplicated delivery.

- Suspected or confirmed abuse in a pregnant patient is reported with code(s) from subcategory O9A.- sequenced first, followed by the appropriate codes to identify any injury or perpetrator of abuse as documented.

Trimester Coding

The episode of care during which the patient receives treatment is not an axis of classification in ICD-10-CM. Instead, the trimester in which the condition occurred is reported.

ICD-9-CM Episode of Care

ICD-9-CM uses fifth-digit subclassifications to denote the current episode of care. Valid digits for each code were placed in brackets. A valid fifth-digit box was placed at the beginning of the code sections with definitions for each digit. For example:

Ø	unspecified as to episode of care or not applicable
1	delivered, with or without mention of antepartum condition
2	delivered, with mention of postpartum condition
3	antepartum condition or complication
4	postpartum condition or complication

651.Ø   **Twin pregnancy**
[Ø,1,3]

ICD-10-CM Trimester Reporting

In a concept similar to that of ICD-9-CM, the final character of many ICD-10-CM chapter 15 codes reports the trimester of care (often the fifth or sixth character). The assignment of the fifth character for trimester of both pre-existing conditions and those that occur during pregnancy are based on the trimester for the current admission/encounter.

In ICD-10-CM, certain obstetric conditions or complications are classified as unique to specific trimesters of pregnancy, where applicable. Therefore, the options for reporting the applicable trimester are tailored to each code. If the indication of current trimester is not a component of a code, either the condition is classified to occur during a specific trimester or the concept of the trimester of pregnancy is not applicable to the code. Where trimester reporting is not applicable, the option to report the trimester is not available in the classification. The rationale for code relevance to certain trimesters is that not all codes apply to all trimesters, although certain conditions may occur in more than one trimester.

ICD-10-CM lists complete code descriptions with each code. It is not necessary for the coder to refer back to the beginning of a code section to check the definitions of the valid characters. Instructional note at the beginning of chapter 15 defines trimesters as follows:

> **NOTE** Trimesters are counted from the first day of the last menstrual period. They are defined as follows:
> 1st trimester – less than 14 weeks Ø days
> 2nd trimester – 14 weeks Ø days to less than 28 weeks Ø days
> 3rd trimester – 28 weeks Ø days until delivery

For example:

Final characters available for each trimester of pregnancy:

O12.ØØ **Gestational edema, unspecified trimester**

O12.Ø1 **Gestational edema, first trimester**

O12.Ø2 **Gestational edema, second trimester**

O12.Ø3 **Gestational edema, third trimester**

Final characters are not applicable to trimester, and instead designate other timeframes of pregnancy, which is predefined at the category or subcategory level:

O99.81 **Abnormal glucose complicating pregnancy, childbirth and the puerperium**

    O99.81Ø Abnormal glucose complicating pregnancy

    O99.814 Abnormal glucose complicating childbirth

    O99.815 Abnormal glucose complicating the puerperium

Final characters designating trimester are not available. The concept of trimester does not apply:

O61 **Failed induction of labor**

    O61.Ø Failed medical induction of labor

    O61.1 Failed instrumental induction of labor

    O61.8 Other failed induction of labor

    O61.9 Failed induction of labor, unspecified

Final characters designating trimester are not available. Certain trimesters are not applicable, as the timeframe of the condition is predefined at the subcategory level:

O2Ø **Hemorrhage in early pregnancy**
    Hemorrhage before completion of 2Ø weeks gestation

    O2Ø.Ø Threatened abortion

    O2Ø.8 Other hemorrhage in early pregnancy

    O2Ø.9 Hemorrhage in early pregnancy, unspecified

In addition to reporting the trimester of care, use additional code from category Z3A Weeks of gestation, to identify the specific week of the pregnancy:

Diagnosis: Hyperemesis gravidarum at 11 weeks gestation

| O21.0 | Mild hyperemesis gravidarum |
| Z3A.11 | 11 weeks gestation of pregnancy |

Identification of Affected Fetus

At certain obstetric code categories, a seventh character is required to identify the affected fetus in a multiple gestation code. An instructional note at the category level instructs the coder to assign a seventh character to each code within a category. This note states to assign a seventh character 0 for:

- Single gestations

- For multiple gestations when the fetus is unspecified

- When it is not clinically possible to determine which fetus is affected

Characters 1 through 9 identify the specific fetus in a multiple gestation pregnancy for which the code applies. The appropriate code from category O30 Multiple gestation, must also be assigned when assigning reporting a code with a seventh character of 1 through 9. For example:

O31 Complications specific to multiple gestation

0	not applicable or unspecified
1	fetus 1
2	fetus 2
3	fetus 3
4	fetus 4
5	fetus 5
9	other fetus

Diagnosis: Second trimester supervision of monochorionic/diamniotic twin pregnancy complicated by polyhydramnios twin 1, oligohydramnios, twin 2

O40.2XX1	Polyhydramnios, second trimester, fetus 1
O41.02X2	Oligohydramnios, second trimester, fetus 2
O30.032	Twin pregnancy, monochorionic/diamniotic, second trimester

Encounter for Routine Delivery

Code O80 reports a full-term normal delivery of a single, healthy infant without antepartum, delivery, or postpartum complications. Code O80 is always listed as the principal diagnosis during the admission for the delivery episode, and is invalid if used with any other code from chapter 15. However, additional codes from other chapters may be reported if they are in no way related to the pregnancy. The only valid outcome of delivery code assignment reported with code O80 is Z37.0 Single live birth. For example:

ICD-9-CM

| 650 | Normal delivery |

ICD-10-CM

| O80 | Encounter for full-term uncomplicated delivery |

Code O82 reports a cesarean delivery without mention of indication (e.g., cephalopelvic disproportion). Report this code with caution, as medical documentation should support the necessity of cesarean section delivery. If the documentation is lacking or otherwise unclear, query the provider.

ICD-9-CM

669.7 Cesarean delivery, without mention of indication
[0,1]

ICD-10-CM

O82   **Encounter for cesarean delivery without indication**

Multiple Coding

ICD-10-CM chapter 15 contains hundreds of codes that encompass a wide range of diverse obstetrical conditions. Many combination codes are available that associate a specific condition with certain associated complications, secondary conditions, or infections. However, many codes require multiple coding in which more than one code is necessary to report a diagnosis in its entirety. Such diagnostic coding can be complex in nature, as multiple codes are usually reported in a specific sequence. For example:

Diagnosis: Bladder infection in dichorionic/diamniotic multiple gestation (twin) pregnancy at 28 weeks complicated by mild pre-eclampsia

O23.12   **Infections of bladder in pregnancy, second trimester**

O30.042   **Twin pregnancy, dichorionic/diamniotic, second trimester**

O14.02   **Mild to moderate pre-eclampsia, second trimester**

Z3A.28   **28 weeks gestation of pregnancy**

In this example, the reason for the encounter is sequenced first (bladder infection), comorbid conditions (multiple gestation, pre-eclampsia) and other health status (weeks gestation) are reported as additional diagnoses. The *ICD-10-CM Draft Official Guidelines for Coding and Reporting* provides sequencing instruction for specific types of encounters, including prenatal visits, encounters for complications of pregnancy and deliveries. Instructional notes throughout the text prompt for the use of multiple codes and assist with code sequence.

Etiology/manifestation coding is not included among the coding conventions in this chapter, however, because the chapter 15 obstetric codes take sequencing priority. Yet, chapter 15 contains multiple instructional notes that are essential to ensuring correct coding practices.

Code First/Use Additional Code

These notes tell the coder that although certain conditions may occur independently of each other, multiple codes may be necessary to report associated conditions or designate underlying cause, as appropriate. For example:

O34   **Maternal care for abnormality of pelvic organs**
                 Code first any associated obstruction of labor (O65.5)
                 Use additional code for specific condition

O3.87   **Sepsis following complete or unspecified spontaneous abortion**
                 Use additional code to identify infectious agent (B95–B97)
                 Use additional code to identify severe sepsis, if applicable (R65.2-)

Code Also

Code also notes alert the coder that more than one code may be necessary to report the condition in its entirety. Code sequencing is discretionary. Factors that may determine sequencing include severity and reason for the encounter. For example:

> **O3Ø   Multiple gestation**
> Code also any complications specific to multiple gestation

Chapter 15 Coding Exercises

Assign the appropriate ICD-10-CM diagnoses codes for all reportable diagnoses, excluding external causes of morbidity (VØØ–Y99).

Answers to coding exercises are listed in the back of the book.

1.   Spontaneous abortion, with retained products of conception _____

_____

2.   Supervision of diet-controlled gestational diabetes, first trimester _____

_____

3.   Threatened abortion, 19-weeks' gestation _____

_____

4.   Threatened premature labor at 36-weeks' gestation, undelivered _____

_____

5.   Second trimester pregnancy complicated by dichorionic/diamniotic twin gestation and mild pre-eclampsia _____

_____

6.   Full-term delivery of single liveborn complicated by prolonged second stage of labor and first degree perineal laceration _____

_____

Chapter 15 Coding Scenarios

Assign the appropriate ICD-10-CM diagnoses codes for all reportable diagnoses, excluding external causes of morbidity (VØØ–Y99).

Answers to coding exercises are listed in the back of the book.

1.   A 22-year-old Gravida 1 Para 0 patient is admitted in active labor at 39-weeks' gestation. The first trimester of pregnancy was complicated by *E. coli* urinary tract infection, which was treated with ampicillin. The second trimester of pregnancy was complicated by a cervical spine sprain suffered during a minor motor vehicle collision. Ultrasound was negative for abruption or evidence of fetal injury. The patient responded well to conservative therapy. On admission to the hospital, the patient was dilated to 6 cm on admission, and progressed to complete dilation approximately six hours after admission. The patient spontaneously delivered a healthy infant in cephalic presentation with Apgar scores of 8 and 10 with manual assistance.

_____

_____

2. A 38-year-old Gravida 2 Para 1 gestational diabetic patient is admitted in active labor at 38-weeks' gestation with a footling breech fetus by most recent ultrasound. Attempts at version have been unsuccessful, and a cesarean delivery was scheduled for next week. The fetus remains in a footling breech position, and the patient now presents in active, obstructed labor due to fetal malposition and macrosomia. Attempts at external version were unsuccessful. The patient agreed to delivery by cesarean section. A large, healthy, full-term single liveborn with Apgar scores of 9 and 9, was delivered by low transverse cesarean section without incident.

    _____

    _____

3. A patient presents five-weeks postpartum with fever and right upper quadrant pain and tenderness. History is consistent with chronic hepatitis B, which remained inactive on lamivudine during the last eight weeks of her pregnancy. She was diagnosed as HIV seropositive upon routine prenatal workup for management of this pregnancy. Clinical workup revealed elevated liver enzymes. Diagnosis is consistent with evidence of the maternal immune system suppression resulting in a relapse of chronic viral hepatitis B infection.

    _____

    _____

Chapter 16. Certain Conditions Originating in the Perinatal Period (P00–P96)

Chapter 16 contains 12 coding families, with the first character "P." The 12 coding families classified to chapter 16 are:

P00–P04	Newborn affected by maternal factors and by complications of pregnancy, labor, and delivery
P05–P08	Disorders of newborn related to length of gestation and fetal growth
P09	Abnormal findings on neonatal screening
P10–P15	Birth trauma
P19–P29	Respiratory and cardiovascular disorders specific to the perinatal period
P35–P39	Infections specific to the perinatal period
P50–P61	Hemorrhagic and hematological disorders of newborn
P70–P74	Transitory endocrine and metabolic disorders specific to newborn
P76–P78	Digestive system disorders of newborn
P80–P83	Conditions involving the integument and temperature regulation of newborn
P84	Other problems with newborn
P90–P96	Other disorders originating in the perinatal period

In ICD-10-CM, chapter 16, "Certain Conditions Originating in the Perinatal Period," immediately follows the chapter that classifies conditions in pregnancy, childbirth, and the puerperium. Chapter 17, "Congenital Malformations, Deformations and Chromosomal Abnormalities," immediately follows this chapter, providing what many consider to be a more logical flow to the classification.

ICD-9-CM

Chapter 10. Diseases of the Genitourinary System (580–629)

Chapter 11. Complications of Pregnancy, Childbirth and the Puerperium (630–679)

Chapter 12. Diseases of the Skin and Subcutaneous Tissue (680–709)

Chapter 13. Diseases of the Musculoskeletal System and Connective Tissue (710–739)

Chapter 14. Congenital Anomalies (740–759)

Chapter 15. Certain Conditions Originating in the Perinatal Period (760–779)

Chapter 16. Symptoms, Signs, and Ill-Defined Conditions (780–799)

ICD-10-CM

Chapter 14. Diseases of the Genitourinary System (N00–N99)

Chapter 15. Pregnancy, Childbirth and the Puerperium (O00–O9A)

Chapter 16. Certain Conditions Originating in the Perinatal Period (P00–P96)

Chapter 17. Congenital Malformations, Deformations and Chromosomal Abnormalities (Q00–Q99)

Chapter 18. Symptoms, Signs and Abnormal Clinical and Laboratory Findings, Not Elsewhere Classified (R00–R99)

ICD-10-CM Section and Category Restructuring

Chapter 16 of ICD-10-CM has been restructured to bring together related condition into distinct code blocks. For example, ICD-9-CM groups conditions into only the two subchapters as shown below, whereas ICD-10-CM separates the classification into the 12 distinct, aforementioned code blocks, each containing related code categories.

ICD-9-CM Subchapters

760–763   **Maternal Causes of Perinatal Morbidity and Mortality**

764–779   **Other Conditions Originating in the Perinatal Period**

The two ICD-9-CM subchapters contain a total of 20 code categories that contain subcategories and subclassification codes.

The ICD-10-CM code blocks contain a total of 59 separate three-character code categories that contain subcategories or specific codes, which reflect code classification refinement. For example, ICD-9-CM category 779 included central nervous system, digestive, cardiovascular, and other drug-induced conditions not classifiable elsewhere. ICD-10-CM separates these conditions by type, and reclassifies them into distinct code blocks and categories:

ICD-9-CM Category

779   **Other and ill-defined conditions originating in the perinatal period**

ICD-10-CM Categories

P29   **Cardiovascular disorders originating in the perinatal period**

P90   **Convulsions of newborn**

P91   **Other disturbances of cerebral status of newborn**

P92   **Feeding problems of newborn**

P94   **Disorders of muscle tone of newborn**

P96   **Other conditions originating in the perinatal period**

Category Title Changes and Organizational Adjustments

A number of category title revisions were made in chapter 16. Titles were changed to better reflect categorical content, which was often necessary when specific types of diseases were given their own block, a new category was created, or an existing category was redefined. For example, ICD-9-CM category 770 included multiple types of respiratory conditions, whereas the ICD-10-CM code block groups respiratory conditions together, but refines the specificity of the code categories to separate respiratory conditions by type. The distinct code categories include specific codes of similar type.

ICD-9-CM

769   **Respiratory distress syndrome**

770   **Other respiratory conditions of fetus and newborn**

ICD-10-CM

Respiratory and Cardiovascular Disorders Specific to the Perinatal Period (P19–P29)

P19	Metabolic academia in newborn
P22	Respiratory distress of newborn
P23	Congenital pneumonia
P24	Neonatal aspiration
P25	Interstitial emphysema and related conditions originating in the perinatal period
P26	Pulmonary hemorrhage originating in the perinatal period
P27	Chronic respiratory disease originating in the perinatal period
P28	Other respiratory conditions originating in the perinatal period

The expansion of conditions classified to the subsequent chapter 17, "Congenital Malformations, Deformations and Chromosomal Abnormalities (Q00–Q99)," has resulted in some conditions being reclassified accordingly. For example, in ICD-10-CM, fetal alcohol syndrome has been reclassified to chapter 17 and retitled accordingly. This reclassification occurred due to the recognition that fetal alcohol syndrome is a nonreversible condition associated with an array of mental and physical defects and anomalies.

ICD-9-CM

760.71	Noxious influences affecting fetus or newborn via placenta or breast milk, alcohol

ICD-10-CM

Q86.0	Fetal alcohol syndrome (dysmorphic)

ICD-9-CM code descriptions that contain the phrase "fetus or newborn" have been revised in ICD-10-CM. Instead, the term "newborn" is used consistently in the code descriptions for chapter 16. The intent is to clarify that these codes are for use on the newborn record only—never on the maternal record. For example:

ICD-9-CM

760	Fetus or newborn affected by maternal conditions which may be unrelated to present pregnancy

ICD-10-CM

P00	Newborn (suspected to be) affected by maternal conditions that may be unrelated to present pregnancy

Chapter 16 Coding Guidance

Official Guidelines and Conventions

In general, coding advice as published in section C16 of the "ICD-10-CM Draft Official Guidelines for Coding and Reporting" parallels that of ICD-9-CM, though the systematic restructuring of certain conditions resulted in significant revisions. The underlying concepts, however, remain the same. Key concepts include:

- The perinatal period is defined as before birth through the 28th day following birth.

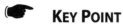 **KEY POINT**

The codes in chapter 16 should only be used on the newborn's record and not the mother's record.

- Chapter 16 codes are never reported on the maternal record.
- Chapter 16 codes may be used throughout the life of the patient if the condition is still present. For example:

Diagnosis: A 14-year-old patient presents for a school physical for participation in sports. Physical exam and history reveal weakness and decreased range of motion of left upper extremity consistent with history of known Erb's palsy from shoulder dystocia birth injury.

Z02.5	**Encounter for examination for participation in sport**
P14.0	**Erb's paralysis due to birth injury**

- A category Z38.- code is always sequenced first on the newborn record, when coding the birth episode. Code Z38.- is assigned only once, and is invalid for transfer admissions or any subsequent encounter. For example:

Diagnosis: A single liveborn infant is born at 35-weeks' gestation via cesarean section at hospital A with transient tachypnea of newborn (TTN)

Z38.01	**Single liveborn infant, delivered by cesarean**
P22.1	**Transient tachypnea of newborn**

Diagnosis: The infant is transferred to the NICU at hospital B for continued care of the TTN and monitoring

P22.1	**Transient tachypnea of newborn**

Diagnosis: A single, liveborn infant is delivered vaginally at home, and is taken to the hospital for signs of respiratory distress. The patient is diagnosed with transient TTN and admitted for treatment and respiratory support.

P22.1	**Transient tachypnea of newborn**

- Codes from other chapters may be reported with chapter 16 codes to provide detail, as appropriate.
  - Codes for signs and symptoms may be assigned in lieu of an established diagnosis.
- Chapter 16 codes are assigned by default if a condition cannot be determined as community acquired or due to the birth process. However, if the condition is community acquired, a chapter 16 code should not be assigned.
- All clinically significant conditions should be coded and reported, including any of those that require:
  - clinical evaluation
  - therapeutic treatment
  - diagnostic procedures
  - extended length of hospital stay
  - increased nursing care and/or monitoring
  - future health care need implications
- When identified signs or symptoms are present, they should be coded instead of the (ruled out) suspected condition.
- Do not assign a code for prematurity unless a diagnosis of prematurity is documented by the provider.

- Categories PØ5 Disorders related to slow fetal growth and fetal malnutrition, and PØ7 Disorders of newborn related to short gestation and low birth weight, not elsewhere classified, are assigned based on the documentation.
  - Category PØ5 codes cannot be assigned with category PØ7 codes.
  - Assign codes from subcategories P07.2 or P07.3 with a code from category P05 to specify weeks of gestation as documented by the provider.
  - Report both birth weight and gestational age codes from category PØ7, as appropriate. Sequence the birth weight code first. For example:

Diagnosis: A premature live born twin infant (twin B) was delivered vaginally at 35 completed week's gestation with low birth weight at 2325 grams

Z38.3Ø	Twin live born infant, delivered vaginally
P07.18	Other low birth weight newborn, 2ØØØ–2499 grams
P07.38	Preterm newborn, gestational age 35 completed weeks

- Codes from category PØ7 may be assigned for a child or adult who was premature or had low birth weight as a newborn, if it is documented as affecting the patient's current health status. For example:

Diagnosis: A two-year-old "ex-35-week preemie" presents with acute recurrent suppurative otitis media, right ear

| H66.ØØ4 | Acute suppurative otitis media without spontaneous rupture of ear drum, recurrent, right ear |
| PØ7.38 | Preterm newborn, gestational age 35 completed weeks |

- A category P36 Bacterial sepsis of newborn, code is assigned by default if a perinate with sepsis is not documented as having either community-acquired or congenital sepsis. Code also severe sepsis (R65.2-), as appropriate and the causal organism (B35-, B36-) if the organism is not specified in the P36 code description. For example:

Diagnosis: A single, full-term infant was delivered by cesarean section with severe sepsis due to maternal group streptococcus chorioamnionitis

Z38.Ø1	Single live born infant, delivered by cesarean
P36.Ø	Sepsis of newborn due to streptococcus, group B
R65.2Ø	Severe sepsis without septic shock
PØ2.7	Newborn (suspected to be) affected by chorioamnionitis

- P95 Stillbirth, is for use only when institutions maintain separate records for stillbirths. This code should never be reported on the mother's record.

Refer to the "ICD-10-CM Draft Official Guidelines for Coding and Reporting" in appendix A of this book for additional information.

Instructional Notes

Chapter 16 contains many important instructional notes to provide definitions, ensure clarification of the intended use of the codes, or to provide guidance for complete and accurate coding and sequencing practices. The Optum *ICD-10-CM—The Complete Official Draft Code Set* highlights these crucial coding instructions in red font for ease of reference. Instructional notes appear at

---

CODING AXIOM

Perinatal conditions classified to this chapter have their origin in the fetal or perinatal period, which is defined as before birth through the first 28 days of life, even if the illness, disease or other condition manifests at a later time.

---

the section, category, subcategory, and individual code levels throughout the tabular list. Notes at the beginning of the chapter apply to all codes in within the chapter. Notes at the beginning of the code block apply to conditions within that block. Notes at the category level apply to the codes within the three-character category. Notes at the subcategory apply to all codes within the subcategory. Notes listed at individual codes apply only to that code.

Notes

Certain instructional notes are preceded by the label "NOTE," whereas others appear throughout the text, where applicable. These notes often appear at the beginning of a category, chapter, or section and apply to all subsequent codes. The term "note" often serves as an alert to highlight coding instruction, but may also provide necessary definitions, ensure clarification of the intended use of the codes, or provide other guidance for complete and accurate coding and sequencing practices as shown in the following:

- Note at beginning of chapter that applies to all chapter 16 codes:

Chapter 16. Certain Conditions Originating in the Perinatal Period (P00–P96)

NOTE Codes from this chapter are for use on newborn records only, never maternal records.

- Note at beginning of code block that applies to all codes within that code block:

Newborn Affected by Maternal Factors and by Complications of Pregnancy, Labor and Delivery (P00–P04)

NOTE These codes are for use when the listed maternal conditions are specified as the cause of confirmed morbidity or potential morbidity which have their origin in the perinatal period (before birth through the first 28 days after birth). Codes from these categories are also for use for newborns who are suspected of having an abnormal condition resulting from exposure from the mother or the birth process, but without signs, symptoms, and, which after examination and observation, is found not to exist. These codes may be used even if treatment is begun for a suspected condition that is ruled out.

- Note at the beginning of a code category that applies to all codes within that category:

P07 Disorders of newborn related to short gestation and low birth weight, not elsewhere classified

NOTE When both birth weight and gestational age of the newborn are available, both should be coded with birth weight sequenced before gestational age.

As per ICD coding conventions, instructional notes appear throughout the text to provide sequencing instruction when more than one code is necessary to report a diagnosis in its entirety. These conditions may be identified with notations prompting the coder to "code first," certain conditions or to "use an additional code" to provide additional information.

Code First

Maternal conditions specified as the cause of confirmed morbidity or potential morbidity and originating in the perinatal period are reported with a code from categories P00–P04. The physiologic effects, disease, or manifestation in the newborn, if classifiable separately, may be sequenced first. For example, categories P00–P04 list instructional notes to this effect at the beginning of the category:

P00 **Newborn (suspected to be) affected by maternal conditions that may be unrelated to present pregnancy**
Code first any current condition in newborn

P01 **Newborn (suspected to be) affected by maternal complications of pregnancy**
Code first any current condition in newborn

P02 **Newborn (suspected to be) affected by complications of placenta, cord and membranes**
Code first any current condition in newborn

P03 **Newborn (suspected to be) affected by other complications of labor and delivery**
Code first any current condition in newborn

For example:

Diagnosis: Single liveborn infant delivered vaginally by forceps assisted extraction. Exam reveals an asymmetrical appearance of the face noted when the baby cries. The physician documents a suspected facial nerve injury due to instrumentation. The patient will be monitored and evaluated for treatment versus expected spontaneous resolution.

Z38.00 **Single liveborn infant, delivered vaginally**

P11.3 **Birth injury to facial nerve**

P03.1 **Newborn (suspected to be) affected by other malpresentation, malposition and disproportion during labor and delivery**

Similarly, certain conditions classified to chapter 16, which are drug or chemical induced, may require multiple coding. Combination codes include the causal drug, chemical, or external agent and the external cause (e.g., therapeutic use).

Effects of drugs are sequenced according to instruction in the ICD-10-CM text. Note that chapter 19 codes, which classify adverse effects of drugs in therapeutic use, are sequenced secondary to the nature of the condition, manifestation, or affect (e.g., inflammation, fibrosis), whereas in poisonings, overdoses, and other circumstances, the chapter 19 code is sequenced first. Code section T36–T50 includes poisoning by, adverse effects of, and underdosing of drugs, medicaments, and biological substances, whereas section T51–T65 includes toxic effects of substances chiefly nonmedicinal as to source. For example, subcategory P58.4 provides specific codes that identify neonatal jaundice due to drugs or toxins transmitted from the mother versus drugs or toxins given directly to the newborn. For example:

P58.4 **Neonatal jaundice due to drugs or toxins transmitted from mother or given to newborn**
Code first poisoning due to drug or toxin, if applicable, (T36–T65 with fifth or sixth character 1–4 or 6)
Use additional code for adverse effect, if applicable, to identify drug (T36–T50 with fifth or sixth character 5)

P58.41 **Neonatal jaundice due to drugs or toxins transmitted from mother**

CODING AXIOM

Conditions classified to code categories P00–P04 may be reported either as the cause of confirmed morbidity or *potential* morbidity in the newborn. These codes may also be used for newborns who are observed or treated for suspicion of the listed conditions, which after study, are found not to exist (are ruled out).

P58.42   Neonatal jaundice due to drugs or toxins given to the newborn

Use Additional Code

These notations tell the coder that although certain conditions may occur independently of each other, multiple codes may be necessary to report a condition or the spectrum of a disease or disorder in its entirety. Certain conditions in chapter 16 prompt the coder to assign additional codes to identify:

- Associated signs, symptoms, and conditions

- Infectious organism

- Secondary manifestations of disease (e.g., pulmonary hypertension)

- Severe sepsis

- Specific type or site of infection

  For example:

  Diagnosis: Congenital mycoplasma pneumonia

  P23.6 Congenital pneumonia due to other bacterial agents
          Use additional code (B95–B96) to identify organism
  B96.Ø Mycoplasma pneumoniae [M. pneumoniae] as the cause of diseases classified elsewhere

Chapter 16 Coding Exercises

Assign the appropriate ICD-10-CM diagnoses codes for all reportable diagnoses, excluding external causes of morbidity (VØØ–Y99).

Answers to coding exercises are listed in the back of the book.

1. Single live vaginal birth with cephalohematoma due to instrumentation at delivery _____

    _____

2. Premature birth at 28 weeks of liveborn infant, 1400 grams _____

    _____

3. Premature infant (exercise 2 above) is transferred to another hospital for NICU admission and supervision. The infant was treated with phototherapy for jaundice of prematurity. _____

    _____

4. A 16-week-old infant presents for monitoring and treatment of transitory neonatal hypoglycemia, ex-intrauterine growth restriction (IUGR) with continued slow progress _____

    _____

5. A 14-day-old infant presents with *Klebsiella pneumoniae* pneumonia

    _____

    _____

Chapter 16 Coding Scenarios

Assign the appropriate ICD-10-CM diagnoses codes for all reportable diagnoses, excluding external causes of morbidity (V00–Y99).

Answers to coding exercises are listed in the back of the book.

1. A 34-year-old female presents for treatment of infertility due to a congenital uterine anomaly. The patient was exposed to DES (diethylstilbestrol) in utero, during her mother's pregnancy when she was prescribed DES by her obstetrician.

    _____

    _____

2. A 24-day-old, pale, agitated infant presents with breathing difficulty, poor feeding, and fever. Physical exam is significant for cyanosis around the mouth and extremities, nostril flaring, grunting, and rapid, labored breathing with periods of apnea. The patient was admitted and placed on respiratory support and antishock prophylaxis. Diagnostic labs included blood cultures that were positive for group B streptococcus. The infant is diagnosed with severe bacterial sepsis of newborn.

    _____

    _____

3. Twin full-term liveborn infants were delivered at term via cesarean section. Twin A was small for gestational age at 2345 grams, but healthy with Apgar scores of 8 and 9. Twin B was slightly larger, with a birth weight of 2595 grams. Twin B had signs of fetal distress in utero due to cord compression and aspiration of amniotic fluid, resolved upon cord reduction at delivery. Distress resolved postsuctioning with no subsequent respiratory symptoms. Twin B Apgar scores were 5 and 9. Assign codes for both twin A and twin B.

    Twin A: _____

    _____

    Twin B: _____

    _____

Chapter 17. Congenital Malformations, Deformations and Chromosomal Abnormalities (Q00–Q99)

Chapter 17 contains the following 11 coding families with first character "Q." The coding families classified to chapter 17 are:

Q00–Q07	Congenital malformations of the nervous system
Q10–Q18	Congenital malformations of eye, ear, face and neck
Q20–Q28	Congenital malformations of the circulatory system
Q30–Q34	Congenital malformations of the respiratory system
Q35–Q37	Cleft lip and cleft palate
Q38–Q45	Other congenital malformations of the digestive system
Q50–Q56	Congenital malformations of genital organs
Q60–Q64	Congenital malformations of the urinary system
Q65–Q79	Congenital malformations and deformations of the musculoskeletal system
Q80–Q89	Other congenital malformations
Q90–Q99	Chromosomal abnormalities, not elsewhere classified

Note that the chapter title has been revised to include updated clinical terminology that more accurately reflects advances in our understanding of diseases.

ICD-9-CM

Chapter 14. Congenital Anomalies (740–759)

ICD-10-CM

Chapter 17. Congenital Malformations, Deformations and Chromosomal Abnormalities (Q00–Q99)

In ICD-10-CM, chapter 17 immediately follows chapter 16, "Certain Conditions Originating in the Perinatal Period (P00–P96)," which is preceded by the chapter classifying conditions in pregnancy, childbirth, and the puerperium. This chapter resequencing provides what many consider to be a more logical flow to the classification.

ICD-10-CM Category Restructuring

Chapter 17 of ICD-10-CM has been structured in such a way as to group together congenital anomalies into code blocks by affected anatomic site. For example, ICD-9-CM has no separate subchapters for the above conditions. However, in ICD-10-CM, the 11 previously mentioned distinct blocks have been created.

Category Title Changes

A number of category title revisions were made in chapter 17. Titles were revised in order to better reflect the categorical content, which was often necessary when specific types of diseases were given their own block, a new category was created, or an existing category was redefined. For example, code block Q00–Q07 separates two ICD-9-CM categories into eight distinct code categories with descriptive titles. For example:

 KEY POINT

The following chapters are placed sequentially in ICD-10-CM:

- Chapter 14. Diseases of the Genitourinary System (N00–N99)
- Chapter 15. Pregnancy, Childbirth and the Puerperium (O00–O9A)
- Chapter16. Certain Conditions Originating in the Perinatal Period (P00–P96)
- Chapter 17. Congenital Malformations, Deformations and Chromosomal Abnormalities (Q00–Q99)

ICD-9-CM

741	Spina bifida
742	Other congenital anomalies of nervous system

ICD-10-CM

Congenital Malformations of the Nervous System (Q00–Q07)

Q00	Anencephaly and similar malformations
Q01	Encephalocele
Q02	Microcephaly
Q03	Congenital hydrocephalus
Q04	Other congenital malformations of brain
Q05	Spina bifida
Q06	Other congenital malformations of spinal cord
Q07	Other congenital malformations of nervous system

Organizational Adjustments

When comparing ICD-9-CM to ICD-10-CM, some codes have been added, deleted, combined, or moved. For example, the code for persistent fetal circulation is classified to code 747.83 in ICD-9-CM. This condition has been relocated in ICD-10-CM to chapter 16, "Certain Conditions Originating in the Perinatal Period (P00–P96)." For example:

ICD-9-CM

747.83	Persistent fetal circulation

ICD-10-CM

P29.3	Persistent fetal circulation

Level of Detail in Coding

As in ICD-9-CM, diagnosis codes are to be used and reported to the highest degree of specificity available. ICD-10-CM provides, in the majority of cases, an exponentially increased level of specificity than ICD-9-CM. In chapter 17, this code expansion is intended to facilitate identification of specific types of anomalies, deformities, and chromosomal anomalies, many of which include codes that specify anatomic site and laterality. These changes are largely due to advances in our understanding of diseases, to provide necessary data to support epidemiology and research efforts, or have been made in accordance with updates of currently applicable clinical terminology. As such, new ICD-10-CM codes have been created for specific diseases or disorders not previously identifiable with unique codes in ICD-9-CM. Most chromosomal abnormalities are classified to category 758 in ICD-9-CM. However, ICD-10-CM includes nine separate expanded categories that classify chromosomal abnormalities (not elsewhere classified) by specific type and associated features, where possible. Note the code description (code title) changes. For example:

ICD-9-CM

758.1	Patau's syndrome
	Trisomy:
	13
	D_1

ICD-10-CM

Q91.4   **Trisomy 13, nonmosaicism (meiotic nondisjunction)**

Q91.5   **Trisomy 13, mosaicism (mitotic nondisjunction)**

Q91.6   **Trisomy 13, translocation**

Q91.7   **Trisomy 13, unspecified**

Similarly, codes that classify certain congenital anomalies of reproductive organs have been revised or expanded. These changes reflect advances in genetics technology. Similarly, certain codes have been revised or created to separately identify and report conditions by type or sex, where applicable. For example:

Code expansion by inclusion of sex:

ICD-9-CM

752.7   **Indeterminate sex and pseudohermaphroditism**
Gynandrism
Hermaphroditism
Ovotestis
Pseudohermaphroditism (male) (female)
Pure gonadal dysgenesis

ICD-10-CM

Q56   **Indeterminate sex and pseudohermaphroditism**

Q56.Ø   **Hermaphroditism, not elsewhere classified**
Ovotestis

Q56.1   **Male pseudohermaphroditism, not elsewhere classified**
46, XY with streak gonads
Male pseudohermaphroditism NOS

Q56.2   **Female pseudohermaphroditism, not elsewhere classified**
Female pseudohermaphroditism NOS

Q56.3   **Pseudohermaphroditism, unspecified**

Q56.4   **Indeterminate sex, unspecified**
Ambiguous genitalia

Code expansion by refinement of classification and specific type of condition:

ICD-9-CM		ICD-1Ø-CM	
757.1	Ichthyosis congenita	Q8Ø.Ø	Ichthyosis vulgaris
		Q8Ø.1	X-linked ichthyosis
		Q8Ø.2	Lamellar ichthyosis
		Q8Ø.3	Congenital bullous ichthyosiform erythroderma
		Q8Ø.4	Harlequin fetus
		Q8Ø.8	Other congenital ichthyosis
		Q8Ø.9	Congenital ichthyosis, unspecified

Many chapter 17 codes have been expanded to include greater anatomic specificity, and laterality of site, where applicable. For example:

Code expansion of anatomic site classifications:

ICD-9-CM		ICD-10-CM	
742.0	Encephalocele	Q01.0	Frontal encephalocele
		Q01.1	Nasofrontal encephalocele
		Q01.2	Occipital encephalocele
		Q01.8	Encephalocele of other sites
		Q01.9	Encephalocele unspecified

Code expansion by inclusion of laterality classification:

ICD-9-CM		ICD-10-CM	
754.30	Congenital dislocation of hip, unilateral	Q65.00	Congenital dislocation of unspecified hip, unilateral
		Q65.01	Congenital dislocation of right hip, unilateral
		Q65.02	Congenital dislocation of left hip, unilateral
		Q65.1	Congenital dislocation of hip, bilateral
		Q65.2	Congenital dislocation of hip, unspecified

Chapter 17 Coding Guidance

Official Guidelines

Coding advice as published in the "ICD-10-CM Draft Official Guidelines for Coding and Reporting" parallels that of ICD-9-CM. Key concepts include:

- Chapter 17 codes may be listed as the principal/first listed diagnosis or as a secondary diagnosis.

- When there is no unique code available, assign additional codes for any manifestations or associated conditions present that are not inherent components of the chapter 17 condition.

- Manifestations that are an inherent component of a chapter 17 code are not reported separately.

- Chapter 17 codes may be used throughout the life of the patient, as appropriate. Although present at birth, chapter 17 conditions may not be identified until later in life.

- Personal history of a *corrected* congenital anomaly are not classified to chapter 17. Rather, report the appropriate personal history status code.

- Congenital anomalies identified at the time of birth are reported as secondary diagnoses. Sequence the appropriate Z38 code as the principal diagnosis for the birth admission.

Refer to the "ICD-10-CM Draft Official Guidelines for Coding and Reporting" in appendix A of this book for additional information.

Multiple Coding

ICD-10-CM chapter 17 contains a wide range of congenital malformations, deformations, and chromosomal abnormalities that are arranged by affected body system, with residual categories for other specified and unspecified conditions. Instructional notes are listed throughout the chapter where certain conditions may require more than one code to report the condition in its entirety. Optum's *ICD-10-CM—The Complete Official Draft Code Set* highlights these crucial coding instructions in red font for ease of reference. These notes appear at the section, category, subcategory, and individual code levels throughout the tabular list.

Code First/Use Additional Code

These notes direct the coder that although certain conditions may occur independently of each other, multiple codes may be necessary to report associated conditions or designate an underlying cause, as appropriate. For example:

- Use additional code:

    Cleft lip and cleft palate (Q35–Q37)
    Use additional code to identify associated malformation of the nose (Q30.2)

- Code first:

    Q55.3   Atresia of vas deferens
    Code first any associated cystic fibrosis (E84.-)

Code Also

Code also notes alert the coder that more than one code may be necessary to report the condition in its entirety. Code sequencing is discretionary. Factors that may determine sequencing include severity and reason for the encounter. For example:

    Q93.7   Deletions with other complex rearrangements
    Code also any associated duplications due to unbalanced translocations, inversions and insertions (Q92.5)

Chapter 17 Coding Exercises

Assign the appropriate ICD-10-CM diagnoses codes for all reportable diagnoses, excluding external causes of morbidity (V00–Y99).

Answers to coding exercises are listed in the back of the book.

1. Lumbar spina bifida with incomplete paraplegia _____

   _____

2. Cleft soft palate with unilateral cleft lip _____

   _____

3. Patent foramen ovale _____

   _____

4. Marfan's syndrome with aortic dilation and multiple skeletal deformities

   _____

   _____

Chapter 17 Coding Scenarios

Assign the appropriate ICD-10-CM diagnoses codes for all reportable diagnoses, excluding external causes of morbidity (VØØ–Y99).

Answers to coding exercises are listed in the back of the book.

1. A full-term, male liveborn was delivered vaginally. Upon examination, the infant was noted to have multiple anomalous features including bilateral abdominal cryptorchism, wide-set eyes (hypertelorism), low-set ears, and excess nuchal skin. Pediatric cardiology was consulted and diagnostic imaging revealed pulmonary valve stenosis. Diagnosis was documented as consistent with Noonan Syndrome.

   _____

   _____

2. A 40-year-old man presents with numbness, tingling, and painful tumors in his left arm. Family history is noncontributory. MRI of the head revealed no intracranial tumors, including vestibular schwannoma (VS), whereas MRI of the left arm showed well-defined densely enhancing lesions in the medial compartment adjacent to the brachial artery and vein consistent with schwannoma arising from the median nerve.

   _____

   _____

CHAPTER 18. SYMPTOMS, SIGNS AND ABNORMAL CLINICAL AND LABORATORY FINDINGS, NOT ELSEWHERE CLASSIFIED (RØØ–R99)

Chapter 18 contains 14 coding families, with first character of "R." The 14 coding families classified to chapter 9 are:

RØØ–RØ9	**Symptoms and signs involving the circulatory and respiratory systems**
R1Ø–R19	**Symptoms and signs involving the digestive system and abdomen**
R2Ø–R23	**Symptoms and signs involving the skin and subcutaneous tissue**
R25–R29	**Symptoms and signs involving the nervous and musculoskeletal systems**
R3Ø–R39	**Symptoms and signs involving the genitourinary system**
R4Ø–R46	**Symptoms and signs involving cognition, perception, emotional state and behavior**
R47–R49	**Symptoms and signs involving speech and voice**
R5Ø–R69	**General symptoms and signs**
R7Ø–R79	**Abnormal findings on examination of blood, without diagnosis**
R8Ø–R82	**Abnormal findings on examination of urine, without diagnosis**
R83–R89	**Abnormal findings on examination of other body fluids, substances and tissues, without diagnosis**
R9Ø–R94	**Abnormal findings on diagnostic imaging and in function studies, without diagnosis**
R97	**Abnormal tumor markers**
R99	**Ill-defined and unknown cause of mortality**

ICD-10-CM Category Restructuring

After reviewing the different disease categories, developers of ICD-10 restructured some of them to bring together those groups that are related in some way. For example, in ICD-9-CM, all symptoms are grouped together under one subchapter. In ICD-10-CM, separate blocks have been created (similar to the separate code categories within ICD-9-CM) and the disorders sequenced according to affected body system, where possible.

Category Title Changes

A number of category title revisions were made in chapter 18. Titles were modified to more accurately reflect categorical content, which was often necessary when specific types of diseases were given their own block, a new category was created, or an existing category was redefined. For example:

ICD-9-CM

786 **Symptoms involving respiratory system and other chest symptoms**

ICD-10-CM

RØ5	**Cough**
RØ6	**Abnormalities of breathing**
RØ7	**Pain in throat and chest**
RØ9	**Other symptoms and signs involving the circulatory and respiratory system**

Organizational Adjustments

When comparing ICD-9-CM to ICD-10-CM, some codes have been added, deleted, combined, or moved. For example, the code for gangrene is listed in

 KEY POINT

Note that not all signs and symptoms are classified to this chapter. Those that point definitively to a given diagnosis have been assigned to a category in other chapters of the classification. For example, a mass or lump in the breast is classified to chapter 14, "Diseases of the Genitourinary System."

chapter 16, "Symptoms, Signs, and Ill-Defined Conditions (780–799)," in ICD-9-CM. This condition has now been reassigned in ICD-10-CM to chapter 9, "Diseases of the Circulatory System (100–199)." For example:

ICD-9-CM

Chapter 16. Symptoms, Signs, and Ill-Defined Conditions (780–799)

785   Symptoms involving cardiovascular system

    785.4   Gangrene

ICD-10-CM

Chapter 9. Diseases of the Circulatory System (100–199)

Other and unspecified disorders of the circulatory system (195–199)

196   Gangrene, not elsewhere classified

Within this chapter classification, the code for elevated prostate specific antigen (PSA) has been moved to a different category in ICD-10-CM. This condition is now classified to the category for other abnormal tumor markers (R97). For example:

ICD-9-CM

790   Nonspecific findings on examination of blood

    790.93   Elevated prostate specific antigen [PSA]

ICD-10-CM

R97   Abnormal tumor markers

    R97.2   Elevated prostate specific antigen [PSA]

Level of Detail in Coding

As in ICD-9-CM, diagnosis codes are to be used and reported to the highest degree of specificity available. ICD-10-CM provides, in the majority of cases, an exponentially increased level of specificity than ICD-9-CM. In chapter 18, this code expansion is intended to facilitate identification of specific symptoms and signs. Refinements in the data granularity between the ICD systems are intended to enhance understanding of diseases and to provide necessary data to support epidemiology and research efforts. Similarly, certain changes have been made in accordance with updated use of currently applicable clinical terminology.

As such, new ICD-10-CM codes have been created for specific conditions not previously identifiable with unique codes in ICD-9-CM. For example:

ICD-9-CM		ICD-10-CM	
782.0	Disturbance of skin sensation	R20.0	Anesthesia of skin
		R20.1	Hypoesthesia of skin
		R20.2	Paraesthesia of skin
		R20.3	Hyperesthesia
		R20.8	Other disturbances of skin sensation
		R20.9	Unspecified disturbances of skin sensation

ICD-9-CM		ICD-10-CM	
784.99	Other symptoms involving head and neck	R06.5	Mouth breathing
		R06.7	Sneezing
		R06.89	Other abnormalities of breathing
		R19.6	Halitosis
787.3	Flatulence eructation and gas pain	R14.0	Abdominal distension (gaseous)
		R14.1	Gas pain
		R14.2	Eructation
		R14.3	Flatulence

Many chapter 18 codes have been expanded to include enhanced anatomic specificity, and laterality of site, where applicable. For example:

Code expansion of anatomic site classifications by site and laterality:

ICD-9-CM		ICD-10-CM	
782.2	Localized superficial swelling, mass, or lump	R22.0	Localized swelling, mass and lump, head
		R22.1	Localized swelling, mass and lump, neck
		R22.2	Localized swelling, mass and lump, trunk
		R22.30	Localized swelling, mass and lump, unspecified upper limb
		R22.31	Localized swelling, mass and lump, right upper limb
		R22.32	Localized swelling, mass and lump, left upper limb
		R22.33	Localized swelling, mass and lump, upper limb, bilateral
		R22.40	Localized swelling, mass and lump, unspecified lower limb
		R22.41	Localized swelling, mass and lump, right lower limb
		R22.42	Localized swelling, mass and lump, left lower limb
		R22.43	Localized swelling, mass and lump, lower limb, bilateral
		R22.9	Localized swelling, mass and lump, unspecified

Note the significant expansion of abnormal finding codes. Whereas, ICD-9-CM codes report abnormality by specimen, the ICD-10-CM equivalent codes further specify the type of abnormality (e.g., hormone levels, presence of drugs, cytology, histology).

ICD-9-CM		ICD-10-CM	
790.99	Other nonspecific findings on examination of blood	R70.1	Abnormal plasma viscosity
		R77.0	Abnormality of albumin
		R77.1	Abnormality of globulin
		R77.2	Abnormality of alphafetoprotein
		R77.8	Other specified abnormalities of plasma proteins
		R77.9	Abnormality of plasma protein, unspecified
		R78.1	Finding of opiate drug in blood
		R78.2	Finding of cocaine in blood
		R78.3	Finding of hallucinogen in blood
		R78.4	Finding of other drugs of addictive potential in blood
		R78.5	Finding of other psychotropic drug in blood
		R78.6	Finding of steroid agent in blood
		R78.89	Finding of other specified substances, not normally found in blood
		R78.9	Finding of unspecified substance, not normally found in blood
		R79.89	Other specified abnormal findings of blood chemistry

ICD-9-CM		ICD-10-CM	
792.0	Nonspecific abnormal findings in cerebrospinal fluid	R83.0	Abnormal level of enzymes in cerebrospinal fluid
		R83.1	Abnormal level of hormones in cerebrospinal fluid
		R83.2	Abnormal level of other drugs, medicaments and biological substances in cerebrospinal fluid
		R83.3	Abnormal level of substances chiefly nonmedicinal as to source in cerebrospinal fluid
		R83.4	Abnormal immunological findings in cerebrospinal fluid
		R83.5	Abnormal microbiological findings in cerebrospinal fluid
		R83.6	Abnormal cytological findings in cerebrospinal fluid
		R83.8	Other abnormal findings in cerebrospinal fluid
		R83.9	Unspecified abnormal finding in cerebrospinal fluid

Coma

Code classifications for coma have been expanded to reflect clinical severity in accordance with the Glasgow clinical coma scaling used in assessing trauma. One code from each R40.2- subcategory is required to report coma. Instruction notations have been included to direct the coder to sequence first the associated trauma or fracture. Seventh characters describe the circumstances of coma at the time of encounter for health care services. These seventh characters must match for all three subcategory R40.2- codes.

ICD-9-CM

780.01   Coma

ICD-10-CM

R40.2   Coma

Codes first any associated:
coma in fracture of skull (S02.-)
coma in intracranial injury (S06.-)

> The appropriate 7th character is to be added to each code from subcategory R40.21-, R40.22-, R40.23-.
>
> **0   unspecified time**
> **1   in the field [EMT or ambulance]**
> **2   at arrival to emergency department**
> **3   at hospital admission**
> **4   24 hours or more after hospital admission**

NOTE These codes are intended primarily for trauma registry and research use but may be utilized by all users of the classification who wish to collect this information
A code from each subcategory is required to complete the coma scale.

R40.20   Unspecified coma

R40.21   Coma scale, eyes open

    R40.211   Coma scale, eyes open, never

    R40.212   Coma scale, eyes open, to pain

    R40.213   Coma scale, eyes open, to sound

    R40.214   Coma scale, eyes open, spontaneous

R40.22   Coma scale, best verbal response

    R40.221   Coma scale, best verbal response, none

    R40.222   Coma scale, best verbal response, incomprehensible words

    R40.223   Coma scale, best verbal response, inappropriate words

    R40.224   Coma scale, best verbal response, confused conversation

    R40.225   Coma scale, best verbal response, oriented

R40.23   Coma scale, best motor response

    R40.231   Coma scale, best motor response, none

    R40.232   Coma scale, best motor response, extension

    R40.233   Coma scale, best motor response, abnormal

    R40.234   Coma scale, best motor response, flexion withdrawal

    R40.235   Coma scale, best motor response, localizes pain

    R40.236   Coma scale, best motor response, obeys commands

R40.24   Glasgow coma scale, total score[END BOLD]
Use codes R40.21- through R40.23- only when the individual score(s) are documented

    R40.241   Glasgow coma scale score 13-15

    R40.242   Glasgow coma scale score 9-12

    R40.243   Glasgow coma scale 3-8

    R40.244   Other coma, without documented Glasgow coma scale score, or with partial score reported

Chapter 18 Coding Guidance

Official Guidelines

The "ICD-10-CM Draft Official Guidelines for Coding and Reporting" section C.18 provides essential instructions, that serve to reinforce coding conventions and principles regarding the appropriate coding, sequencing, and reporting of symptom, sign, and abnormal result codes. No chapter-specific guidelines are included in the current ICD-9-CM official guidelines. However, the underlying concepts of the chapter 18 ICD-10-CM guidelines are consistent with advice as published in the official ICD-9-CM general guidelines I.B.6–8, II E and section III.B, regarding symptoms, signs, and abnormal findings. These underlying concepts remain the same. Key concepts include:

- Chapter 18 codes are intended to report symptoms, signs, and abnormal results of diagnostic procedures for which no definitive classifiable diagnosis has been established or confirmed by the provider.

- Signs and symptoms inherent in conditions classifiable elsewhere are not separately reported, unless otherwise prompted by instructional notes in the text. For example:

  Diagnosis: Acute cholecystitis with right upper quadrant pain

  (The right upper quadrant pain is *not* reported.)

  K81.0   **Acute cholecystitis**

- Signs and symptoms may be reported in addition to a related definitive diagnosis when not routinely associated with that diagnosis; however, the definitive diagnosis should be sequenced first. For example:

  Diagnosis: COPD with hypoxia

  J44.9   **Chronic obstructive pulmonary disease, unspecified**

  R09.02   **Hypoxemia**

- When a symptom is followed by comparing/contrasting diagnoses, the symptom code is sequenced first.

- When reporting a combination code in which common symptoms are associated with a definitive diagnosis, do not assign an additional code for the symptom.

- Report code R29.6 Repeated falls, when the reason for a recent fall is being investigated.

- Report code Z91.81 History of falling, when the documentation states that the patient has fallen in the past and is at risk for future falls.

- Codes R29.6 and Z91.81 may be reported together, when appropriate.

- Coma scale codes (R40.2-) may be sequenced as a secondary diagnosis in conjunction with traumatic brain injury (TBI), acute cerebrovascular disease, or sequelae of cerebrovascular disease.

  - A code from each coma scale subcategory (R40.21-, R40.22-, and R40.23-) is necessary to complete the coma scale classification. The seventh character should match for all three codes.

    For example:

    Diagnosis: At arrival to the emergency department (ER) the patient had the following coma scale documented by the ER physician: Eyes open to sound, inappropriate words, abnormal motor response.

> **R40.2132** **Coma scale, eyes open, to sound, at arrival to emergency department (ED)**
>
> **R40.2232** **Coma scale, best verbal response inappropriate words, at arrival to ED**
>
> **R40.2332** **Coma scale, best motor response abnormal, at arrival to ED**

- Report the initial score documented upon arrival to the facility; however, data may be collected on multiple coma scale scores.

- Report subcategory R40.24- codes when only the total score is documented, with no documentation of the individual scores.

- Code R53.2 Functional quadriplegia, should not be assigned for cases of neurologic quadriplegia. Assign only if specifically documented by the provider.

- When SIRS is documented with a noninfectious condition, report the underlying causal condition (e.g., injury) first, followed by code R65.1-, as appropriate. For example:

Diagnosis: Acute alcoholic pancreatitis with SIRS

> **K85.2** **Alcohol induced acute pancreatitis**
>
> **R65.10** **Systemic inflammatory response syndrome (SIRS) of noninfectious origin without acute organ dysfunction**

Note: In the example above, the coder would assign additional codes for the alcohol abuse or dependence and any associated organ dysfunction, if documented.

- Code R99 Ill-defined and unknown cause of mortality, is limited to facilitate reporting of a patient who expired prior to arrival at the facility, or is pronounced dead upon arrival. Code R99 does not represent the discharge disposition of "expired."

Refer to the "ICD-10-CM Draft Official Guidelines for Coding and Reporting" in appendix A of this book for additional information.

Drug- or Chemical-Induced Conditions

Combination codes include the causal drug, chemical, or external agent and the external cause (e.g., therapeutic use). Effects of drugs are sequenced according to instruction in the ICD-10-CM text. Note that chapter 19 codes, which classify adverse effects of drugs in therapeutic use, are sequenced secondary to the nature of the condition, manifestation, or affect (e.g., inflammation, fibrosis), whereas in poisonings, overdoses, and other circumstances, the chapter 19 code is sequenced first. Code section T36–T50 includes poisoning by, adverse effects of, and underdosing of drugs, medicaments, and biological substances. For example:

- Drug-induced condition in therapeutic use (T36–T50):

> **R33.0** **Drug-induced retention of urine**
> Use additional code for adverse effect, if applicable, to identify drug (T36–T50 with fifth or sixth character 5)

Diagnosis: Urinary retention due to therapeutic use of Spiriva for COPD

R33.Ø   **Drug induced retention of urine**
> Use additional code for adverse effect, if applicable, to identify drug (T36–T5Ø with fifth or sixth character 5)

T44.3X5A   **Adverse effect of other parasympatholytics [anticholinergics and antimuscarinics] and spasmolytics, initial encounter**

J44.9   **Chronic obstructive pulmonary disease, unspecified**

Multiple Coding

Chapter 18 contains multiple instructional notes that are essential to ensuring correct coding practices when reporting symptoms, signs, and other ill-defined conditions. Optum's *ICD-10-CM—The Complete Official Draft Code Set* highlights these crucial coding instructions in red font for ease of reference. These notes appear at the section, category, subcategory, and individual code levels throughout the tabular list.

Code First/Use Additional Code

These notes tell the coder that although certain conditions may occur independently of each other, multiple codes may be necessary to report associated conditions or designate underlying cause, as appropriate. For example:

- Code first:

  R13.1   **Dysphagia**
  > Code first, if applicable, dysphagia following cerebrovascular disease (I69. with final characters -91)

Diagnosis: Oropharyngeal dysphagia status post intracerebral hemorrhage

I69.191   **Dysphagia following nontraumatic intracerebral hemorrhage**
> Use additional code to identify the type of dysphagia, if known (R13.1-)

R13.12   **Dysphagia, oropharyngeal phase**

- Use additional code:

  R63.6   **Underweight**
  > Use additional code to identify body mass index (BMI), if known (Z68-)

Diagnosis: Encounter for school sports physical, 14-year-old patient underweight with BMI in less than fifth percentile

Z02.5   **Encounter for examination for participation in sport**

R63.6   **Underweight**

Z68.51   **Body mass index (BMI), pediatric, less than 5th percentile for age**

Chapter 18 Coding Exercises

Assign the appropriate ICD-10-CM diagnoses codes for all reportable diagnoses, excluding external causes of morbidity (VØØ–Y99).

Answers to coding exercises are listed in the back of the book.

1. Nausea and vomiting _____

   _____

2. Ovarian carcinoma with malignant ascites _____

   _____

3. Localized mass, right upper arm _____

   _____

4. Anterior chest wall pain _____

   _____

5. Recurrent convulsions _____

   _____

6. Menopausal hot flashes with night sweats _____

   _____

Chapter 18 Coding Scenarios

Assign the appropriate ICD-10-CM diagnoses codes for all reportable diagnoses, excluding external causes of morbidity (VØØ–Y99).

Answers to coding exercises are listed in the back of the book.

1. A patient presents to the outpatient clinic for diagnostic EEG and lab tests upon referral by her private physician to investigate a recent onset of mental status changes. The patient has a history of TIA. The physician order lists mental status changes and history of TIA.

   _____

   _____

2. A 32-day-old infant with no prior significant medical history was admitted to the PICU in acute respiratory failure with idiopathic pulmonary hemorrhage. Physical exam upon admission was positive for hemoptysis with frank blood in the airway and infiltrates on chest x-ray. The patient was intubated and placed on mechanical ventilation. The physician documents respiratory failure and AIPHI.

   _____

   _____

3. A 38-year-old female presents to her physician for evaluation of fecal urgency and smearing. History is significant for third-degree obstetric perineal laceration with possible resultant rectal muscle damage. She will be referred for surgical evaluation.

   _____

   _____

CHAPTER 19. INJURY, POISONING AND CERTAIN OTHER CONSEQUENCES OF EXTERNAL CAUSES (SØØ–T88)

Chapter 19 groups together injuries by anatomic site of injury (SØØ–S99) or by related injuries and conditions that are further categorized by specific affected anatomic site or type. This chapter has been widely expanded from the ICD-9-CM equivalent classifications, primarily due to the refinement of specificity within the code set that includes the following variables, where applicable:

- Anatomic site of injury (e.g., first metatarsal, second metatarsal, great toe, lesser toes)

- Inclusion of laterality (e.g., right, left, unspecified)

- Type of injury (e.g., fracture: segmental, oblique, type I, type II)

- Severity (e.g., displaced, nondisplaced, superficial, deep, minor, major)

- Complications (e.g., delayed healing, malunion, nonunion)

- Causal substance (e.g., venom: wasp, snake, scorpion; pesticides: insecticides, rodenticides)

- Episode of care (e.g., initial, subsequent, sequelae)

- External cause of effects of substances formerly identified by supplementary classification (e.g., self-harm, adverse effect, accidental)

Chapter 19 contains 22 code families (code blocks), with the first characters "S" or "T." The S section includes classifications for different types of injuries related to single body regions. The T section classifies injuries to unspecified body regions as well as poisoning and certain other consequences of external causes.

The code families are:

SØØ–SØ9	Injuries to the head
S1Ø–S19	Injuries to the neck
S2Ø–S29	Injuries to the thorax
S3Ø–S39	Injuries to the abdomen, lower back, lumbar spine, pelvis, and external genitals
S4Ø–S49	Injuries to the shoulder and upper arm
S5Ø–S59	Injuries to the elbow and forearm
S6Ø–S69	Injuries to the wrist and hand
S7Ø–S79	Injuries to the hip and thigh
S8Ø–S89	Injuries to the knee and lower leg
S9Ø–S99	Injuries to the ankle and foot
TØ7	Unspecified multiple injuries
T14	Injury of unspecified body region
T15–T19	Effects of foreign body entering through natural orifice
T2Ø–T25	Burns and corrosions of external body surface, specified by site
T26–T28	Burns and corrosions confined to eye and internal organs
T3Ø–T32	Burns and corrosions of multiple and unspecified body regions
T33–T34	Frostbite

T36–T50	**Poisoning by adverse effects of drugs and underdosing of medicaments and biological substances**
T51–T65	**Toxic effects of substances chiefly nonmedicinal as to source**
T66–T78	**Other and unspecified effects of external causes**
T79	**Certain early complications of trauma**
T80–T88	**Complications of surgical and medical care, not elsewhere classified**

The following instructional notes appear at the beginning of chapter 19 and apply to the entire chapter:

- Use secondary code(s) from chapter 20 External causes of morbidity, to indicate the cause of injury.

- Codes within the T section that include the external cause do not require an additional external cause code.

- Use an additional code to identify any retained foreign body, if applicable (Z18.-).

At the beginning of certain categories, there is an instructional note to use an additional code to identify any associated wound infection of an open wound.

Seventh Characters

The majority of codes within this chapter require seventh characters. Confirm each code in the tabular list. Refer back to the beginning of the code category, where necessary, for the definitions of each applicable seventh character. Certain seventh characters are applicable only to specific categories of codes. For example, the following seventh characters are required with categories S00–S01, yet category S02 requires a different set of seventh characters. The instructional note at the category level prompts the coder for the addition of valid characters which are required within the specified category. For example:

- Seventh character that indicates the episode of care:

  S01   Open wound of head

  > The appropriate 7th character is to be added to each code from category S01.
  >
  > A   initial encounter
  > B   subsequent encounter
  > C   sequela

- Seventh character that indicates routine versus delayed healing and complications:

  S02   Fracture of skull and facial bones

  > The appropriate 7th character is to be added to each code from category S02.
  >
  > A   initial encounter for closed fracture
  > B   initial encounter for open fracture
  > D   subsequent encounter for fracture with routine healing
  > G   subsequent encounter for fracture with delayed healing
  > K   subsequent encounter for fracture with nonunion
  > S   sequela

- Seventh character that indicates the type of fracture, with or without complication:

S52   Fracture of forearm

The appropriate 7th character is to be added to each code from category S52.

  A   initial encounter for closed fracture
  B   initial encounter for open fracture type I or II
  C   initial encounter for open fracture type IIIA, IIIB, or IIIC
  D   subsequent encounter for closed fracture with routine healing
  E   subsequent encounter for open fracture type I or II with routine healing
  F   subsequent encounter for open fracture type IIIA, IIIB, or IIIC with routine healing
  G   subsequent encounter for closed fracture with delayed healing
  H   subsequent encounter for open fracture type I or II with delayed healing
  J   subsequent encounter for open fracture type IIIA, IIIB, or IIIC with delayed healing
  K   subsequent encounter for closed fracture with nonunion
  M   subsequent encounter for open fracture type I or II with nonunion
  N   subsequent encounter for open fracture type IIIA, IIIB, or IIIC with nonunion
  P   subsequent encounter for closed fracture with malunion
  Q   subsequent encounter for open fracture type I or II with malunion
  R   subsequent encounter for open fracture type IIIA, IIIB, or IIIC with malunion
  S   sequela

The following definitions apply to the assignment of certain seventh characters:

- Initial encounter extensions are used while the patient is receiving active treatment for the injury. Active treatment includes surgical treatment, emergency department encounters and evaluation and management by a *new* physician.

- Subsequent encounter characters are used for encounters *after* the patient has received active treatment, and is receiving routine care during the healing or recovery phase. Examples include:

  - cast change or removal
  - follow-up visits following injury treatment
  - medication adjustment
  - removal of internal or external fixation device
  - other aftercare

- Sequela (S) represents after effects, late effects, or other adverse conditions that occur subsequent to the healing and recovery phase of the injury. This character is used for complications or conditions which arise as a direct result of injury. Report two codes: the injury that precipitated the sequela and the sequela itself. The S is added only to the injury code, not the sequela code. The specific sequela (after effect, late effect condition) is sequenced first, followed by the injury code with the seventh character S. For example:

Diagnosis: Right claw hand deformity due to old (healed) upper arm median nerve injury

M21.511   **Acquired claw hand, right hand**

S44.11XS   **Injury of median nerve at upper arm level, right arm, sequela**

ICD-10-CM Category Restructuring

Chapter 19 is organized by site, rather than by type of injury. The first code block is SØØ–SØ9, which classifies injuries to the head. The S section then progresses down the body to code block S9Ø–S99 Injuries to the ankle and toes. Each injury section by anatomic site is then further organized by type of injury, beginning with minor injuries, then progressing in severity.

The primary axis of classification for code sections SØØ–S99 is organized anatomically (ICD-10-CM) instead of by the type of injury (ICD-9-CM). ICD-9-CM subchapters designate anatomic site, whereas ICD-10-CM classifies the body region as primary, with code categories that further specify the type of injury. For example:

ICD-9-CM

Chapter 17. Injury and Poisoning (8ØØ–999)

Fractures (8ØØ–829)
Fracture of Skull (8ØØ–8Ø4)

ICD-10-CM

Chapter 19. Injury, Poisoning and Certain Other Consequences of External Causes (SØØ–T88)

Injuries to head (SØØ–SØ9)

SØØ   **Superficial injury of head**

In ICD-9-CM, "Fractures" is the first subchapter in the injury and poisoning chapter. The secondary axis of classification is affected anatomic site, (e.g., vault of skull, base of skull). In ICD-10-CM, the first subchapter axis of classification is for injuries to the head (the body region), with the subsequent axis of type of injury (e.g., superficial injury of head, open wound of head). Note how the code categories generally progress from minor to major in severity within these ICD-10-CM code blocks.

ICD-9-CM

Chapter 17. Injury and Poisoning (8ØØ–999)

Fracture of Skull (8ØØ–8Ø4)

8ØØ   **Fracture of vault of skull**

8Ø1   **Fracture of base of skull**

8Ø2   **Fracture of face bones**

| 803 | Other and unqualified skull fractures |
| 804 | Multiple fractures involving skull or face with other bones |

ICD-10-CM

Chapter 19. Injury, Poisoning and Certain Other Consequences of External Causes (S00–T88)

Injuries to the Head (S00–S09)

S00	Superficial injury of head
S01	Open wound of head
S02	Fracture of skull and facial bones
S03	Dislocation and sprain of joints and ligaments of head
S04	Injury of cranial nerve
S05	Injury of eye and orbit
S06	Intracranial injury
S07	Crushing injury of head
S08	Avulsion and traumatic amputation of part of head
S09	Other and unspecified injuries of head

ICD-10-CM further enhances this restructuring by adding characters to designate laterality and severity. Seventh characters report expanded types of injury (where applicable), associated complications, and status of the encounter. For example:

- Seventh characters indicate complications and status of encounter:

| S42 | Fracture of shoulder and upper arm |

> The appropriate 7th character is to be added to all codes from category S42.
>
> | A | initial encounter for closed fracture |
> | B | initial encounter for open fracture |
> | D | subsequent encounter for fracture with routine healing |
> | G | subsequent encounter for fracture with delayed healing |
> | K | subsequent encounter for fracture with nonunion |
> | P | subsequent encounter for fracture with malunion |
> | S | sequela |

- Expanded classifications that include laterality and severity (displaced vs. nondisplaced):

S42.021	Displaced fracture of shaft of right clavicle
S42.022	Displaced fracture of shaft of left clavicle
S42.023	Displaced fracture of shaft of unspecified clavicle
S42.024	Nondisplaced fracture of shaft of right clavicle
S42.025	Nondisplaced fracture of shaft of left clavicle
S42.026	Nondisplaced fracture of shaft of unspecified clavicle

Category Title Changes

A number of category title revisions were made in chapter 19 due to the restructuring described above. Titles were changed to better reflect categorical content, which was often necessary when specific types of injury or other conditions were given their own block, a new category was created, or an existing category was redefined. For example, frostbite is classified to a unique code block consisting of the three-character categories T33–T34. Severity is built into the code structure, in that category T33 classifies superficial frostbite, whereas category T34 classifies frostbite with tissue necrosis. These categories include expanded subcategories and classification codes that specify the affected anatomic site and laterality, where applicable. Furthermore, these diagnosis codes have been expanded in structure from four-character subclassification codes to seven-character codes. The required seventh character reports status of encounter (e.g., initial, subsequent, sequelae). Note the category title changes that have occurred as a result of this expansion. For example:

ICD-9-CM

Chapter 17. Injury and Poisoning

Other and Unspecified Effects of External Causes (990–995)

991 **Effects of reduced temperature**
- **991.0** **Frostbite of face**
- **991.1** **Frostbite of hand**
- **991.2** **Frostbite of foot**
- **991.3** **Frostbite of other and unspecified sites**

ICD-10-CM

Chapter 19. Injury, Poisoning and Certain Other Consequences of External Causes

Frostbite (T33–T34)

T33 **Superficial frostbite**

> The appropriate 7th character is to be added to each code from T33.
> - **A** **initial encounter**
> - **B** **subsequent encounter**
> - **S** **sequelae**

- **T33.0** **Superficial frostbite of head**
    - **T33.01** **Superficial frostbite of ear**
        - **T33.011** **Superficial frostbite of right ear**
        - **T33.012** **Superficial frostbite of left ear**
        - **T33.019** **Superficial frostbite of unspecified ear**
    - **T33.02** **Superficial frostbite of nose**
    - **T33.09** **Superficial frostbite of other part of head**

T34 **Frostbite with tissue necrosis**

> The appropriate 7th character is to be added to each code from T34.
> - **A** **initial encounter**
> - **B** **subsequent encounter**
> - **S** **sequelae**

- **T34.0** **Frostbite with tissue necrosis of head**
    - **T34.01** **Frostbite with tissue necrosis of ear**
        - **T34.011** **Frostbite with tissue necrosis of right ear**
        - **T34.012** **Frostbite with tissue necrosis of left ear**
        - **T34.019** **Frostbite with tissue necrosis of unspecified ear**
    - **T34.02** **Frostbite with tissue necrosis of nose**
    - **T34.09** **Frostbite with tissue necrosis of other part of head**

 KEY POINT

Chapter 19 classifies injuries related to single body systems to the S section, whereas the T section is used to classify injuries to unspecified and multiple body regions, as well as poisoning, burns, and certain other consequences of external causes.

Organizational Adjustments

When comparing ICD-9-CM to ICD-10-CM, many codes have been added, deleted, combined, or moved. For example, the code for cataract fragments in the eye following cataract surgery is found in the injury and poisoning chapter in ICD-9-CM. However, these conditions have been reclassified in ICD-10-CM to chapter 7, "Diseases of the Eye and Adnexa," as many postoperative complication codes have been moved to complication-specific code categories at the end of the individual body system chapters.

ICD-9-CM

Chapter 17. Injury and Poisoning (800–999)

Other and Unspecified Effects of External Causes (990–995)

998   Other complications of procedures, not elsewhere classified

     998.8   Other complications of procedures, not elsewhere classified

         998.82   Cataract fragments in eye following cataract surgery

ICD-10-CM

Chapter 7. Diseases of the Eye and Adnexa (H00–H59)

Other disorders of eye and adnexa (H55–H59)

H59   Intraoperative and postprocedural complications and disorder of eye and adnexa, not elsewhere classified

     H59.0   Disorders of the eye following cataract surgery

         H59.02   Cataract (lens) fragments in eye following cataract surgery

             H59.021   Cataract (lens) fragments in eye following cataract surgery, right eye

             H59.022   Cataract (lens) fragments in eye following cataract surgery, left eye

             H59.023   Cataract (lens) fragments in eye following cataract surgery, bilateral

             H59.029   Cataract (lens) fragments in eye following cataract surgery, unspecified eye

ICD-10-CM provides an exponentially increased level of specificity than ICD-9-CM; however, certain conditions have been reclassified to nonspecific residual subcategories. For example, note that the specific code for nonhealing surgical wound has been deleted in ICD-10-CM. At the time of this publication, this condition is classified to the residual subcategory for other complications of procedures, not elsewhere classified.

ICD-9-CM

998.83   Non-healing surgical wound

ICD-10-CM

T81.89XA   Other complications of procedures, not elsewhere classified, initial encounter

T81.89XD   Other complications of procedures, not elsewhere classified, subsequent encounter

T81.89XS   Other complications of procedures, not elsewhere classified, sequela

In the example above, a placeholder "X" is required to fill the sixth-character position when the code is not a full six characters in length, yet a seventh character is required. When a seventh character is required, it must always be populated in the seventh character data field.

Complications

In ICD-10-CM, many postoperative complications have been moved to complication-specific code categories at the end of the individual body system chapters. However, chapter 19 includes categories T80–T88, which include codes that report complications of surgical and medical care, not elsewhere classified. Instructional notes appear at the beginning of the code block which prompts the coder to use an additional code to specify the condition resulting from the complication and to identify devices and circumstances involved, as appropriate. This code block lists multiple Excludes 2 conditions. An Excludes 2 note indicates that it may be acceptable to use an applicable code(s) together with the excluded codes if supported by the medical documentation.

Complications of surgical and medical care, not elsewhere classified (T80–T88)

Use additional code for adverse effect, if applicable, to identify drug (T36–T50 with fifth or sixth character 5)

Use additional code(s) to identify the specified condition resulting from the complication

Use additional code (Y62–Y82) to identify devices involved and details of circumstances

EXCLUDES 2 *any encounters with medical care for postprocedural conditions in which no complications are present, such as:*
> *artificial opening status (Z93.-)*
> *closure of external stoma (Z43.-)*
> *fitting and adjustment of external prosthetic device (Z44.-)*
> *burns and corrosions from local applications and irradiation (T20–T32)*
> *complications of surgical procedures during pregnancy, childbirth and the puerperium (O00–O9A)*
> *mechanical complication of respirator [ventilator] (J95.850)*
> *poisoning and toxic effects of drugs and chemicals (T36–T65 with final characters 1–4 or 6)*
> *postprocedural fever (R50.82)*
> *specified complications classified elsewhere, such as:*
>> *cerebrospinal fluid leak from spinal puncture (G97.0)*
>> *colostomy malfunction (K94.0-)*
>> *disorders of fluid and electrolyte imbalance (E86–E87)*
>> *functional disturbances following cardiac surgery (I97.0–I97.1)*
>> *intraoperative and postprocedural complications of specified body systems (D78.-, E36.-, E89.-, G97.3-, G97.4, H59.3-, H59.-, H95.2-, H95.3, I97.4-, I97.5, J95.6-, J95.7, K91.6-, L76.-, M96.-, N99.-)*
>> *ostomy complications (J95.0-, K94.-, N99.5-)*
>> *postgastric surgery syndromes (K91.1)*
>> *postlaminectomy syndrome NEC (M96.1)*
>> *postmastectomy lymphedema syndrome (I97.2)*
>> *postsurgical blind-loop syndrome (K91.2)*
>> *ventilator associated pneumonia (J95.851)*

Chapter 19 Coding Guidance

Official Guidelines and Conventions

In general, coding advice as published in the "ICD-10-CM Draft Official Guidelines for Coding and Reporting" parallels that of ICD-9-CM, except where the changes in the classification have resulted in revision of the guidelines. Many underlying concepts, however, remain similar. Key concepts include:

- Burns and corrosions:
  - When reporting multiple burns, sequence first the burn of highest severity.
  - When reporting both internal and external burns, the circumstances of admission govern sequencing.
  - When reporting burns and other related conditions, the circumstances of admission govern sequencing.
  - The "rule of nines" is used when assigning codes for extent of body surface involved (T31, T32).
- Complications of care:
  - Code assignment is based on the provider's documentation of the relationship between the condition and the procedure.
  - Two codes are required to report transplant complications: the appropriate subcategory T86 code followed by a secondary code that identifies the complication.
    - A subcategory T86.1 code should not be assigned for post-kidney transplant patients with CKD, unless the transplant complication (failure, rejection) is documented.
- Injury and fracture:
  - A fracture not specified as open or closed should be coded as closed.
  - Separate codes for injuries or fractures (by type, site, etc.) should be assigned unless a combination code is available. If a combination code is available that completely satisfies the diagnostic statement, assign the combination code.
  - Do not assign a code for unspecified multiple injuries or fractures if information for more specific code assignment is available.
  - Sequence the most serious injury or fracture first, as determined by the provider and focus of treatment.
  - Care for complications of surgical treatment for fracture repair during the healing or recovery phase should be reported with the appropriate complication codes.
  - Report the appropriate category M80 code for patients with known osteoporosis who suffer a fracture due to trauma that would not typically cause a break in a normal, healthy bone.
- Poisoning:
  - Poisoning by and adverse effects of drugs (also medicaments and biological substances)are defined as follows:

- Poisoning—includes overdose of substances and wrong substance given or taken in error, (also includes interactions of drug and alcohol). Sequence first the chapter 19 combination code that includes the causal substance and intent. Use additional codes to report manifestations. Code also any substance abuse or dependence, if documented.

- Adverse effect—includes hypersensitivity or other adverse reaction to correct substances properly administered. Sequence first the condition which reports the nature of the adverse effect. The chapter 19 code that reports the causal substance and intent should have a fifth or sixth character 5.

— When no intent of poisoning is indicated, code to "accidental."

— Undetermined intent is only for use when there is specific documentation in the record that the intent cannot be determined. Do not assume "undetermined intent."

— Assign as many codes as necessary to report all the causal substances involved.

— Report toxic effect codes T51–T65 for ingestion or contact with harmful substances. Intent is incorporated into the classification categories.

Chapter 19 Coding Concepts

Coding concepts unique to ICD-10-CM chapter 19 include:

- Abuse, neglect and other maltreatment:

  — Sequence first the category T74.- (confirmed) or T76.- (suspected) code, as appropriate, followed by additional codes to identify injury as supported by the documentation or diagnostic statement. For example:

    Diagnosis: Multiple contusions of buttock and lower back, suspected child abuse, subsequent encounter

    T76.12XD   Child physical abuse, suspected

    S3Ø.ØXXD   Contusion of lower back and pelvis, subsequent encounter

  - Report the appropriate external cause (X92–YØ8) and perpetrator (Y07) codes for cases of confirmed abuse or neglect.

  - Report suspected abuse, neglect, or mistreatment ruled out during an encounter with codes ZØ4.71 (adult) or ZØ4.72 (child). Report suspected sexual abuse ruled out during an encounter with codes Z04.41 (adult) and Z04.42 (child). Do not report a category T76 code in these circumstances.

- Burns and corrosions:

  — ICD-10-CM distinguishes between burns and corrosions, yet the guidelines for burns and corrosions apply to both conditions.

    - Burns—includes thermal burns (except sunburn) that are caused by a heat source, including electricity and radiation

    - Corrosions—burns due to chemicals. Corrosions require toxic effect codes from categories T51–T65 to report the chemical and intent of injury. Sequence the toxic effect code first, followed by the corrosion code (by degree of burn) and the total body surface code. For example:

T20.6   Corrosion of second degree of head, face and neck
Code first (T51–T65) to identify chemical and intent
Use additional external cause code to identify place (Y92)

Diagnosis: Accidental hydrochloric acid splash with a small (<10 percent area) second-degree corrosion of chin, initial encounter, factory worker, occupational injury

T54.2X1A Toxic effect of corrosive acids and acid-like substances, accidental (unintentional) initial encounter

T20.63XA Corrosion of second degree of chin, initial encounter

T32.0   Corrosions involving less than 10% of body surface

Y92.63   Factory as the place of occurrence of the external cause

Y99.0   Civilian activity done for income or pay

In the example above, a category Y93 activity code should be assigned to report the activity of the patient at the time of injury. However, since the activity is unknown, it is inappropriate to assign Y93.9 Unspecified activity.

See chapter 20, "External Causes of Morbidity" for detailed instruction regarding assignment of external cause codes V00–Y99.

- Complications of care:

  - Certain intraoperative and postprocedural complication codes have been reclassified to the specific body system chapters. When reporting one of these codes, the complication code should be sequenced first, followed by an additional code(s) for the specific complication(s).

  - Pain associated with medical devices, implants, or grafts left in a surgical site is reported with the appropriate chapter 19 T-section code. Use additional codes to report the pain: G89.18 (acute) or G89.28 (chronic). For example:

    Diagnosis: Chronic pain due to internal joint prosthesis, left knee, subsequent encounter

    T84.84XD Pain due internal orthopedic prosthetic devices, implants and grafts, subsequent encounter

    G89.28   Other chronic postprocedural pain

  - When a complication of care code is a combination code that represents the nature of the complication and type of procedure that caused the complication, report only the combination code. No additional external cause code is necessary to indicate the type of procedure.

- Injury and fracture:

  - Care for complications of fractures (e.g., malunions, nonunion) are reported with the appropriate seventh characters for subsequent care of fracture. For example:

    S59.012K Salter-Harris Type I physeal fracture of the lower end of ulna, left arm, subsequent encounter for fracture with nonunion

  - A fracture not specified as displaced or nondisplaced should be coded to displaced.

  - Aftercare Z codes should not be reported for aftercare of injuries. Instead, report the acute injury code with the seventh character "D" for subsequent encounter.

- Poisoning:

  - Combination code in categories T36–T65 include the substances related to the conditions as well as the external cause (intent). No additional external cause code is required unless associated with other injury, status, or circumstances.

  - Underdosing is defined as taking less of a medication that is prescribed or instructed by the manufacturer, whether inadvertently or deliberately.

    - Underdosing codes should never be assigned as principal or first-listed codes. Sequence the medical condition first.

    - Report noncompliance or complication of care codes, as appropriate to indicate intent. For example:

      Diagnosis: Intractable epilepsy, subtherapeutic Dilantin levels due to noncompliance, initial encounter. The patient is suddenly refusing medication for stated religious reasons.

      G40.919 Epilepsy, unspecified, intractable, without status epilepticus

      T42.0X6A Underdosing of hydantoin derivatives, initial encounter

      Z91.128 Patient's intentional underdosing of medication regimen for other reason

Refer to the "ICD-10-CM Draft Official Guidelines for Coding and Reporting" in appendix A of this book for additional information.

Combination Codes

Certain injury classifications have been expanded in ICD-10-CM by use of combination codes, which facilitate reporting of both the injury and any associated complications, conditions, manifestations, intent, or other external factors within a single code. As such, code to the highest level of specificity as documented in the record. For example:

- Combination codes that identify causal substance, intent, and status of encounter in a single code.

  Note that these conditions previously required two codes to report: the poisoning code followed by an external cause (E code). The status of encounter (seventh character) was not included in the ICD-9-CM classifications in the same manner (exception: late effects).

ICD-9-CM		ICD-10-CM	
969.72	Poisoning by amphetamines	T43.621A	Poisoning by amphetamines, accidental (unintentional), initial encounter
		T43.621D	Poisoning by amphetamines, accidental (unintentional), subsequent encounter
		T43.621S	Poisoning by amphetamines, accidental (unintentional), sequela
		T43.622A	Poisoning by amphetamines, intentional self-harm, initial encounter
		T43.622D	Poisoning by amphetamines, intentional self-harm, subsequent encounter
		T43.622S	Poisoning by amphetamines, intentional self-harm, sequela
		T43.623A	Poisoning by amphetamines, assault, initial encounter
		T43.623D	Poisoning by amphetamines, assault, subsequent encounter
		T43.623S	Poisoning by amphetamines, assault, sequela
		T43.624A	Poisoning by amphetamines, undetermined, initial encounter
		T43.624D	Poisoning by amphetamines, undetermined, subsequent encounter
		T43.624S	Poisoning by amphetamines, undetermined, sequela

- Combination codes that identify specific complications.

Note that these conditions previously required two codes to report: the complication code followed by a specific code from other chapters to identify the complication. The status of encounter (seventh character) was not included in the ICD-9-CM classifications in the same manner (exception: late effects).

ICD-9-CM		ICD-10-CM	
996.71	Other complications, due to heart valve prosthesis	T82.817	Embolism of cardiac prosthetic devices, implants and grafts
		T82.818	Embolism of vascular prosthetic devices, implants and grafts
		T82.827	Fibrosis of cardiac prosthetic devices, implants and grafts
		T82.828	Fibrosis of vascular prosthetic devices, implants and grafts
		T82.837	Hemorrhage of cardiac prosthetic devices, implants and grafts
		T82.838	Hemorrhage of vascular prosthetic devices, implants and grafts
		T82.847	Pain from cardiac prosthetic devices, implants and grafts
		T82.848	Pain from vascular prosthetic devices, implants and grafts
		T82.857	Stenosis of cardiac prosthetic devices, implants and grafts,
		T82.858	Stenosis of vascular prosthetic devices, implants and grafts
		T82.867	Thrombosis of cardiac prosthetic devices, implants and grafts
		T82.868	Thrombosis of vascular prosthetic devices, implants and grafts
		The appropriate 7th character is to be added to each code from category T82.	
		A	initial encounter
		D	subsequent encounter
		S	sequela

Level of Detail in Coding

As in ICD-9-CM, diagnosis codes are to be used and reported to the highest level of specificity available. ICD-10-CM provides, in the majority of cases, an exponentially increased level of specificity than ICD-9-CM. In chapter 19, this code expansion is intended to facilitate identification of specific anatomic sites, laterality of paired sites and organs, and types or causes of injury. Many of these changes are intended to provide the refined data necessary to support epidemiology and research efforts and improve patient outcomes initiatives. Additionally, some changes have been made in accordance with updates to currently applicable clinical terminology. As such, new ICD-10-CM codes have been created for specific anatomic sites or types of injuries not previously identifiable with unique codes in ICD-9-CM. For example:

- Anatomic site and laterality specificity:

ICD-9-CM		ICD-10-CM	
842.13	Sprain and strain of interphalangeal joint	S63.621	Sprain of interphalangeal joint of right thumb
		S63.622	Sprain of interphalangeal joint of left thumb
		S63.629	Sprain of interphalangeal joint of unspecified thumb
		S63.630	Sprain of interphalangeal joint of right index finger
		S63.631	Sprain of interphalangeal joint of left index finger
		S63.632	Sprain of interphalangeal joint of right middle finger
		S63.633	Sprain of interphalangeal joint of left middle finger
		S63.634	Sprain of interphalangeal joint of right ring finger
		S63.635	Sprain of interphalangeal joint of left ring finger
		S63.636	Sprain of interphalangeal joint of right little finger
		S63.637	Sprain of interphalangeal joint of left little finger
		S63.638	Sprain of interphalangeal joint of other finger
		S63.639	Sprain of interphalangeal joint of unspecified finger
		The appropriate 7th character is to be added to each code from category S63.	
		A	initial encounter
		D	subsequent encounter
		S	sequela

- Type of injury:

  Note that in this example, the anatomic site is less specific than ICD-9-CM. Classifications for uncomplicated open wound of the nasal cavity, sinus, and septum are included in the anatomic site "nose" in ICD-10-CM. Instead, the type of open wound is specified as laceration, puncture, open bite, or unspecified open wound. ICD-9-CM required a separate external cause code to report the type of bite (e.g., human, animal) to identify the open wound specifically as a bite. For example:

Diagnosis: Open wound of nose, dog bite

ICD-9-CM

873.22	**Open wound of nasal cavity without mention of complication**
E906.0	**Dog bite**

ICD-10-CM

The external cause (nonvenomous animal bite) is also reportable in ICD-10-CM from code block W50–W64 Exposure to animate mechanical forces. The instructional note at the beginning of chapter 19 prompts the use of secondary chapter 20 codes to indicate the cause of injury where not included in the code description.

Since two codes are still required to report an open (dog) bite wound of the nose, this represents a code refinement, not the creation of a combination code, per se. For example:

> The appropriate 7th character is to be added to each code from category S63.
>
> **A   initial encounter**
> **D   subsequent encounter**
> **S   sequela**

S01.25	**Open bite of nose**

Complete code assignment (one of the following would be assigned, depending on the episode of encounter):

S01.25XA	**Open bite of nose, initial encounter**
S01.25XD	**Open bite of nose, subsequent encounter**
S01.25XS	**Open bite of nose, sequela**

> The appropriate 7th character is to be added to each code from category W54.
>
> **A   initial encounter**
> **D   subsequent encounter**
> **S   sequela**

W54.0	**Bitten by dog**

Complete code assignment (one of the following would be assigned, depending on the episode of encounter):

W54.0XXA	**Bitten by dog, initial encounter**
W54.0XXD	**Bitten by dog, subsequent encounter**
W54.0XXS	**Bitten by dog, sequela**

In the example above, a placeholder "X" is required to fill fifth- and sixth-character positions when the code is not a full six characters in length, and yet a seventh character is required. The seventh character is always required in the seventh-character position within a valid code.

Multiple Coding

ICD-10-CM chapter 19 contains a wide range of injuries, poisoning, effects of other external causes, and certain complications of trauma, procedures, and medical care. This chapter includes many notes which prompt the assignment of additional codes to report certain external causes, effects, or other specific associated conditions. Instructional notes appear throughout the text to provide sequencing instruction when more than one code is necessary to report a diagnosis in its entirety.

Such diagnostic coding can be complex in nature, often requiring multiple codes in a specific sequence. As such, chapter 19 contains multiple instructional notes which are essential to ensuring correct coding practices. Optum's *ICD-10-CM—The Complete Official Draft Code Set* highlights these crucial coding instructions in red font for ease of reference. These notes appear at the section, category, subcategory and individual code levels throughout the tabular list.

Code First/Use Additional Code

These notes direct the coder that although certain conditions may occur independently of each other, multiple codes may be necessary to report associated conditions or designate underlying cause, as appropriate. For example:

- Code first:

  S04   Injury of cranial nerve
  Code first any associated intracranial injury (S06.-)

- Use additional code:

  T84.6 Infection and inflammatory reaction due to internal fixation device
  Use additional code to identify infection

Code Also

This note alerts the coder that more than one code may be necessary to report the condition in its entirety. Code sequencing is discretionary. Factors that may determine sequencing include severity and reason for the encounter. For example:

S84   Injury of nerves at lower leg level
Code also any associated open wound (S81.-)

Diagnosis: Open wound, right lower leg with injury of tibial nerve, initial encounter

S84.01XA Injury of tibial nerve at lower leg level, right leg, initial encounter

S81.812A Laceration without foreign body, right lower leg, initial encounter

Chapter 19 Coding Exercises

Assign the appropriate ICD-10-CM diagnosis codes for all reportable diagnoses. Assign external causes of morbidity (V00–Y99) codes, where applicable, as prompted by the text.

Answers to coding exercises are listed in the back of the book.

1. Bimalleolar fracture of the right ankle, initial encounter_____
    _____

2. Aftercare of nondisplaced fracture of left femoral epiphysis, with delayed healing_____
    _____

3. Whiplash, initial encounter_____

_____

4. Puncture wound with nail embedded in plantar aspect of foot, initial encounter _____

_____

5. Acute toxic hepatitis and convulsions due to suicide attempt by overdose of acetaminophen _____

_____

6. Displacement of right shoulder prosthesis, subsequent encounter _____

_____

Chapter 19 Coding Scenarios

Assign the appropriate ICD-10-CM diagnosis codes for all reportable diagnoses. Assign external causes of morbidity (VØØ–Y99) codes, where applicable, as prompted by the text.

Answers to coding exercises are listed in the back of the book.

1. A patient presents with an infected wound of the right palm with cellulitis of the hand. The patient was working in the field of the family farm two days prior, when she accidentally cut her hand on barbed wire.

_____

_____

2. A patient with sickle-cell anemia develops tachycardia, tachypnea, and hypotension following blood transfusion. The transfusion was aborted. The patient was placed on IV saline, furosemide, and low-dose dopamine to improve renal support and prevent shock due to acute hemolytic transfusion reaction. Donor blood was re-typed and crossed, resulting in identification of ABO incompatibility clerical error at the blood bank, resulting in mislabeling.

_____

_____

3. An intoxicated, shirtless 25-year-old male presents after contact with flare of flames from the gas barbecue grill in his yard resulted in multiple first- and second-degree burns to the face and neck and multiple sites of upper extremities, including both hands and wrists, with approximately 25 percent of body area affected. Blood alcohol level measured 0.025% = 25 mg/100 ml.

_____

_____

Chapter 20. External Causes of Morbidity (VØØ-Y99)

Chapter 20 contains 29 code families with the first characters of "V," "W," "X," and "Y." The coding families classified to chapter 20 are:

VØØ–VØ9	Pedestrian injured in transport accident
V1Ø–V19	Pedal cycle rider injured in transport accident
V2Ø–V29	Motorcycle rider injured in transport accident
V3Ø–V39	Occupant of three-wheeled motor vehicle injured in transport accident
V4Ø–V49	Car occupant injured in transport accident
V5Ø–V59	Occupant of pick-up truck or van injured in transport accident
V6Ø–V69	Occupant of heavy transport vehicle injured in transport accident
V7Ø–V79	Bus occupant injured in transport accident
V8Ø–V89	Other land transport accidents
V9Ø–V94	Water transport accidents
V95–V97	Air and space transport accidents
V98–V99	Other and unspecified transport accidents
WØØ–W19	Slipping, tripping, stumbling and falls
W2Ø–W49	Exposure to inanimate mechanical forces
W5Ø–W64	Exposure to animate mechanical forces
W65–W74	Accidental non-transport drowning and submersion
W85–W99	Exposure to electric current, radiation and extreme ambient air temperature and pressure
XØØ–XØ8	Exposure to smoke, fire and flames
X1Ø–X19	Contact with heat and hot substances
X3Ø–X39	Exposure to forces of nature
X52–X58	Accidental exposure to other specified factors
X71–X83	Intentional self-harm
X92–YØ9	Assault
Y21–Y33	Event of undetermined intent
Y35–Y38	Legal intervention, operations of war, military operation, and terrorism
Y62–Y69	Misadventures to patients during surgical and medical care
Y7Ø–Y82	Medical devices associated with adverse incidents in diagnostic and therapeutic use
Y83–Y84	Surgical and other medical procedures as the cause of abnormal reaction of the patient, or of later complication, without mention of misadventure at the time of the procedure
Y9Ø–Y99	Supplementary factors related to causes of morbidity classified elsewhere

 KEY POINT

Where multiple sites of injury are specified in the titles, the word "with" indicates involvement of both sites, and the word "and" indicates involvement of either or both sites.

Although chapter 20 codes may be used to report the circumstances of any health care condition in the ICD-10-CM range of AØØ.Ø–T88.9 and ZØØ–Z99, external cause codes are intended to provide data for injury research and evaluation of injury prevention strategies. The cause, intent, place of occurrence, and the patient's status (e.g., civilian or military) are part of the environmental event and circumstance data which describes the cause of injury or other adverse effects. An instructional note at the beginning of this chapter declares that these codes are intended to be reported as additional (secondary) codes to explain the external causes of conditions classifiable to other chapters (1–18); however, they are most commonly reported in addition to chapter 19 Injury, poisoning and certain other consequences of external causes (S00–T88) codes.

ICD-10-CM Category Restructuring

In ICD-9-CM, the supplementary classification of external causes of injury and poisoning (E codes) is organized as the last chapter of the tabular list. In ICD-10-CM, these codes follow chapter 19, "Injury, Poisoning and Certain Other Consequences of External Causes," and precede the final chapter, chapter 20, "Factors Influencing Health Status and Contact with Health Services." In addition, the transport accident section has been completely revised and extended, with blocks of categories identifying the victim's mode of transport.

It is also important to note that after the tragic events of September 11, 2001, the National Center for Health Statistics (NCHS) recognized the need for classification codes to report health conditions related to acts of terrorism. NCHS developed a set of codes within the framework of ICD-10, the classification presently used for mortality reporting, and ICD-9-CM, used for morbidity, to facilitate reporting of these circumstances when they result in illness, injury, or other health care intervention. Terrorism-specific external cause codes (E codes) were introduced into ICD-9-CM in 2002.

ICD-9-CM

In ICD-9-CM, the main axis is whether the event is a traffic or nontraffic accident.

Supplementary Classification of External Causes of Injury and Poisoning (E800–E999)

E800–E807	Railway Accidents
E810–E819	Motor Vehicle Traffic Accidents
E820–E825	Motor Vehicle Nontraffic Accidents
E826–E829	Other Road Vehicle Accidents

ICD-10-CM

In ICD-10-CM, the main axis is the injured person's mode of transport. For land transport accidents (categories V01–V89), the vehicle of which the injured person is an occupant is identified in the first two characters as it is considered an essential issue for prevention purposes.

External Causes of Morbidity (V00–Y99)

V00–V99	Transport accidents
V00–V09	Pedestrian injured in transport accident
V10–V19	Pedal cycle rider injured in transport accident
V20–V29	Motorcycle rider injured in transport accident
V30–V39	Occupant of three-wheeled motor vehicle injured in transport accident
V40–V49	Car occupant injured in transport accident
V50–V59	Occupant of pick-up truck or van injured in transport accident
V60–V69	Occupant of heavy transport vehicle injured in transport accident
V70–V79	Bus occupant injured in transport accident
V80–V89	Other land transport accidents
V90–V94	Water transport accidents

KEY POINT

This chapter, which in previous revisions of ICD constituted a supplementary classification, permits the classification of environmental events and circumstances as the cause of injury, poisoning, and other adverse effects. When a code from this section is applicable, it is to be sequenced in addition to a code from other sections of the classification when indicating the nature of the condition.

KEY POINT

In ICD-10-CM, sequelae of external cause is indicated by using the seventh character "S":

V95.01XS	Helicopter crash injuring occupant, sequelae
W23.0XXS	Caught, crushed, jammed, or pinched between moving objects, sequelae
X15.0XXS	Contact with hot stove (kitchen), sequelae
X76.XXXS	Intentional self-harm by smoke, fire and flames, sequelae
Y28.0XXS	Contact with sharp glass, undetermined intent, sequelae

CODING AXIOM

ICD-10-CM uses a placeholder character "X" as a fifth- or sixth-character placeholder in certain codes to allow for future expansion. Where a placeholder exists, the X must be used for the code to be considered a valid code.

| V95–V97 | Air and space transport accidents |
| V98–V99 | Other and unspecified transport accidents |

Category Title Changes

A number of category title revisions were made in chapter 20. Titles were changed to better reflect categorical content, which was often necessary when specific types of diseases were given their own block, a new category was created, or an existing category was redefined.

ICD-9-CM

| E917 | Striking against or struck accidentally by objects or persons |

ICD-10-CM

W21	Striking against or struck by sports equipment
W22	Striking against or struck by other objects
W50	Accidental hit, strike, kick, twist, bite or scratch by another person
W51	Accidental striking against or bumped into by another person
W52	Crushed, pushed or stepped on by crowd or human stampede

Organizational Adjustments

When comparing ICD-9-CM to ICD-10-CM, some codes have been added, deleted, combined, or moved. For example, the late effect codes for external causes are located in various subchapters throughout the supplementary classification in ICD-9-CM. However, in ICD-10-CM, late effects of external causes (e.g., accidents, suicide) can be classified as such by reporting the seventh character for sequela (S), where applicable.

ICD-9-CM

E929	Late effects of accidental injury
E959	Late effects of self-inflicted injury
E969	Late effects of injury purposely inflicted by other person
E977	Late effects of injuries due to legal intervention
E989	Late effects of injury, undetermined whether accidentally or purposely inflicted
E999	Late effect of injury due to war operations and terrorism

ICD-10-CM

V00.02XS	Pedestrian on foot injured in collision with skateboarder, sequelae
W50.4XXS	Accidental scratch by another person, sequelae
X71.0XXS	Intentional self-harm by drowning and submersion while in bathtub, sequelae
Y02.8XXS	Assault by pushing or placing victim in front of other moving object, sequelae
Y24.8XXS	Other firearm discharge, undetermined intent, sequelae

The external cause codes which classify the accidental circumstances of poisoning by drugs, medicinal substances, and biologicals (E850–E858) and by other solid and liquid substances, gases, and vapors (E860–E869), have been reclassified in ICD-9-CM to chapter 19, "Injury, Poisoning and Certain Other Consequences of External Causes." The specific substance is identified as part of the combination code from the T36–T50 range for poisoning by and adverse

KEY POINT

Contents of this chapter are similar to the "E codes" chapter in ICD-9-CM supplementary classification. With ICD-10-CM, there are four alphabetic characters (V, W, X, and Y) that make up the next-to-last chapter of the classification.

effects of drugs, medicaments, and biological substances, or the T51–T65 range for toxic effects of substances chiefly nonmedicinal, which reports the equivalent of both the poisoning or toxic effect (injury codes), and the circumstances or intent of the external cause (E codes). Note that these conditions required two separate codes to report in ICD-9-CM, whereas ICD-10-CM uses single combination codes. For example:

ICD-9-CM

Two codes required:

960.9   **Poisoning by antibiotics, unspecified antibiotic**

E856   **Accidental poisoning by antibiotics**

Two codes required:

980.3   **Toxic effect of fusel oil**

E860.4   **Accidental poisoning by fusel oil**

ICD-10-CM

One combination code:

T36.0X1A   **Poisoning by penicillins, accidental (unintentional), initial encounter**

One combination code:

T51.3X1A   **Toxic effect of fusel oil, accidental (unintentional), initial encounter**

There is no specific code in ICD-9-CM for exposure to radon. However, a code has been added to ICD-10-CM to classify this health risk factor, used with seventh characters to identify initial encounter, subsequent encounter, and sequelae.

ICD-10-CM

X39.01XA   **Exposure to radon, initial encounter**

X39.01XD   **Exposure to radon, subsequent encounter**

X39.01XS   **Exposure to radon, sequelae**

Chapter 20 Coding Guidance

Official Guidelines and Conventions

In general, coding advice as published in the "ICD-10-CM Draft Official Guidelines for Coding and Reporting" parallels that of ICD-9-CM, except where the changes in the classification have resulted in revision of the guidelines. Many underlying concepts, however, remain similar. Key concepts include:

- An external cause code can never be a first-listed or principal diagnosis, and cannot be reported alone, without a diagnosis for the resulting injury or condition.

- Use the Alphabetic Index of External Causes and instructions in the tabular list to ensure accurate assignment of external cause codes.

- A chapter 20 code may be used in conjunction with any injury, disease, or other health condition code included in this classification (A00.0–T88.9, Z00–Z99) as necessary or appropriate to report the circumstances of the condition.

- Although most commonly applicable to injury, external cause codes are applicable to other healthcare conditions due to external causes. For example:

  Diagnosis: Syncope, overexertion due to running

  R55   **Syncope and collapse**

  Y93.02 Activity, running

- Report as many external cause codes as necessary to report the circumstances in its entirety.

  - Sequence first the external cause most directly related to the first-listed or principal diagnosis.

- Sequence the place of occurrence, activity, and status codes after the other main external cause codes. For example:

  Diagnosis: Initial encounter for open wound of hand due to laceration of left hand with wood carving tool during hobby-related activity in patient's garage at home

  S61.412A Laceration without foreign body of left hand, initial encounter

  W27.8XXA Contact with other nonpowered hand tool, initial encounter

  Y92.015 Private garage of single-family (private) house as the place of occurrence of the external cause

  Y93.D9   Activity, other involving arts and handcrafts

  Y99.8   Other external cause status

  - Place priority on the reporting of the external cause codes most closely related to the principal diagnosis if space prohibits reporting the entire spectrum of applicable external cause codes.

  - See official guidelines 1.C.20.f, for sequencing hierarchy of external cause codes, by type.

- If the intent of an external cause is undetermined or unspecified, assume accidental intent.

  - Undetermined intent can only be reported if it is specifically stated as such in the documentation.

- Assault external codes are applicable to report the intent of an adult or child abuse injury.

- Only one Y92 code should be reported on a medical record—on the initial encounter for treatment.

  - Category Y92 codes are to be used in conjunction with an activity code, when appropriate.

  - Do not report Y92.9 if the place of occurrence is not stated or not applicable.

- Activity codes (Y93) may be used to report activities resulting in acute injury, cumulative, long-term effects of an activity, or as additional codes to provide further information with other external cause codes. For example:

  Diagnosis: A medical transcriptionist presents with a bilateral carpal-tunnel compression syndrome due to occupational repetitive motion injury due to excessive, long-term keyboarding.

G56.01   **Carpal tunnel syndrome, right upper limb**

G56.02   **Carpal tunnel syndrome, left upper limb**

Y93.C1   **Activity, computer keyboarding**

Y99.0   **Civilian activity done for income or pay**

- Report an activity code only once, on the initial encounter for treatment.
- Do not report activity codes for poisonings, adverse effects, misadventures, or late effects.
- Do not report Y93.9 if the activity is not stated.

- External cause status codes (Y99) are assigned for use with other external cause codes to report the occupational, military, or other status of the patient at the time the injury occurred.

  - Do not report external status codes alone without other external cause codes which report cause and activity.
  - Do not report Y99.9 if the status is not stated.

- Do not report a late effect external cause code with a related current injury.

  - Report late effect external cause codes for subsequent visits in which the late effect of injury is being treated (excluding follow-up or rehabilitative care).

- The cause of an injury as terrorism must be determined by the federal government (FBI), in order to report an external cause from category Y38.

  - Do not report "suspected" terrorism as confirmed.

Chapter 20 Coding Concepts

Coding concepts unique to ICD-10-CM chapter 20 include:

- External cause codes are intended for use as secondary codes in any health care setting.

- Report an external cause code, with the appropriate seventh character, for each encounter for which the injury or condition is being treated.

- Late effects of external causes are identified by the seventh character S, sequela. For example:

Diaganosis: Police officer presents with pain and paresthesia due to right brachial plexus injury, at site of previous gunshot wound sustained while on patrol

M79.601   **Pain in right arm**

R20.2   **Paresthesia of skin**

S14.3XXS   **Injury of brachial plexus**

Y35.001S   **Legal intervention involving unspecified firearm discharge, law enforcement official injured**

Note: The activity code and place of occurrence are not assigned, as they are reported only once, at the initial encounter for treatment of the injury.

- A transport accident is defined as one in which the vehicle involved must be moving or running or in use for transport at the time of the accident.

  - Transport vehicle definitions are provided at the beginning of chapter 20.

- No external cause code is needed when the cause and intent are included in a code from anther chapter (e.g., poisonings, adverse effects of drugs).

Refer to the "ICD-10-CM Draft Official Guidelines for Coding and Reporting" in appendix A of this book for additional information.

Multiple Coding

ICD-10-CM chapter 20 contains a wide range of external causes, factors, and circumstances of injury or other health conditions. This chapter includes many notes which prompt the assignment of additional codes to report place of occurrence, activity, or other circumstances, as appropriate. Instructional notes appear throughout the text to provide sequencing instruction when more than one code is necessary to report a cause, situation, or circumstance in its entirety. External cause coding can be complex in nature, often requiring multiple codes in a specific sequence. As such, chapter 20 contains multiple instructional notes which are essential to ensuring correct coding practices. Optum's *ICD-10-CM—The Complete Official Draft Code Set* highlights these crucial coding instructions in red font for ease of reference. These notes appear at the section, category, subcategory, and individual code levels throughout the tabular list.

Code First/Use Additional Note

These notes direct the coder that although certain conditions may occur independently of each other, multiple codes may be necessary to report associated conditions or designate underlying cause, as appropriate. For example:

- Code first:

  W2Ø   Struck by thrown, projected or falling object
  Code first any associated:
  cataclysm (X34–X39)
  lightning strike (T75.ØØ)

- Use additional code:

  W21.4   Striking against diving board
  Use additional code for subsequent falling into water, if applicable (W16.-)

Chapter 20 Coding Exercises

Assign only the appropriate ICD-10-CM external cause codes (V00–Y99) based on the information provided. Assume initial encounter unless otherwise stated.

Answers to coding exercises are listed in the back of the book.

1. Cat bite _____

2. Fall from bicycle (single cyclist) on bike path _____

3. Accidental cut with paring knife, in apartment kitchen while slicing vegetables _____

4. Burn by hot liquid (oil) while working in restaurant _____

Chapter 20 Coding Scenarios

Assign the only appropriate ICD-10-CM external cause codes (V00–Y99) based on the information provided, unless otherwise noted. Assume initial encounter unless otherwise stated.

Answers to coding scenarios are listed in the back of the book.

1. Injury due to being struck by a horse while taking shelter in a barn during a tornado

2. A 17-year-old driver of a sport utility vehicle (SUV) collides with the rear end of another motor vehicle stopped at a residential traffic light while texting on her cell phone.

CHAPTER 21. FACTORS INFLUENCING HEALTH STATUS AND CONTACT WITH HEALTH SERVICES (ZØØ–Z99)

Chapter 21 contains 14 code families, with the first character "Z." The coding families classified to chapter 21 are:

ZØØ–Z13	**Persons encountering health services for examinations**
Z14–Z15	**Genetic carrier and genetic susceptibility to disease**
Z16	**Resistance to antimicrobial drugs**
Z17	**Estrogen receptor status**
Z18	**Retained foreign body fragments**
Z2Ø–Z28	**Persons with potential health hazards related to communicable diseases**
Z3Ø–Z39	**Persons encountering health services in circumstances related to reproduction**
Z4Ø–Z53	**Encounters for other specific health care**
Z55–Z65	**Persons with potential health hazards related to socioeconomic and psychosocial circumstances**
Z66	**Do not resuscitate status**
Z67	**Blood type**
Z68	**Body mass index (BMI)**
Z69–Z76	**Persons encountering health services in other circumstances**
Z77–Z99	**Persons with potential health hazards related to family and personal history and certain conditions influencing health status**

An instructional note at the beginning of chapter 21 defines the use of these codes accordingly, as:

- Reasons for encounters
- Reasons for procedures—a procedure code must accompany these codes
- Circumstances other than disease, injury, or external cause as classified to categories AØØ–Y89 that are documented as "diagnoses" or "problems"
- Encounters for health services for some specific purpose, limited care, or other problem (e.g., immunization, donation)
- Circumstances or problems which influence the patient's health status

ICD-10-CM Subchapter and Category Restructuring

In ICD-9-CM, the "Supplementary Classification of Factors Influencing Health Status and Contact with Health Services" (V codes) was organized as the next-to-last chapter in the tabular list. In ICD-10-CM, these codes follow chapter 20, "Factors Influencing Health Status and Contact with Health Services," and instead, comprise the final chapter of the classification.

Many classifications have been expanded, including personal and family history codes. Certain classifications which do not exist in ICD-9-CM have been built into the ICD-10-CM classification. For example, category Z67 identifies the patient's blood type.

Note how the following ICD-9-CM subchapter title sections show certain reorganizations when compared with the ICD-10-CM classification blocks at the beginning of chapter 21, which are listed above.

ICD-9-CM

Supplementary Classification of Factors Influencing Health Status and Contact with Health Services (VØØ–V91)

V01–V06	Persons with Potential Health Hazards Related to Communicable Disease
V07–V09	Persons with Need for Isolation, Other Potential Health Hazards and Prophylactic Measures
V10–V19	Persons with Potential Heath Hazards Related to Personal and Family History
V20–V29	Persons Encountering Health Services in Circumstances Related to Reproduction and Development
V30–V39	Liveborn Infants According to Type of Birth
V40–V49	Persons with a Condition Influencing Their Health Status
V50–V59	Persons Encountering Health Services for Specific Procedures and Aftercare
V60–V69	Persons Encountering Health Services for Other Circumstances
V70–V82	Persons without Reported Diagnosis Encountered During Examination and Investigation of Individuals and Populations
V83–V84	Genetics
V85	Body Mass Index
V86	Estrogen Receptor Status
V87	Other Specified Personal Exposures and History Presenting Hazards to Health
V88	Acquired Absence of Other Organs and Tissue
V89	Other Suspected Conditions Not Found
V90	Retained Foreign Body
V91	Multiple Gestation Placenta Status

In ICD-10-CM, certain nonspecific Z code categories have undergone classification refinement and reduction in number. Those nonspecific categories that remain are likely to be limited for use in those circumstances in which the documentation fails to support more precise coding. For example:

Z02.9	Encounter for administrative examinations, unspecified
Z04.9	Encounter for examination and observation for unspecified reason
Z13.9	Encounter for screening, unspecified
Z41.9	Encounter for procedure for purposes other than remedying health state, unspecified
Z52.9	Donor or unspecified organ or tissue
Z88.9	Allergy status to unspecified drugs, medicaments and biological substances status
Z92.0	Personal history of contraception

In ICD-9-CM, the code categories for problems related to household, economic, family, and other psychosocial circumstances are classified under the subchapter for persons encountering health services in other circumstances (V60–V69). The categories for these types of problems have been moved to code block Z55–Z65 Persons with potential health hazards related to socioeconomic and psychosocial circumstances, in ICD-10-CM. Retained foreign body status has been moved from a unique classification subchapter in

---

ICD-9-CM (V90) to code block Z18 Retained foreign body fragments, in ICD-10-CM.

Certain factors have been moved elsewhere in the classification. For example, the multiple gestation placental status has been reclassified to obstetric combination codes in ICD-10-CM category O30 Multiple gestation, within chapter 15, "Pregnancy, Childbirth and the Puerperium (O00–O9A)."

ICD-9-CM

V91.00	Twin gestation, unspecified number of placenta, unspecified number of amniotic sacs
V91.01	Twin gestation, monochorionic/monoamniotic (one placenta, one amniotic sac)
V91.02	Twin gestation, monochorionic/diamniotic (one placenta, two amniotic sacs)
V91.03	Twin gestation, dichorionic/diamniotic (two placentae, two amniotic sacs)
V91.09	Twin gestation, unable to determine number of placenta and number of amniotic sacs

ICD-10-CM

O30.001	Twin pregnancy, unspecified number of placenta and unspecified number of amniotic sacs, first trimester
O30.011	Twin pregnancy, monochorionic/monoamniotic, first trimester
O30.021	Conjoined twins, first trimester
O30.031	Twin pregnancy, monochorionic/diamniotic, first trimester
O30.041	Twin pregnancy, dichorionic/diamniotic, first trimester
O30.091	Twin pregnancy, unable to determine number of placenta and number of amniotic sacs, first trimester

Category Title Changes

A number of category title revisions were made in chapter 21. Titles were changed to better reflect the categorical content, which was often necessary when specific types of diseases were given their own block, a new category was created, or an existing category was redefined. For example:

ICD-9-CM

V60	Housing, household, and economic circumstances
V61	Other family circumstances
V62	Other psychosocial circumstances

ICD-10-CM

Z59	Problems related to housing and economic circumstance
Z60	Problems related to social environment
Z62	Problems related to upbringing
Z63	Other problems related to primary support group, including family circumstances
Z64	Problems related to certain psychosocial circumstances
Z65	Problems related to other psychosocial circumstances

📖 **DEFINITIONS**

Z codes. Used to report reasons for encounters in ICD-10-CM. A corresponding procedure code should accompany a Z code if a procedure is performed.

When comparing ICD-9-CM to ICD-10-CM, some codes have been added, deleted, combined, or moved. As such, the title revisions reflect those changes. For example, supervision of high-risk pregnancy (V23) has been moved in ICD-10-CM to chapter 15, "Pregnancy, Childbirth and the Puerperium."

ICD-9-CM

V23.0   **Pregnancy with a history of infertility**

ICD-10-CM

O09.00   **Supervision of pregnancy with history of infertility, unspecified trimester**

O09.01   **Supervision of pregnancy with history of infertility, first trimester**

O09.02   **Supervision of pregnancy with history of infertility, second trimester**

O09.03   **Supervision of pregnancy with history of infertility, third trimester**

In ICD-10-CM, orthopaedic aftercare (ICD-9-CM: V54.0–V54.9) is classified to category Z47. Aftercare for healing fracture has been eliminated from this category since fracture codes require seventh characters such as subsequent encounter (D) or sequela (S). In ICD-10-CM, the aftercare codes are not used to report aftercare of injury. Instead, the acute injury code is assigned with the appropriate seventh character.

ICD-9-CM

V54.0   **Aftercare involving internal fixation device**
V54.1   **Aftercare for healing traumatic fracture**
V54.2   **Aftercare for healing pathologic fracture**
V54.8   **Other orthopedic aftercare**
V54.9   **Unspecified orthopedic aftercare**

ICD-10-CM

Z47.1   **Aftercare following joint replacement surgery**
Z47.2   **Encounter for removal of internal fixation device**

Similarly, ICD-9-CM category V57 Care involving use of rehabilitation procedures, is not reported in the same manner in ICD-10-CM. Instead, encounters for rehabilitative therapy are reported by the underlying condition for which the therapy is being provided (e.g., injury) with the appropriate seventh character.

Chapter 21 Coding Guidance

Official Guidelines and Conventions

In general, coding advice as published in the "ICD-10-CM Draft Official Guidelines for Coding and Reporting" parallels that of ICD-9-CM, except where the changes in the classification have resulted in revision of the guidelines. Many underlying concepts, however, remain similar. Key concepts include:

- Z codes are for use in any health care setting.

- Certain Z codes report the reason for an encounter or procedure. The appropriate procedure codes must accompany a Z code to report any procedure performed.

- Z codes may be reported as the principal diagnosis in the inpatient setting, where appropriate, or as secondary diagnoses.
- Certain Z codes may only be reported as a first-listed diagnosis, yet other codes should not be reported as first-listed codes.
  - Consult the official guidelines 1.C.21.3-16 for additional, specific sequencing information.
- Categories of Z codes with specific guidelines for use and sequencing include:
  - contact/exposure
  - inoculations and vaccinations
  - status
  - history of (personal and family)
  - screening
  - observation
  - aftercare
  - follow-up
  - donor
  - counseling
  - encounters for obstetrical and reproductive services
  - newborns and infants
  - routine and administrative examinations
  - miscellaneous Z codes
  - nonspecific Z codes
  - Z codes that may only be sequenced as principal/first-listed diagnosis

Refer to the "ICD-10-CM Draft Official Guidelines for Coding and Reporting" in appendix A of this book for additional information.

Multiple Coding

ICD-10-CM chapter 21 contains a wide range of codes which represent reasons for encounters or provide additional important information about a patient's health status and the necessity for certain services or levels of care. This chapter includes many notes which prompt the coder to review the assignment of additional codes to report additional significant findings, testing, health status, and relevant historical information. Instructional notes appear throughout the text to provide sequencing instruction when more than one code is necessary to report a cause, situation, or circumstance in its entirety. Multiple codes may be necessary to report in a specific sequence. As such, chapter 21 contains multiple instructional notes which are essential to ensuring correct coding practices. Optum's *ICD-10-CM—The Complete Official Draft Code Set* highlights these crucial coding instructions in red font for ease of reference. These notes appear at the section, category, subcategory, and individual code levels throughout the tabular list.

Code First/Use Additional Code

These notes inform the coder that although certain conditions may occur independently of each other, multiple codes may be necessary to report associated conditions or designate an underlying cause, as appropriate. For example:

- Code first:

  Z16   **Resistance to antimicrobial drugs**
  Code first the infection

  Z17   **Estrogen receptor status**
  Code first malignant neoplasm of breast (C5Ø.-)

  Z23   **Encounter for immunization**
  Code first any routine childhood examination

- Use additional code:

  ZØ8   **Encounter for follow-up examination after completed treatment for malignant neoplasm**
  Use additional code to identify any acquired absence of organs (Z9Ø.-)
  Use additional code to identify the personal history of malignant neoplasm (Z85.-)

  Z47.1   **Aftercare following joint replacement surgery**
  Use additional code to identify the joint (Z96.6-)

  Z71.3   **Dietary counseling and surveillance**
  Use additional code for any associated underlying medical condition
  Use additional code to identify body mass index (BMI), if known (Z68.-)

Chapter 21 Coding Exercises

Assign the appropriate ICD-10-CM diagnoses codes for all reportable diagnoses, excluding external causes of morbidity (VØØ–Y99).

Answers to coding exercises are listed in the back of the book.

1. Newborn health check, 14-day-old infant _____

   _____

2. Single liveborn, delivered vaginally in the hospital, blood type O negative

   _____

   _____

3. Yearly GYN examination with HPV screening and vaginal PAP smear

   _____

   _____

Chapter 21 Coding Scenarios

Assign the appropriate ICD-10-CM diagnoses codes for all reportable diagnoses, excluding external causes of morbidity (VØØ–Y99):

Answers to coding scenarios are listed in the back of the book.

1. An otherwise healthy post-menopausal 60-year-old female with endometrial hyperplasia presents for repeat endometrial biopsy. She has a history of estrogen therapy, which has been discontinued in recent years.

    _____

    _____

2. A patient presents for management of insulin-dependent secondary diabetes status post partial pancreatectomy for benign insulinoma.

    _____

    _____

3. A 5-year-old adoptee presents for a preschool admission examination. Upon review of record, the physician documents under-immunization status and orders antibody testing.

    _____

    _____

Coding Exercise Answers

Note: Official guidelines noted in rationale are in reference to the "ICD-10-CM Draft Official Guidelines for Coding and Reporting," 2013 version. The current version of the guidelines is available on the NCHS website at: http://www.cdc.gov/nchs/icd/icd10cm.htm.

ANSWERS TO CHAPTER 1 CODING EXERCISES

1. **N3Ø.ØØ**   **Acute cystitis without hematuria**
   B96.2Ø   **Unspecified Escherichia coli [E. coli] as the cause of diseases classified elsewhere**

   The "use additional code" note at category N3Ø prompts the coder that an additional code is required to identify the infectious agent (organism). The instructional note at code sections B95–B97 explain that the codes included in that block are intended to be sequenced as supplementary or additional codes.

2. **AØ8.39**   **Other viral enteritis**

   The main term "Coxsackie" lists "enteritis" as a subterm with reference to code AØ8.39. In the tabular list, "coxsackie virus enteritis" is listed as an inclusion term with code AØ8.39. This provides confirmation of code assignment. However, since the inclusion terms are not considered exhaustive, code assignment can be made upon the direction of the alphabetic index without information to the contrary in the tabular list.

3. **G51.Ø**   **Bell's palsy**
   B94.8   **Sequelae of other specified infectious and parasitic diseases**

   The instructional note at code section B9Ø–B94 states, "Code first condition resulting from (sequelae) the infectious or parasitic disease." Therefore, the residual Bell's palsy is sequenced first, followed by the late effect (sequela) code.

4. **M41.54**   **Other secondary scoliosis, thoracic region**
   B91   **Sequelae of poliomyelitis**

   The instructional note at code section B9Ø–B94 states, "Code first condition resulting from (sequelae) the infectious or parasitic disease." Therefore, the residual secondary kyphoscoliosis is sequenced first, followed by the late effect (sequela) code.

5. **B2Ø**   **Human immunodeficiency virus [HIV] disease**
   G94   **Other disorders of brain in diseases classified elsewhere**

   ICD-10-CM guidelines state to assign code B2Ø sequenced first when a patient presents for an HIV-related condition. Assign additional codes for all HIV-related conditions.

6.   **Z21**   **Asymptomatic human immunodeficiency virus [HIV] infection status**

Code Z21 is assigned for patients without any documented symptoms or history of HIV-related illness, yet is documented as "HIV positive" or with similar status-without-active disease diagnosis.

7.   **A41.52**   **Sepsis due to Pseudomonas**
     N39.Ø   **Urinary tract infection, site not specified**
     B96.5   **Pseudomonas as the cause of diseases classified elsewhere**

Code A41.52 is assigned to report the underlying systemic infection by specific organism. A code from subcategory R65.2 is not assigned in the absence of diagnosis of severe sepsis, or notation of associated acute organ dysfunction. Although Pseudomonas is identified in both the blood and urine, code B96.5 identifies the UTI causal organism.

8.   **A4Ø.3**   **Sepsis due to Streptococcus pneumoniae**
     R65.2Ø   **Severe sepsis without septic shock**
     J13   **Pneumonia due to Streptococcus pneumoniae**
     N17.9   **Acute kidney failure, unspecified**

Code A4Ø.3 is assigned for the systemic infection and sequenced first. Code R65.2Ø is assigned secondary to report the diagnosis of severe sepsis. Code N17.9 is reported as an additional diagnosis to report the specific type of organ dysfunction associated with the severe sepsis.

9.   **A41.Ø2**   **Sepsis due to Methicillin resistant Staphylococcus aureus**

Assign only A41.Ø2 based on the diagnosis provided. Do not report a separate code (Z16.11) for the drug-resistant status, since that information is provided in the code description.

Answers to Chapter 1 Coding Scenarios

1.   **B97.6**   **Parvovirus B19**
     MØ1.X9   **Direct infection of multiple joints in infectious and parasitic diseases classified elsewhere**

The ICD-10-CM index lists "Arthritis, due to or associated with, human parvovirus" with reference to code B97.6. An instructional note, "see also category MØ1," directs the coder to select the appropriate code within this category to report the affected anatomic site. Multiple sites were involved, which is reported with the fifth character 9. At category MØ1 the note, "Code first underlying disease," instructs that the underlying condition be sequenced first.

2.   **B2Ø**   **Human immunodeficiency virus [HIV] disease**
     B59   **Pneumocystosis**

Code B2Ø is assigned and sequenced first since the patient has documentation of an HIV-related illness. Code B59 is assigned as an additional diagnosis to identify the HIV-associated manifestation.

3. **A41.51**   **Sepsis due to Escherichia coli [E. coli]**
    R65.21   **Severe sepsis with septic shock**
    J96.00   **Acute respiratory failure**
    S61.012D **Laceration without foreign body of left thumb without damage to nail**
    L08.9   **Local infection of the skin and subcutaneous tissue, unspecified**
    E11.9   **Type 2 diabetes mellitus without complications**

    Code A41.51 is assigned for the systemic infection and sequenced first. Code R65.21 is reported since septic shock indicates the presence of severe sepsis. Code J96.00 is reported as an additional diagnosis to report the specific type of acute organ dysfunction associated with the severe sepsis. Code S61.012D is assigned to report the wound, present on examination. Code L08.9 indicates the open wound is infected. Code E11.9 is reported for the diabetes mellitus. Since the type of diabetes was not further specified, it is coded to type 2 disease by default, without mention of complication.

ANSWERS TO CHAPTER 2 CODING EXERCISES

1. **C20**   **Malignant neoplasm of rectum**

    Consult the ICD-10-CM Neoplasm Table under the main term "Neoplasm, neoplastic." The first column lists subterms by anatomic site. The subterm "rectum" lists code C20 under the second column "Malignant primary." Confirm code assignment in the tabular list.

2. **D24.9**   **Benign neoplasm of unspecified breast**

    Consult the ICD-10-CM Neoplasm Table under the main term "Neoplasm, neoplastic." The first column lists subterms by anatomic site. The subterm "breast" lists multiple specific anatomic sites. Notice that the fifth column "Benign" lists D24.- for all benign neoplasms of the breast, except skin. Confirm code assignment in the tabular list. Since laterality is not specified, fourth character .9 is assigned.

3. **C7A.011** **Malignant carcinoid tumor of the jejunum**

    The ICD-10-CM Neoplasm Table provides a cross-reference for carcinoid tumors, "see Tumor, carcinoid." In the alphabetic index, the main term "Tumor" and subterm "carcinoid" lists additional subterms by behavior and site. See the subterm "malignant" for behavior and "jejunum" as the anatomic site for reference to code C7A.011. Confirm code assignment in the tabular list.

4. **C7B.04** **Secondary carcinoid tumors of peritoneum**

    The ICD-10-CM Neoplasm Table provides a cross-reference for carcinoid tumors, "see Tumor, carcinoid." In the alphabetic index, the main term "Tumor" and subterm "carcinoid" lists additional subterms by behavior and site. See the subterm "mesentery metastasis" for reference to code C7B.04. Confirm code assignment in the tabular list.

5. **C92.10 Chronic myeloid leukemia, BCR/ABL-positive, not having achieved remission**

    In the alphabetic index, the main term "Leukemia" lists the subterm "chronic, myeloid" with reference to code C92.1-. The dash (-) indicates an additional character is required. Confirm code assignment in the tabular list. Note that code C92.0 Acute myeloblastic leukemia, excludes acute exacerbation of chronic myeloid leukemia (C92.10).

6. **C81.92 Hodgkin lymphoma, unspecified, intrathoracic lymph nodes**

    In the alphabetic index, the main term "Lymphoma" lists the subterm "Hodgkin" with a default code of C81.9-. The dash (-) indicates an additional character is required. Confirm code assignment in the tabular list. The intrathoracic anatomic site is identified by fifth character .2.

7. **Z51.11 Encounter for antineoplastic chemotherapy**
    C56.9 Malignant neoplasm of ovary, unspecified side

    Encounters for therapy are reported with the appropriate encounter for therapy (Z51 Encounter for other aftercare) code listed first, followed by the code for the neoplasm. An instructional note at category Z51 prompts the coder to "code also condition requiring care."

8. **C61 Malignant neoplasm of prostate**
    C79.51 Secondary malignant neoplasm of bone

    Assign codes for both the primary and secondary sites. Sequencing is dependent upon the circumstances of the encounter and focus of treatment.

9. **C53.8 Malignant neoplasm of overlapping sites of cervix uteri**

    Neoplasms overlapping the boundaries of one or more contiguous sites are reported with a fourth character .8 for overlapping sites.

10. **D05.11 Intraductal carcinoma in situ of the right breast**

    Consult the ICD-10-CM Neoplasm Table under the main term "Neoplasm, neoplastic." The first column lists subterms by anatomic site. The subterm "breast" lists multiple specific anatomic sites. Notice that the fifth column, "Ca in situ," references D05.- for all ca in situ neoplasms of the breast, except skin. Confirm code assignment in the tabular list. Intraductal ca in situ is classified to subcategory D05.1 with the fifth character 1 (right) that specifies laterality.

Answers to Chapter 2 Coding Scenarios

1. **Z51.11 Encounter for antineoplastic chemotherapy**
    Z51.12 Encounter for antineoplastic immunotherapy
    C50.412 Malignant neoplasm of upper-outer quadrant of left female breast

    Encounters for therapy are reported with the appropriate encounter for therapy (Z51) code listed first, followed by the code for the neoplasm. If the documentation supports that the patient's surgical resection was a mastectomy resulting in removal of the breast, code Z90.12 Acquired absence of left breast and nipple, would be assigned as an additional diagnosis.

2. **R11.2**   **Nausea with vomiting, unspecified**
   T45.1X5A **Adverse effect of antineoplastic and immunosuppressive drugs, initial encounter**
   C34.11   **Malignant neoplasm of upper lobe, right bronchus or lung**

   When an encounter is for management of an adverse effect of cancer therapy, sequence the appropriate codes to specify the nature of the adverse effect first, followed by the appropriate *adverse effect* code (T36–T5Ø) with the fifth or sixth character of 5. Code the neoplasm as an additional diagnosis.

3. **Z51.Ø**   **Encounter for antineoplastic radiation therapy**
   C61   **Malignant neoplasm of prostate**
   C79.51   **Secondary malignant neoplasm of bone**

   Encounters for therapy are reported with the appropriate encounter for therapy (Z51 Encounter for other aftercare) code listed first, followed by the code for the neoplasm. Code C79.51 was assigned to report the additional metastatic site.

4. **C78.7**   **Secondary malignant neoplasm of liver and intrahepatic bile duct**
   Z85.Ø38 **Personal history of other malignant neoplasm of large intestine**
   Z9Ø.49   **Acquired absence of other specified parts of digestive tract**

   Primary malignancies previously excised for which there is no treatment are reported with the appropriate Z85 personal history of malignant neoplasm code. The secondary neoplasm is sequenced first as the reason for the encounter. The history of colon resection (acquired absence of organ) is reported as an additional diagnosis.

5. **C7B.Ø2**   **Secondary carcinoid tumor of liver**
   C7A.Ø21 **Malignant carcinoid tumor of the cecum**

   If the treatment or admission of a patient with an existing primary malignancy is focused on a secondary neoplasm (metastatic site), the secondary neoplasm is sequenced first.

6. **D49.81**   **Neoplasm of unspecified behavior of retina and choroid**

   Consult the ICD-10-CM Neoplasm Table under the main term "Neoplasm, neoplastic." The first column lists subterms by anatomic site including the subterms "choroid" and "retina." The seventh column, "Unspecified Behavior," lists D49.81 for all sites. Confirm code assignment in the tabular list. This neoplasm was not classified to "uncertain behavior" since the definition remains consistent between classification systems. These codes are assigned when neither behavior of the tumor nor morphology is specified in the diagnostic statement. A patient referral to another medical care site for further diagnostic studies is commonplace with these diagnoses. These diagnosis codes are common in the outpatient setting to report a working diagnosis.

ANSWERS TO CHAPTER 3 CODING EXERCISES

1. **D52.Ø   Dietary folate deficiency anemia**

    The alphabetic index lists the main term "Anemia" with subterms "deficiency," "folate," and "dietary" with reference to code D52.Ø. Confirm code assignment in the tabular list.

2. **D57.412   Sickle-cell thalassemia with splenic sequestration**

    In the alphabetic index the main term "Thalassemia," subterm "sickle cell" is cross-referenced to the main term "Disease" and subterms "sickle cell" and "thalassemia." These terms are indexed to code D57.4Ø. Subterms "with crisis" and "splenic sequestration" specify code D57.412. Confirm code assignment in the tabular list.

3. **D58.2   Other hemoglobinopathies**

    ICD-10-CM contains many commonly used abbreviations. For example, the main term "Disease" lists the subterm "hemoglobin or HB," and subsequently "HB-C" with reference to code C58.2. In the absence of further diagnostic specification, the code assignment is confirmed in the tabular list.

4. **D61.1   Drug-induced aplastic anemia**
    T45.1X5A Adverse effect of antineoplastic and immunosuppressive drugs, initial encounter

    An instructional note at code D61.1 in the tabular list states to use the appropriate additional code from categories T36–T5Ø Poisoning by, adverse effects of and underdosing of drugs, medicaments, and biological substances. The fifth or sixth character "5" identifies the condition as an adverse effect of drug in therapeutic use. The anemia is listed first.

5. **D61.818   Other pancytopenia**

    The alphabetic index lists the main term "Pancytopenia" with reference to code D61.818. The nonessential modifier in parentheses assists in clarification that the code reference is an acquired form of the disorder. In the absence of further diagnostic specification, the code assignment is confirmed in the tabular list. Note that code D61.81 lists multiple exclusions. Pancytopenia due to or with certain conditions is more appropriately classified elsewhere.

6. **D46.9   Myelodysplastic syndrome, unspecified**
    D64.1   Secondary sideroblastic anemia due to disease

    An instructional note at code D64.1 states to code first the underlying disease. As such, the myelodysplastic syndrome is sequenced first. Note that category D46 Myelodysplastic syndromes, lists several specific subclassifications. Report D46.9 Myelodysplastic syndrome, unspecified, only if the condition can not be further specified by type.

7. **D7Ø.8   Other neutropenia**
    R5Ø.81   Fever presenting with conditions classified elsewhere

    The alphabetic index references code D7Ø.9 for neutropenia by default. In the absence of a subterm specifically for "toxic," confirmation of the code category in the tabular list provides an option to classify neutropenia otherwise specified to a fourth character of .8. Instructional notes within the text provide essential coding and sequencing instruction. The note at code R50.81 states to code first the underlying condition when associated fever is present. Examples of such conditions are provided such as neutropenia (D70.-). An instructional note at category D70 states to use an additional code for any associated condition including fever (R50.81).

8. **D80.1   Nonfamilial hypogammaglobulinemia**

The alphabetic index references code D80.1 for the main term diagnosis of "hypogammaglobulinemia" by default. Note that a cross-reference is provided for a similar term. In the absence of further specification, confirmation of the code in the tabular list verifies that hypogammaglobulinemia not otherwise specified (NOS) or unspecified according to type is classified to code D80.1.

9. **D86.0   Sarcoidosis of lung**

Note that in ICD-9-CM sarcoidosis was classified to chapter 1, "Infectious and Parasitic Diseases (001–139)." However, ICD-10-CM has reclassified the disease to chapter 3 with expansion of the code category to include specification of anatomic site (e.g., lung, lymph nodes, and skin) and certain specific manifestations of disease (e.g., meningitis, pyelonephritis, myocarditis). Sarcoidosis is now attributed to an abnormal immune response that can trigger manifestations in multiple body systems. Disease manifestations vary, depending on affected organs, severity, and onset of disease.

ANSWERS TO CHAPTER 3 CODING SCENARIOS

1. **D61.82   Myelophthisis**
   E75.22   Gaucher disease

   An instructional note at code D61.82 states to code the underlying disorder as an additional diagnosis.

2. **D69.51   Posttransfusion purpura**

   In the alphabetic index the main term "Purpura" lists the subterm "posttransfusion," which references code D69.51. Alternately, the main term "Thrombocytopenia, thrombocytopenic" lists subterms for "due to" and "extracorporeal circulation of blood." These terms reference code D69.5-, that when confirmed in the tabular list, can be further specified within the category hierarchy to include purpura by classification to D69.51.

3. **T86.09A   Other complication of bone marrow transplant, initial encounter**
   D89.810   Acute graft-versus-host disease
   R19.7   Diarrhea, unspecified
   L30.8   Other specified dermatitis
   R50.81   Fever presenting with conditions classified elsewhere
   R10.30   Lower abdominal pain, unspecified

   Code D89.81 lists multiple instructional notes for accurate code assignment. The note, "Code first underlying cause," prompts the coder to sequence the transplant complication first. The note, "Use additional code to identify associated manifestations," instructs to report diarrhea, dermatitis, fever, and abdominal pain as secondary diagnoses.

ANSWERS TO CHAPTER 4 CODING EXERCISES

1. **E03.1   Congenital hypothyroidism without goiter**

   The alphabetic index lists the main term "Hypothyroidism" with subterm "congenital" and nonessential modifier "without goiter" with reference to code E03.1. The code is confirmed in the tabular list.

2. **E11.00   Type 2 diabetes mellitus with hyperosmolarity without nonketotic hyperglycemic-hyperosmolar coma (NKHHC)**

   The alphabetic index lists the main term "Diabetes, diabetic" with main terms to designate type and or complications. The "type 2" subterm lists an additional subterm for "hyperosmolarity" which references code E11.00. The code is confirmed in the tabular list.

3. **E27.1   Primary adrenocortical insufficiency**

   The alphabetic index lists the main term "Insufficiency" and subterms "adrenocortical" and "primary," which reference code E27.1. Additionally, Addison's in the alphabetic index has a subterm, "disease (bronze) or syndrome E27.1." The code is confirmed in the tabular list.

4. **E53.8   Deficiency of other specified B group vitamins**

   The alphabetic index lists the main term "Deficiency" and subterms "vitamin" and "B12" with reference to code E53.8. By confirmation of the code in the tabular list, vitamin B12 deficiency is listed as an inclusion term for code E53.8.

5. **E10.11   Type 1 diabetes mellitus with ketoacidosis with coma**

   The alphabetic index lists the main term "Diabetes, diabetic" with subterms to designate type and or complications. The "type 1" subterm lists additional subterms for "ketoacidosis" and "with coma," which reference code E10.11. The code is confirmed in the tabular list.

6. **E05.01   Thyrotoxicosis with diffuse goiter with thyrotoxic crisis or storm**

   The alphabetic index provides multiple listings by which to reference this diagnosis. For example, the main term "Disease" and subterm "Graves" lists a cross-reference to see the main term "Hyperthyroidism, with goiter (diffuse)." Similarly, the main term "Crisis" lists subterms "thyroid" and "thyrotoxic," which provide cross-references to see the index terms "Thyrotoxicosis, with thyroid storm." As such, the main term "Thyrotoxicosis" is listed with subterms "with," "goiter," and "with thyroid storm," or "with" and "thyroid storm." Both index options reference code E05.01 for the condition. Confirmation of the code in the tabular list confirms Graves' disease as an inclusion term for subcategory E05.0. Fifth characters distinguish between the presence or absence of thyrotoxic crisis/storm.

ANSWERS TO CHAPTER 4 CODING SCENARIOS

1. **E34.51   Complete androgen insensitivity syndrome**

   The alphabetic index provides multiple terms by which to reference this code. A cross-reference at the main term "Androgen insensitivity syndrome" states to see also "Syndrome, androgen insensitivity." The main term "Insensitivity" also lists the subterm "androgen," which is further indexed by type (e.g., unspecified, complete or partial). The tabular list confirms code assignment.

2. **E1Ø.621   Type 1 diabetes mellitus with foot ulcer**
   L97.412   Non-pressure chronic ulcer of right heel and midfoot with fat layer exposed
   E1Ø.51   Type 1 diabetes mellitus with diabetic peripheral angiopathy without gangrene
   E1Ø.4Ø   Type 1 diabetes mellitus with diabetic neuropathy, unspecified

   When multiple body system complications coexist (EØ8–E13), all associated manifestations or complications are reported as documented. Assign as many codes as necessary and appropriate to describe the complications of the disease. Therefore, the diabetic ulcer, vascular disease, and neuropathy are reported separately. An instructional note at code E1Ø.621 states to use an additional code to identify the site of the ulcer (L97.4-, L97.5-).

3. **C73   Malignant neoplasm of thyroid gland**
   E31.22   Multiple endocrine neoplasia [MEN] type IIA
   E21.1   Secondary hyperparathyroidism, not elsewhere classified
   I15.2   Hypertension secondary to endocrine disorders
   Z83.41   Family history of multiple endocrine neoplasia [MEN] syndrome

   MEN is specified as type II A in this scenario. MEN type IIA is closely associated with certain types of thyroid cancer, with resultant hypertension and hyperparathyroidism. An instructional note at subcategory E31.2 states to code any associated malignancies and other conditions associated with the syndromes. The thyroid neoplasm is sequenced as the first-listed diagnosis based on the circumstances of the encounter, with secondary hyperparathyroidism and secondary hypertension and multiple endocrine neoplasia assigned as additional diagnoses. Chapter 4 codes may be used as additional diagnoses to indicate either functional activity by neoplasms and ectopic endocrine tissue, or associated dysfunction of endocrine glands associated with neoplasms and other conditions classified elsewhere.

4. **E86.9   Volume depletion**
   AØ8.4   Viral intestinal infection, unspecified

   Volume depletion is sequenced as the first-listed diagnosis as the condition necessitating treatment. The underlying infection is listed as an additional diagnosis. The main term "Depletion" in the alphabetic index lists subterm "volume NOS" with a reference to code E86.9. The code is confirmed in the tabular list.

5. **E78.Ø** **Pure hypercholesterolemia**
   E66.3 **Overweight**
   Z68.27 **Body mass index (BMI) 27.Ø–27.9, adult**

   The index references code E66.3 under the main term "Overweight." Confirmation of the code in the tabular list provides an instructional note at category E66 that states to use an additional code to identify the body mass index (BMI), if known (Z68.-).

6. **F5Ø.ØØ** **Anorexia nervosa, unspecified**
   E44.Ø **Moderate protein-calorie malnutrition**
   N91.1 **Secondary amenorrhea**
   I45.81 **Long QT syndrome**
   Z68.51 **Body mass index [BMI] pediatric, less than 5th percentile for age**

   In the alphabetic index, the main term "Anorexia" with subterm "nervosa" is coded to F5Ø.ØØ. Underweight is a chapter 18 sign or symptom code, and as a symptom of anorexia nervosa, it is not reported when integral to a definitive diagnosis. Secondary amenorrhea is reported with N91.1 and although a symptom of anorexia nervosa in females, it is assigned because it is not a chapter 18 code. The main term "Malnutrition" has the following subterms: protein, calories, moderate, which leads to E44.0. With physician documentation of malnutrition and clinical relevance supported, code Z68.51 can be assigned to indicate BMI. Note the difference between adult and pediatric BMI codes. Syncope is a chapter 18 sign or symptom code and is integral to symptomatic prolonged QT interval, I45.81. Prolonged QT interval is a sign of anorexia nervosa but is assigned since it is not a chapter 18 code.

ANSWERS TO CHAPTER 5 CODING EXERCISES

1. **F1Ø.229** **Alcohol dependence with intoxication, unspecified**

   Code F1Ø.229 is a combination code that includes both the alcohol dependence and intoxication status. This condition includes acute drunkenness in alcoholism. Code references are limited under the main term "Alcoholism" in the alphabetic index. Instead, index the main term such as, "Dependence," and subtems "alcohol, with intoxication."

2. **F15.98Ø** **Other stimulant use, unspecified with other stimulant-induced anxiety disorder**

   Caffeine is a psychoactive stimulant. Code F15.98Ø is a combination code that specifies the substance (caffeine), status (use), and associated complications (anxiety disorder). If neither abuse nor dependence are documented, the default category is "use" when associated with a mental or behavioral disorder by the provider.

3. **F33.Ø** **Major depressive disorder, recurrent, mild**

   The alphabetic index references code F32.9 for major depression. However, recurrent major depression may be partially indexed under the subterm "major (recurrent)" at which a cross-reference is listed to see the main term "Disorder" and subterms "depressive" and "recurrent." Code F33.Ø is selected for the severity level specified as mild.

4. **F43.12   Post-traumatic stress disorder, chronic**

Code F43.12 is most directly indexed under the main term "Disorder" and subterms "post-traumatic stress (PTSD)" and "chronic." Confirm the code in the tabular list.

5. **F10.10   Alcohol abuse, uncomplicated**
   F12.90   Cannabis use, unspecified, uncomplicated

Assign the highest degree of pattern of use of the same substance documented for each separate type of psychoactive substance. When more than one degree for the same substance is noted, selection of the highest degree is based on the clinical hierarchy.

6. **F90.0   Attention-deficit hyperactivity disorder, predominately inattentive type**

Note that attention deficit disorder (ADD) and attention deficit hyperactivity disorder (ADHD) are both classified to category F90 in ICD-10-CM, although ADD without hyperactivity is classified to code F90.0 as a predominantly inattentive type. The alphabetic index provides a subterm for "attention-deficit without hyperactivity" under the main term "Disorder," which references code F90.0. Codes within block F90–F98 may be assigned regardless of the age of the patient.

7. **F31.12   Bipolar disorder, current episode manic without psychotic features, moderate**

Bipolar disorder classifications in ICD-10-CM are similar to those within ICD-9-CM, although category and subcategory titles have been revised. Category F31 classifies bipolar disorder by type of episode and severity.

ANSWERS TO CHAPTER 5 CODING SCENARIOS

1. **G40.009   Localization-related (focal) (partial) idiopathic epilepsy and epileptic syndromes with seizures of localized onset, not intractable, without status epilepticus**
   F07.0   Personality change due to known physiological condition

Instructional notes at the F07 category level and at code F07.0 state to code first the underlying physiological condition. Code G40.009 was selected for the localized (temporal lobe) epilepsy without mention of intractable seizures for the diagnosis of temporal lobe epilepsy, not otherwise specified and sequenced as the first-listed diagnosis.

2. **F84.0   Autistic disorder**
   F70   Mild intellectual disabilities
   H90.3   Sensorineural hearing loss, bilateral

Code category F84 lists an instructional note to use an additional code to identify associated medical condition and intellectual disability. An instructional note at code block F70–F79 states to sequence the associated physical or developmental disorder is listed first, followed by the appropriate code from F70–F79.

3. **F15.23**   **Other stimulant dependence with withdrawal**
    F10.929   **Alcohol use, unspecified with intoxication, unspecified**
    Y90.1   **Blood alcohol level of 20–39 mg/100ml**

    In ICD-10-CM, combination codes for drug and alcohol use include associated conditions (e.g., withdrawal, sleep disorders, and psychosis). An additional code is necessary to assign to report blood alcohol level (Y90.-), when documented.

4. **G30.9**   **Alzheimer's disease, unspecified**
    F02.81   **Dementia in other diseases classified elsewhere**
    Z91.83   **Wandering in diseases classified elsewhere**

    Code F02.81 is a manifestation code that requires mandatory dual coding, with sequencing of the etiology first (Alzheimer's disease), followed by the manifestation (dementia). An instructional note at code F02.81 prompts to assign an additional code to report any documented wandering (Z91.83), which poses significant health, safety, and management risks for the patient.

ANSWERS TO CHAPTER 6 CODING EXERCISES

1. **G40.909**   **Epilepsy, unspecified, not intractable, without status epilepticus**

    The alphabetic index lists the main term "Seizure(s)" with subterm "recurrent" with reference to code G40.909. The code is confirmed in the tabular list where "recurrent seizures NOS" is listed as an inclusion term.

2. **G00.2**   **Streptococcal meningitis**
    B95.1   **Streptococcal, group B, as the cause of diseases classified elsewhere**

    An instructional note at code G00.2 states to assign an additional code to further identify the organism (by type).

3. **G21.11**   **Neuroleptic induced Parkinsonism**
    T43.3X5D **Adverse effect of phenothiazine antipsychotics and neuroleptics, subsequent encounter**

    An instructional note at code G21.11 states to use an additional code to report the adverse effect and identify the causal neuroleptic drug (T43.3X5-). If the condition requiring neuroleptic medication is documented, report it as an additional diagnosis.

4. **G30.0**   **Alzheimer's disease with early onset**

    Fourth character .0 designates early onset. Alzheimer's disease unspecified is reported with the fourth character .9. Use an additional code to report any associated delirium, dementia, or behavioral disturbance, if documented.

5. **G43.829**   **Menstrual migraine, not intractable, without status migrainosus**

    The alphabetic index lists the main term "Migraine" with subterm "menstrual" with reference to code G43.829. Subterms further differentiate menstrual migraine with or without status migrainosus. In the absence of documentation of status migrainosus, code G43.829 is assigned.

6. **G40.219** **Localization-related (focal) (partial) symptomatic epilepsy and epileptic syndromes with complex partial seizures, intractable, without status epilepticus**

The alphabetic index provides a cross-reference under the main term "Epilepsy, epileptic, epilepsia" and subterm "with," which references the subterms "localization related" and "symptomatic, with complex partial seizures." The index hierarchy references code G40.209. However, at that index level, subterms exist that differentiate between intractable and not intractable status. Code 40.219 is referenced for intractable status. The code is confirmed in the tabular list.

7. **G45.9** **Transient cerebral ischemic attack, unspecified**

TIA and related syndromes have been reclassified in ICD-10-CM to chapter 6, "Diseases of the Nervous System (G00–G99)," although cerebrovascular disease remains classified to chapter 9, "Diseases of the Circulatory System (I60–I69)." Category G45 includes site and type-specific TIA syndromes including vertebro-basilar artery syndrome (G45.0) and carotid artery syndrome (G45.1). In the alphabetic index, under "Attack, attacks," the subterm "transient ischemic (TIA)" references code G45.9. Confirm in the tabular list.

ANSWERS TO CHAPTER 6 CODING SCENARIOS

1. **G37.3** **Acute transverse myelitis in demyelinating disease of central nervous system**

The alphabetic index lists the main term "Myelitis" with subterm "transverse" with reference to G37.3. The term "transverse" indicates dysfunction at a specific level across the spinal cord with altered function below this level and normal function above it. Note that the parenthetical terms "acute" and "idiopathic" are nonessential modifiers to the main term "Myelitis." This condition, when associated with a demyelinating process is classified to chapter 6, "Diseases of the Nervous System," as opposed to chapter 1 classifications, which are infectious in nature.

2. **G44.40** **Drug-induced headache, not elsewhere classified, intractable**
    T39.1X5A **Adverse effect of 4-Aminophenol derivatives, initial encounter**
    G89.28 **Other chronic postprocedural pain**

The instructional note at subcategory G44.4 states to use an additional adverse effect code (T36–T50) to identify the causal drug. The fifth or sixth character "5" identifies the condition as an adverse effect of drug in therapeutic use. Postoperative pain, specified as chronic, is reported with code G89.28 when not associated with a specific postoperative complication. Note the multiple exclusions at category G89.

3. **G03.0** **Nonpyogenic meningitis**
    G83.22 **Monoplegia of upper limb affecting left dominant side**

Meningitis of unknown etiology, determined to be noninfectious is classified to code G03.0 Nonpyogenic meningitis, which includes aseptic and nonbacterial meningitis. The symptoms are inherent to the inflammatory condition and are not reported separately, with the exception of the upper limb paralysis. Since the patient is left-handed, and the paralysis affects his left arm, it is classified accordingly to the left dominant side.

4. **G04.02   Postimmunization acute disseminated encephalitis, myelitis and encephalomyelitis**
   T50.B95A Adverse effect of other viral vaccines, initial encounter

An instructional note at code G04.02 states to use and additional code from categories T50.A-, T50.B-, and T50.Z- to identify the vaccine. This coding convention instructs the coder to identify and sequence the causal substance secondary to the disease or resultant condition.

Answers to Chapter 7 Coding Exercises

1. **H00.14   Chalazion left upper eyelid**
   H00.15   Chalazion left lower eyelid

Subcategory H00.1 Chalazion, contains subclassification codes that are laterality and anatomic site specific. When bilateral or multiple site classification options are not available, assign as many codes as necessary to report each affected site.

2. **H04.123   Dry eye syndrome of bilateral lacrimal glands**

Subcategory H04.12 contains bilateral classification option H04.123. When a bilateral classification exists and the disease or disorder affects both eyes, do not code each site separately.

3. **T54.3X1A Toxic effect of corrosive alkalis and alkali-like substances, accidental (unintentional), initial encounter**
   H10.211   Acute toxic conjunctivitis, right eye

An instructional note at subcategory H10.21 states to code first the appropriate code from categories T51–T65 to identify the chemical and report intent.

4. **H18.212   Corneal edema secondary to contact lens, left eye**

Sixth character 2 identifies the condition affecting the left eye. Do not report an unspecified eye option 9 when laterality is specified. Note that other corneal disorders due to contact lenses are excluded from subcategory H18.21, and instead classified to H18.82 Corneal disorder due to contact lens.

5. **H25.011   Cortical age-related cataract, right eye**

ICD-10-CM code descriptions for cataract classifications have been updated by replacing the term "senile" with "age-related." The term "age-related" associates a stated condition only with the natural aging process—without implying a change in mental or cognitive status. The alphabetic index lists "senile" as a subterm to the main term "Cataract" with multiple subclassification references. Senile cortical cataract references code H25.01-. Confirmation of the code in the tabular list facilitates selection of the appropriate sixth character to report laterality.

6. **H44.619   Retained (old) magnetic foreign body in anterior chamber, unspecified eye**
    Z18.11   Retained magnetic metal fragments

    Sixth character 9 designates the condition as affecting unspecified eye. Sixth character 9 should only be reported when no documentation is available regarding laterality. Review documentation carefully for specificity or query physician, as appropriate. An instructional note at subcategory H44.6 states to use additional code Z18.11 to identify the magnetic foreign body status.

ANSWERS TO CHAPTER 7 CODING SCENARIOS

1. **H47.033   Optic nerve hypoplasia, bilateral**
    H52.13   Myopia, bilateral

    When bilateral classification options exist, it is inappropriate to report both affected sides individually. For each diagnostic code, the fifth and sixth character 3 designates a bilateral condition.

2. **H26.211   Cataract with neovascularization, right eye**
    H20.041   Secondary noninfectious iridocyclitis, right eye

    The alphabetic index lists the main term "Cataract" with a subterm "with neovascularization" and a cross-reference to "*see* Cataract, complicated." Subterm "complicated" additionally lists "with neovascularization" and references code H26.21-. Confirmation of the code in the tabular list assists with reporting the sixth character 1 to report right affected eye. An instructional note at subcategory H26.21 provides sequencing instruction by the statement "code *also* associated condition, such as chronic iridocyclitis (H20.1-)."

3. **H40.2212   Chronic angle closure glaucoma, right eye, moderate stage**
    H40.2211   Chronic angle closure glaucoma, left eye, mild stage
    H47.011   Ischemic optic neuropathy, right eye

    Glaucoma is documented as the same type (chronic angle closure), but different stages in each eye. Assign the appropriate code for each eye rather than the code for bilateral glaucoma. The right eye is documented as moderate (seventh character 2) and the left eye, mild (seventh character 1). Disease progression in the right eye has caused ischemic optic myopathy in that eye; report code H47.011.

ANSWERS TO CHAPTER 8 CODING EXERCISES

1. **H74. 12   Adhesive left middle ear disease**

    The alphabetic index lists a cross-reference with the main term "Otitis" and subterm "adhesive" to "see subcategory H74.1-." Subcategory H74.1 lists adhesive otitis as an inclusion term. This subcategory includes a fifth character to denote laterality.

2. **H61.22   Impacted cerumen, left ear**

    As in ICD-9-CM, ICD-10-CM provides unique classification codes for the cerumen impaction, with a fifth character that specifies laterality.

3. **H60.329   Hemorrhagic otitis externa, unspecified ear**

ICD-9-CM classified hemorrhagic otitis media to code 380.10 Infective otitis externa, unspecified, with hemorrhagica listed as an inclusion term. ICD-10-CM, however, provides unique classifications for otitis externa specified as hemorrhagic. Sixth character 9 designates the condition as affecting unspecified ear. Sixth character 9 should only be reported when no documentation is available regarding laterality. Review documentation carefully for specificity or query physician, as appropriate.

4. **H83.2X1   Labyrinthine dysfunction, right ear**

When the causal condition of the symptom, vertigo (R42), is specified, report only the causal condition. Subcategory H83.2 Labyrinthine dysfunction, includes a fifth character placeholder "X" for future classification expansion. The sixth character reports laterality. When a placeholder "X" appears in a code, the X must be reported accordingly in order for the code to be considered valid.

5. **H92.02   Otalgia, left ear**
   H91.92   Unspecified hearing loss, left ear

Two codes are necessary to represent the diagnostic statement in its entirety. Code H91.92 Unspecified hearing loss, includes high- and low-frequency deafness and deafness not otherwise specified.

6. **H95.01   Recurrent cholesteatoma of postmastoidectomy cavity, right ear**

The alphabetic index main term "Granuloma" lists a cross-reference under the subterm "ear, middle," to "*see* Cholesteatoma." The main term "Cholesteatoma" lists a cross-reference under subterms "postmastoidectomy cavity" and "recurrent (postmastoidectomy)" to "*see* Complications, postmastoidectomy, recurrent cholesteatoma," which references code H95.0-. Note that the index differentiates between "granulation tissue" and "granuloma." Granuloma is classified as a recurrent cholesteatoma, whereas the presence of granulation tissue described as granulation is classified to H95.12-. The term "Granuloma" also has a subterm for postmastoidectomy cavity, which advises the coder to "*see* Complications, postmastoidectomy, recurrent cholesteatoma."

ANSWERS TO CHAPTER 8 CODING SCENARIOS

1. **H65.01   Acute serous otitis media, right ear**
   H72.01   Central perforation of tympanic membrane, right ear
   Z77.22   Contact with and (suspected) exposure to environmental tobacco smoke (acute) (chronic)

Instructional notes at categories H65 and H72 prompt the coder to also report a perforated tympanum or otitis media, respectively. Similarly, an instructional note at H65 states to use an additional code to identify tobacco exposures and smoking history, when applicable.

2. **H81.10   Benign paroxysmal vertigo, unspecified ear**

When the causal condition of specified symptoms is specified, report only the causal condition. The fifth character 0 designates unspecified laterality.

Report this character only when laterality is not definitively documented or cannot be determined. Query the physician as appropriate.

3. **H60.332** **Swimmer's ear, left ear**
H74.02 **Tympanosclerosis, left ear**
H90.12 **Conductive hearing loss, unilateral, left ear with unrestricted hearing on the contralateral side**

As the primary reason for the encounter, swimmer's ear is sequenced as the first-listed diagnosis with the sixth character 2 to specify laterality. The tympanosclerosis and conductive hearing loss are reported as additional diagnoses. Although the patient has had previous surgery, which may have resulted in tympanosclerosis, the physician does not definitively relate the surgery to the condition in light of the history of recurrent infection. When reporting postoperative complications, code assignment is based on the provider's documentation of the relationship between the condition and the procedure.

ANSWERS TO CHAPTER 9 CODING EXERCISES

1. **I34.1** **Nonrheumatic mitral (valve) prolapse**

The alphabetic index lists the main term "Prolapse" and subterm "mitral (valve)" with reference to code I34.1. Although in some situations ICD-10-CM assumes a rheumatic origin for heart valve pathology, it is not always the case. For example, under the main term "Disorder" and subterm "mitral" a cross-reference states "*see* Endocarditis." The main term "Endocarditis" and subterm "mitral" refer to code I05.9 Rheumatic mitral valve disease unspecified, assuming rheumatic origin. However, further examination of the subterms in the index reveals a listing of multiple code options depending on the essential modifiers (additional descriptive terms) in the diagnosis.

2. **I44.1** **Atrioventricular block, second degree**

Conduction disorders are classified by type in ICD-10-CM. The alphabetic index lists the main term "Block(ed)" and subterms "atrioventricular" and "second degree" or "types I and II" with reference to code I44.1. The code is confirmed in the tabular list, which also lists type I and II block as inclusion terms.

3. **I50.33** **Acute on chronic diastolic (congestive) heart failure**

Similar to ICD-9-CM, category I50 Heart failure, in ICD-10-CM classifies heart failure by type (e.g., left, systolic, diastolic, combined) and severity (e.g., acute, chronic, acute on chronic). Note that congestive heart failure, without further specification, is reported with code I50.9 Heart failure, unspecified. There is no separate designation in ICD-10-CM, however, for *congestive* heart failure as there was in ICD-9-CM (428.0). Instead, "congestive" is a parenthetical term included in the code descriptions of subcategory codes I50.2- through I50.4-.

4. **I61.4   Nontraumatic intracerebral hemorrhage in cerebellum**
    I1Ø   Essential (primary) hypertension

The alphabetic index lists the main term "Stroke" with a cross-reference under the subterm "cerebral hemorrhage." This reference instructs to "code to Hemorrhage, intracranial." The main term "Hemorrhage, hemorrhagic" lists the subterm "intracranial (nontraumatic)," with additional subterms "intracerebral" and "cerebellum," which references code I61.4. Note the instructional notes at the beginning of the code block "Cerebrovascular diseases," which prompts the use of additional codes to identify the presence of certain associated clinical health risks and comorbid conditions. Code I1Ø for hypertension is assigned as an additional diagnosis. If the diagnostic statement associates the hypertension with cerebrovascular disease, the condition is coded with the appropriate code from categories I6Ø–I69 followed by the appropriate hypertension code.

5. **I12.9   Hypertensive chronic kidney disease with stage 1 through stage 4 or unspecified chronic kidney disease**
    N18.3   Chronic kidney disease, stage 3 (moderate)
    I5Ø.9   Heart failure, unspecified

The guidelines in 9.a.1-3 are similar to those in ICD-9-CM for hypertension. As in ICD-9-CM, ICD-10-CM assumes a cause and effect relationship between hypertension and chronic kidney disease, whereas an association between heart disease and hypertension must either be stated (e.g., due to hypertension) or otherwise implied (e.g., hypertensive) to support coding from category I11 Hypertensive heart disease. In the absence of such an association, the heart failure is *not* coded as hypertensive heart disease with failure.

6. **I7Ø.223   Atherosclerosis of native arteries of extremities with rest pain, bilateral legs**
    Z87.891   Personal history of nicotine dependence

Category I7Ø classifies atherosclerotic vascular disease (ASVD) by severity and laterality. ICD-10-CM assumes native artery status unless specified otherwise. The status of the disease arteries should be verified in the documentation. Note the hierarchical structure of the category in which subcategory I7Ø.22 includes ASVD with intermittent claudication. Similarly, the presence of ulceration would require the condition to be coded to I7Ø.23- through I7Ø.25-, as appropriate. Similarly, the presence of gangrene (I7Ø.26-) includes ASVD from with mention of associated conditions classifiable to all preceding categories. An instructional note at category I7Ø prompts to use an additional code to identify the presence of certain associated clinical health risks and comorbid conditions, including history of tobacco use. Note that code N87.891 assumes tobacco dependence, when reporting a history of tobacco use.

7. **I25.711   Atherosclerosis of autologous vein coronary artery bypass graft(s) with angina pectoris with documented spasm**
    I25.111   Atherosclerotic heart disease of native coronary artery with angina pectoris with documented spasm
    I25.83   Coronary atherosclerosis due to lipid rich plaque

ICD-10-CM classifies angina pectoris and atherosclerotic heart disease to combination codes that specify the type of CAD (e.g., native, graft, transplanted) and the type of angina pectoris (e.g., with spasm, unstable, other). A causal relationship between the CAD and angina pectoris is assumed. Inclusion notes have been added to subcategory I25.1 to clarify the classification of these conditions. When disease is present in both native and grafted vessels, two codes are required to identify the disease in each type of affected vessel. An additional code for angina pectoris is not required when reporting conditions classifiable to subcategories I25.1- and I25.7-. An instructional note at both subcategories prompts the use of an additional code to identify lipid rich plaque, when documented.

ANSWERS TO CHAPTER 9 CODING SCENARIOS

1. **I51.81** **Takotsubo syndrome**
   F43.Ø **Acute stress reaction**
   F41.1 **Generalized anxiety disorder**

   The alphabetic index lists the main term "Cardiomyopathy" and subterm "stress induced" with reference to code I51.81. The symptoms inherent in the cardiomyopathy syndrome are not reported separately. However, the patient's coexisting anxiety disorder is listed as additional diagnosis.

2. **I45.81** **Long QT syndrome**

   The alphabetic index lists the main term "Syndrome" and subterm "Romano-Ward" with reference to code I45.81 Long QT syndrome. Note that an Excludes 1 note exists at code R94.31 Abnormal electrocardiogram, which lists long QT syndrome as a mutually exclusive code. An Excludes 1 notation may be translated as "Not coded here." This exclusion indicates that the excluded codes should never be reported together. Additionally, an abnormal EKG is inherent to diagnosis of long QT syndrome.

3. **I21.Ø2** **ST elevation (STEMI) myocardial infarction involving left anterior descending coronary artery**
   I25.11Ø **Atherosclerotic heart disease of native coronary artery with unstable angina pectoris**
   I1Ø **Essential (primary) hypertension**
   I25.2 **Old myocardial infarction**

   ICD-10-CM classifies myocardial infarction as initial or subsequent infarctions. This patient presents with an initial MI (I21.-), and a remote history of an old MI (I25.2). Subcategory I21.Ø provides site-specific subclassification codes for anterior wall MI involving the left main coronary artery (I12.Ø1) or left anterior descending coronary artery (I2Ø.Ø2). ICD-10-CM classifies angina pectoris and atherosclerotic heart disease to combination codes, which specify the type of CAD (e.g., native, graft, transplanted) and the type of angina pectoris (e.g., with spasm, unstable, other). A causal relationship between the CAD and angina pectoris is assumed. At this time, neither ICD-10-CM guidelines nor instructional notes in the text preclude reporting unstable angina pectoris and myocardial infarction during the same episode of care. However, ICD-10-CM guideline, 1.C.9.b, states that when a patient with coronary artery disease is admitted with AMI, the AMI is sequenced first.

ANSWERS TO CHAPTER 10 CODING EXERCISES

1. **JØ1.Ø1** **Acute recurrent maxillary sinusitis**
B95.3 **Streptococcus pneumoniae as the cause of diseases classified elsewhere**

ICD-10-CM category JØ1 Acute sinusitis, includes a fifth character 1 indicating recurrent acute infection. An instructional note at category JØ1 states to use an additional code to identify the infectious agent. Code B95.3 is assigned as a secondary diagnosis to report the *Streptococcus pneumoniae* organism.

2. **JØ5.Ø** **Acute obstructive laryngitis [croup]**
B97.Ø **Adenovirus as the cause of diseases classified elsewhere**

The alphabetic index lists the main term "Croup" and nonessential modifier (infectious) to a default code of JØ5.Ø, without further specification. The code is confirmed in the tabular list, where an instructional note is present at the beginning of the category to use an additional code from B95–B97 to identify the infectious agent. Code B97.Ø identifies adenovirus.

3. **J1Ø.83** **Influenza due to other identified influenza virus with otitis media**

ICD-10-CM provides specific codes for influenza with otitis media under "with other manifestations" subcategories. The alphabetic index lists the main term "Otitis" and subterms "media" and "in (due to) (with), influenza" with a cross-reference to see "Influenza, with, otitis media." The main term "Influenza" and subterms "with, otitis media" reference code J11.83. However, this code classifies "unidentified influenza virus." The subterm entries "identified influenza virus NEC, with otitis media" reference code J1Ø.83. This code is more appropriate, since the type of influenza has been identified in the diagnostic statement as type B. Code to the highest level of specificity as supported by the medical documentation. An instructional note is also present advising the coder to use an additional code to report any associated perforated tympanic membrane (H72.-).

4. **J11.Ø8** **Influenza due to unidentified influenza virus with specified pneumonia**
J15.211 **Pneumonia due to methicillin susceptible Staphylococcus aureus**

Category J11 classifies influenza due to unidentified influenza virus. In the alphabetic index, under the main term "Influenza" there is a subterm "with pneumonia, specified type" that directs the coder to see J11.Ø8. These codes are reported when influenza is specified as the causal infection, but the type is not further specified. Two pneumonia codes are required to report the pneumonia in its entirety. Code also the other specified pneumonia, per the instructional note in the text. The alphabetic index main term "Pneumonia," followed by "in (due to) Staphylococcus aureus (methicillin susceptible)," references code J15.211.

5. **J38.1** **Polyp of vocal cord and larynx**
J38.Ø1 **Paralysis of vocal cords and larynx, unilateral**

Two codes are required to report this condition in its entirety. ICD-10-CM classifies vocal cord paralysis according to laterality. The ICD-9-CM designation of partial or complete does not exist in ICD-10-CM at the time of this publication. Note that adenomatous polyps (D14.1) are excluded from code J38.1.

6. **J45.9Ø2   Unspecified asthma with status asthmaticus**

Category J45 Asthma, includes severity-specific subcategories and fifth character codes. Report subcategory J45.9- Other and unspecified asthma, only when no further documentation is available in the medical record to support a more specific code. Unspecified codes may indicate the need for documentation improvement initiatives to meet the demands of the ICD-10-CM classification for specific coded data.

7. **J44.1   Chronic obstructive pulmonary disease with (acute) exacerbation**

The alphabetic index lists the main term "Disease" with subterms "pulmonary" and "chronic obstructive." An additional subterm lists "with, exacerbation (acute)" with reference to code J44.1. The code is confirmed in the tabular list.

8. **J95.Ø2   Infection of tracheostomy stoma**
   LØ3.221   Cellulitis of neck
   B95.61   Methicillin susceptible Staphylococcus aureus as the cause of diseases classified elsewhere

In ICD-10-CM, postoperative complications have been moved to procedure-specific body system chapters. An instructional note is listed at code J95.Ø2 indicating the need to use an additional code to identify the type of infection. Code LØ3.221 is assigned as a secondary diagnosis to report the site of the cellulitis. An instructional note at the beginning of chapter 12 states to use an additional code (B95–B97) to identify the infectious agent. *Staphylococcus aureus* not otherwise specified defaults to code B95.61, as a methicillin-susceptible (treatable) organism.

ANSWERS TO CHAPTER 10 CODING SCENARIOS

1. **J45.42   Moderate persistent asthma with status asthmaticus**
   J44.1   Chronic obstructive disease with (acute) exacerbation

The Excludes 2 note at category J45 Asthma, indicates that it is appropriate to report both codes if the patient presents for treatment of both conditions. Code J45.42 reports the status asthmaticus and type of asthma, whereas code J44.1 is necessary to report the obstructive component of the conditions and the COPD exacerbation. The note at category J44 states to code also type of asthma, if known.

2. **J14   Pneumonia due to Hemophilus influenzae**
   J44.Ø   Chronic obstructive pulmonary disease with lower respiratory infection
   F17.218   Nicotine dependence, cigarettes, with other nicotine-induced disorders

Code J14 is a valid three-character code in ICD-10-CM. As in ICD-9-CM, a three-digit code is to be used only if it is not further subdivided. It is inappropriate to add placeholder characters or zeros when not required; to do so would result in an invalid code. Bullous emphysema is classified to the residual subcategory .9 Unspecified, in ICD-10-CM. An instructional note at category J44 states to use an additional code to identify tobacco dependence. The pneumonia is sequenced as the first-listed diagnosis as the reason for the encounter. Category J43 Emphysema, excludes emphysema with chronic obstructive bronchitis. Code J44.Ø is assigned to report the chronic obstructive lung disease with acute lower respiratory infection.

3. **J96.Ø1   Acute respiratory failure with hypoxia**
   J44.1   Chronic obstructive pulmonary disease with acute exacerbation

   Category J96 classifies respiratory failure with combination codes that designate not only severity, but the presence of associated symptoms of hypoxia and hypercapnia. Category J44 includes chronic obstructive bronchitis. The fourth character .1 is assigned to report the acute exacerbation. Code J96.Ø1 is sequenced as the first-listed diagnosis, as the reason for the admission. (official guideline 1Ø.b.1)

4. **J34.81   Nasal mucositis (ulcerative)**
   C11.9   Malignant neoplasm of nasopharynx, unspecified

   The alphabetic index lists the main term "Mucositis" and subterm "nasal" with reference to code J34.81. The code is confirmed in the tabular list where instructional notes are listed to code also the type of associated therapy. Code C11.9 is also assigned to report the neoplasm currently under treatment.

   Note: If assigning external cause codes, Y84.2 would be reported as an additional diagnosis.

ANSWERS TO CHAPTER 11 CODING EXERCISES

1. **KØ5.21   Aggressive periodontitis, localized**

   The alphabetic index lists the main term "Abscess" and subterm "periodontal" with reference to code KØ5.21. Note that the term "acute" is listed as an inclusion term at subcategory KØ5.2. Similarly, periodontitis is synonymous with pericoronitis in ICD-10-CM. Subcategory KØ5.2 lists multiple type 1 exclusions for periodontitis and abscess more appropriately classified elsewhere.

2. **K11.22   Acute recurrent sialoadenitis**

   The alphabetic index lists the main term "Parotitis" with a cross-reference to "*see also* Sialoadenitis." The subterms listed to do not provide a default code. The main term "Sialoadenitis" references code K11.2Ø as a default code, with subterms for "acute," "acute, recurrent," and "chronic." The "acute, recurrent" subterms reference code K11.22. The code is confirmed in the tabular list where parotitis is listed as an inclusion term at subcategory K11.2.

3. **K21.Ø   Gastroesophageal reflux disease with esophagitis**

   Category K21 includes unique codes for gastroesophageal reflux disease with or without reflux esophagitis. Esophagitis with gastroesophageal reflux and esophagitis specified as "reflux esophagitis" are excluded from category K2Ø Esophagitis.

4.   K26.4   Chronic or unspecified duodenal ulcer with hemorrhage

Code category K26 Duodenal ulcer, includes combination codes that classify duodenal and postpyloric ulcer by severity of presentation and type of associated complication (e.g., hemorrhage, perforation). The ICD-9-CM classification for ulcer included fifth characters to report obstruction status; however, obstruction is no longer an axis of classification for ulcers in ICD-10-CM.

5.   K29.3Ø   Chronic superficial gastritis without hemorrhage

ICD-10-CM reclassified atrophic (K29.4) and superficial (K29.3) chronic gastritis (common clinical subtypes) from residual classifications in ICD-9-CM to unique code subcategories. Fifth characters indicate the condition with or without hemorrhage as in ICD-9-CM.

6.   K72.11   Chronic hepatic failure with coma

The alphabetic index lists the main term "Encephalopathy" and subterm "hepatic" with a cross-reference to "*see* Failure, hepatic." The main term "Failure" and subterm "hepatic" lists multiple additional subterms that reflect the expansion of hepatic failure classification to include etiology, severity, and hepatic coma. In the tabular list, category K72 lists multiple diagnoses in the includes and excludes notes. The Excludes 1 listed conditions, those due to or associated with certain conditions or causal factors (e.g., alcohol, toxicity, viral infection), are more appropriately classified elsewhere.

Answers to Chapter 11 Coding Scenarios

1.   K80.ØØ   Calculus of gallbladder with acute cholecystitis

There are multiple approaches to indexing this diagnosis. The main term "Calculus" is often a preferred approach when findings are positive for gallstones, since the main term "Cholecystitis" lists cross-references to "*see* Calculus, gallbladder." The alphabetic index lists the main term "Calculus" with subterms "gallbladder, with cholecystitis, acute" with reference to code K80.ØØ. The code is confirmed in the tabular list. An inclusion note at subcategory K80.Ø states the inclusion of any condition listed in code K80.2, with mention of acute cholecystitis.

2.   K80.33   Calculus of bile duct with acute cholangitis with obstruction
K85.1   Biliary acute pancreatitis

ICD-10-CM uses combination codes arranged in a severity-related hierarchy to classify gallbladder disease. Category K8Ø classifies cholelithiasis with associated complications of cholecystitis (acute or chronic) obstruction or cholangitis. Note that category K8Ø.3 includes calculus of bile duct classified to K8Ø.5, with cholangitis. ICD-10-CM also uses specific classifications to distinguish acute pancreatitis by underlying cause (e.g., idiopathic, biliary, alcohol, drug-induced).

3. **K12.31** **Oral mucositis (ulcerative) due to antineoplastic therapy**
   T45.1X5A Adverse effects of antineoplastic and immunosuppressive drugs, initial encounter
   C50.919 Malignant neoplasm of unspecified site of unspecified female breast

Certain conditions due to the effects of chemotherapeutic or radiation therapies require multiple codes, but the chapter 19 code may be sequenced in accordance with the circumstances of the encounter. An instructional note at code K12.31 states to "code also type of associated therapy." The chapter 19 code is sequenced secondary to K12.31 to report the circumstance and substance. The neoplasm, under treatment, is reported as an additional diagnosis.

ANSWERS TO CHAPTER 12 CODING EXERCISES

1. **L02.224** **Furuncle of groin**
   B95.8 **Unspecified staphylococcus as the cause of diseases classified elsewhere**

The alphabetic index lists the main term "Boil" with a cross-reference to "*see also* Furuncle, by site." The main term "Furuncle" and subterm "groin" references code L02.224. The code is confirmed in the tabular list where no additional classification is provided for laterality. An instructional note at the beginning of the code block prompts the coder to report an additional code (B95–B97) to identify the infectious agent.

2. **L05.02** **Pilonidal sinus with abscess**

Category L05 Pilonidal cyst and sinus, is an expanded classification that includes fourth character subcategories that differentiate between pilonidal cyst and sinus, with abscess (L05.0) or without abscess (L05.9). Fifth characters differentiate between types of lesions as cyst (dimple) or sinus (fistula).

3. **L21.0** **Seborrhea capitis**

Seborrheic capitis (dandruff) may be indexed under the main term "Dandruff" with reference to code L21.0 or "Seborrhea, seborrheic" with the subterm "capitis." This code is also used to report cradle cap in infants. Note that code block L20–L30 uses the terms "dermatitis" and "eczema" interchangeably.

4. **L27.0** **Generalized skin eruption due to drugs and medicaments taken internally**
   T36.3X5A Adverse effect of macrolides, initial encounter

The alphabetic index lists the main term "Rash" and subterm "drug (internal use)" with reference to code L27.0. This listing assumes a generalized dermatitis unless otherwise specified as a local eruption. An instructional note at category L27 states to use additional code for adverse effect, if applicable, to identify drug (T36–T50 with fifth or sixth character 5).

5. **L93.1** **Subacute cutaneous lupus erythematosus**

The alphabetic index lists the main term "Lupus" with multiple subterms that differentiate between systemic (M32.-) and local (L93.-) disease. The subterms "erythematosus, subacute cutaneous" reference code L93.1. Note the multiple exclusions in the tabular list for code L93.

6. **L89.529   Pressure ulcer of left ankle, unspecified stage**

The term "healing" does not substantiate the use of sixth character 9 Unspecified. Note that "healing pressure ulcer" appears in the inclusion terms for all subcategory classifications of pressure ulcer. Code to the appropriate stage as documented or query the physician, as appropriate. The unspecified classification is only to be reported when no information is available regarding the stage of ulceration. Category L89.52 incorporates laterality specific to the left side.

7. **L92.3   Foreign body granuloma of the skin and subcutaneous tissue**

The alphabetic index lists the main term "Granuloma" and subterms "skin, from residual foreign body" with reference to code L92.3. An instructional note at code L92.3 prompts the coder to assign an additional code to identify the type of retained foreign body, if known.

ANSWERS TO CHAPTER 12 CODING SCENARIOS

1. **L51.9   Erythema multiforme, unspecified**
    T36.0X5A   Adverse effect of penicillins, initial encounter
    L49.1   Exfoliation due to erythematous condition involving 10–19 percent of body surface
    H66.90   Otitis media, unspecified, unspecified ear

Category L51 lists multiple instructional notes that provide essential coding and sequencing instructions, including the notation use additional code for adverse effect, if applicable, to identify drug (T36–T50 with fifth or sixth character 5) Similarly, category L49 lists notations to code first the erythematous condition causing exfoliation. Erythema multiforme minor, NOS, is listed as an inclusion to code L51.9. Otitis media is reported as an additional diagnosis. Code to the specified type and laterality as supported by the documentation.

2. **E10.621   Type 1 diabetes mellitus with foot ulcer**
    E10.51   Type 1 diabetes mellitus with diabetic peripheral angiopathy without gangrene
    L97.413   Non-pressure chronic ulcer of right heel and midfoot with necrosis of muscle

The notation at category L97 states to sequence the underlying cause of the ulcer first, when known. Both manifestations of diabetes are reported. The ulcer is reported to the anatomic site, laterality and extent of necrosis as documented.

3. **I96   Gangrene**
    L89.153   Pressure ulcer of sacral region, stage 3
    L89.322   Pressure ulcer of the left buttock, stage 2
    L89.211   Pressure ulcer of right hip, stage 1

An instructional note at category L89 states to code first any associated gangrene. The "ICD-10-CM Draft Official Guidelines for Coding and Reporting" state to assign as many codes as necessary from category L89 to identify multiple pressure ulcers, by anatomic site and stage. Additionally,

---

pressure ulcers described as "healing" should be reported with the appropriate code as based on the clinical documentation, which in this scenario is documented as a stage 2 ulcer of the left buttock.

The inclusion notes for stage 1 ulcers list preulcer skin changes. This can be indexed under the main term "Pressure" and subterms "area, skin," which provide a cross-reference to "*see* Ulcer, pressure, by site."

ANSWERS TO CHAPTER 13 CODING EXERCISES

1.   M14.69   Charcot's joint, multiple sites

Subcategory M14.6 includes a code to report multiple affected sites. Report the "multiple sites" designation, when the condition affects more than one site within a classification category. If no "multiple site" designation is available, and multiple sites are involved, report multiple codes, as appropriate.

2.   M10.072   Idiopathic gout, left ankle and foot

The alphabetic index lists the main term "Gout" with the parenthetical term "flare" with reference to code M10.9 by default. However, since the type of gout is specified in the diagnostic statement, the subterm "primary" is listed with the cross-reference "*see* Gout, idiopathic." The subterm "idiopathic" lists multiple subterms by anatomic site, with reference to code subcategory M10.37-. Confirmation of the code in the tabular list provides the sixth character 2, which specifies laterality.

3.   D57.20   Sickle-cell/Hb-C disease without crisis
**   M14.862   Arthropathies in other specified diseases classified elsewhere, left knee**

An instructional note at subcategory M14.8 states to code first the underlying disease; therefore, the sickle-cell disease is sequenced first. The type of sickle-cell disease is specified in the diagnostic statement, without mention of crisis.

4.   M16.11   Unilateral primary osteoarthritis, right hip

The alphabetic index lists the main term "Osteoarthritis" and subterm "hip" with reference to code subcategory M16.1. Confirmation of the code in the tabular list reveals that osteoarthritis, not otherwise specified by type, is classified as primary osteoarthritis NOS, by default. Category M16 Osteoarthritis of the hip, classifies this disease by primary laterality (e.g., unilateral, bilateral), secondary laterality (e.g., right, left, unspecified), and type (e.g., primary, dysplastic, post-traumatic).

5.   M51.16   Intervertebral disc disorders with radiculopathy, lumbar region

The alphabetic index lists the main term "Displacement" and subterms "lumbar region, with" and "neuritis, radiculitis, radiculopathy or sciatica" with references to code M51.16. The code is confirmed in the tabular list. Note that the index directs the coder to classify intervertebral disc disorders by anatomic site (e.g., cervical, lumbar), by severity (e.g., with myelopathy, with radiculopathy), or to type (e.g., displacement, degeneration). The main terms "Degeneration," "Displacement," and "Disorder" list thoracic, thoracolumbar, and lumbosacral intervertebral conditions, including as displacement, degeneration, or disorder NOS to subcategory M51.1 when documented as "with radiculitis or radiculopathy."

6.   **M23.221   Derangement of posterior horn of medial meniscus due to old tear or injury, right knee**

The alphabetic index lists the main term "Tear, torn" with subterms "meniscus, old" with a cross-reference to "*see* Derangement, knee, meniscus due to old tear." The main term "Derangement" lists subterms "meniscus, due to old tear or injury" and "medial, posterior horn" with reference to subcategory code M23.22-. The sixth character 1 reports laterality as the right knee. Note that current injury is excluded from category M23, and instead classified to chapter 19.

7.   **M33.Ø2   Juvenile dermatopolymyositis with myopathy**

ICD-10-CM has expanded classifications for dermatomyositis by type, and included combination codes by which to report associated manifestations of disease. However, these conditions require careful consideration in the alphabetic index. In reference to the main term "Myopathy," polymyositis is not listed as a subterm. The default code is M72.9. In the tabular list, note that category G72 Other and unspecified myopathies, lists polymyositis (M33.2-) as an Excludes 1 condition. Excludes 1 terms indicate that the condition is "not coded here," and that the diagnoses are mutually exclusive. Polymyositis is specified as juvenile type in the diagnostic statement. This code may also be indexed under the main term "Polymyositis," which again references code category M33.2-, yet there is no "juvenile" subterm in the index. Examination of the code subcategories in the tabular list indicates a specific subcategory for juvenile dermatopolymyositis (M33.Ø). Note that the main term "Dermatopolymyositis" lists subterms "juvenile, with myopathy" in reference to code M33.Ø2.

ANSWERS TO CHAPTER 13 CODING SCENARIOS

1.   **M79.A21   Nontraumatic compartment syndrome of right lower extremity**

The alphabetic index lists the main term "Syndrome" and subterms "compartment, nontraumatic, lower extremity" with reference to code M79.A2-. Confirmation of the code in the tabular list provides the sixth character 1 to report laterality as affecting the right leg. Note that traumatic compartment syndrome is excluded from subcategory M79.A, and is instead reported to chapter 19.

2.   **M84.58XA Pathological fracture in neoplastic disease, vertebrae, initial encounter**
     C79.51   Secondary malignant neoplasm of bone
     Z85.3   Personal history of malignant neoplasm of the breast

Code M84.58 is reported with the required sixth character placeholder "X," and seventh character "A" to report the initial encounter for fracture. Per ICD-10-CM coding conventions, the placeholder X must be used to fill empty characters when a seventh character is required in the data field, but the code is not six characters in length. An instructional note at subcategory M84.5 states to code also the underlying neoplasm. The history of breast neoplasm is reported as an additional diagnosis.

3. **T84.051A** **Periprosthetic osteolysis of internal prosthetic left hip joint, initial encounter**
   M89.752 **Major osseous defect left pelvic region and thigh**

The alphabetic index lists the main term "Osteolysis" and subterm "periprosthetic" with a cross-reference to "*see* Complications, joint prosthesis, mechanical, periprosthetic, osteolysis, by site." Following these directives, the index references subcategory code T84.05-. The sixth character 1 reports the affected anatomic site and laterality as the left hip joint. The seventh character A reports the initial encounter for treatment of the osteolysis. An instructional note at subcategory T84.05- prompts the coder to use an additional code to identify the major osseous defect. Similarly, an instructional note at subcategory M89.7 states to code first the underlying disease. Periprosthetic osteolysis is listed, by example, with reference to subcategory code T84.05-. Therefore, the chapter 19 complication code is sequenced as the first-listed diagnosis. Code M89.752 reports the major osseous defect by anatomic site and laterality.

ANSWERS TO CHAPTER 14 CODING EXERCISES

1. **N31.2** **Flaccid neuropathic bladder, not elsewhere classified**
   N39.41 **Urge incontinence**

The alphabetic index lists the main term "Neuropathy, neuropathic" with subterms "bladder, atonic" with reference to code N31.2. (Note that category N31 lists excluded conditions due to spinal cord lesion or disease classified elsewhere.) An instructional note at the category level prompts the use of an additional code to identify associated urinary incontinence. Code N39.41 reports urge incontinence.

2. **N13.2** **Hydronephrosis with renal and ureteral calculous obstruction**

ICD-10-CM includes many combination codes, which identify a condition with secondary disease processes, specific manifestations, or associated complications in a single code. The alphabetic index lists the main term "Calculus" with subterms "ureter" and "with hydronephrosis." Per ICD index conventions, both conditions are listed in reference to a single code, N13.2. If infection was also associated with the calculus and hydronephrosis, the condition would be reported to N13.6, as indicated by the indention levels of the index. The code is confirmed in the tabular list, where an Excludes 1 note directs the coder to N13.6, with the presence of infection. However, this diagnostic statement is completely satisfied with classification to N13.2.

3. **N03.5** **Chronic nephritis syndrome with diffuse mesangiocapillary glomerulonephritis**
   N18.3 **Chronic kidney disease, stage 3 (moderate)**

The main terms "Glomerulonephritis" and "Nephritis" both list subterms "membranoproliferative" with nonessential parenthetical modifiers "diffuse, type 1 or 3" with reference to code N00.5. A cross-reference note is listed to "*see also* N00–N07 with fourth character .5. This note prompts the coder to review the code categories specified in order to report the condition by specified type or severity, as appropriate. The fourth character .5 reports the diffuse mesangiocapillary, or membranoproliferative component of the diagnosis. Since this diagnostic statement specifies severity as chronic, category N03 Chronic nephritis syndrome, is a more appropriate classification than the indexed N05 Unspecified nephritis syndrome. It is important to index terms carefully to ensure complete and accurate code assignment. In this exercise, the kidney disease is diagnosis-specific type (membranoproliferative), and severity (chronic). The most direct path to index this diagnosis is under the main term "Nephritis" with subterms "chronic." Note that the subterms listed do not refer the coder to character .5. The code is confirmed in the tabular list. Review of category NØ3 verifies code NØ3.5 as membranoproliferative (chronic) glomerulonephritis as NOS, type 1 or 3 and without mention of dense deposit (6). Per the instructional note at the beginning of code block NØØ–NØ8, the chronic kidney disease (kidney failure) is listed as an additional diagnosis. However, sequencing may vary depending on the circumstances of the encounter.

4. **N4Ø.1   Enlarged prostate with lower urinary tract symptoms**
   R33.8   Other retention of urine

Similar to ICD-9-CM, an instructional note at code N4Ø.1 directs the coder to assign an additional code to report associated symptoms. The urinary retention is reported as an additional diagnosis. An instructional note at code R33.8 states to code, if applicable, any causal condition first. These instructional notes work in tandem to reinforce complete and accurate multiple code sequencing and reporting.

5. **N52.31   Erectile dysfunction following radical prostatectomy**

ICD-10-CM subcategory N52.3 expands classification of erectile dysfunction, classified as Impotence of organic origin (6Ø7.84) in ICD-9-CM, to include the type of causal surgery. Furthermore, the terminology of category N52 Male erectile dysfunction, has been updated to reflect current clinical language.

6. **N8Ø.1   Endometriosis of ovary**
   N8Ø.2   Endometriosis of fallopian tube

As in ICD-9-CM, where a multiple site classification does not exist, each affected site is reported separately. ICD-10-CM does not provide a multiple site classification option in category N8Ø Endometriosis. Therefore, both affected sites are reported separately.

ANSWERS TO CHAPTER 14 CODING SCENARIOS

1. **N44.Ø2   Intravaginal torsion of spermatic cord**
   N44.2   Benign cyst of testes

Intravaginal torsion describes a twisting of the spermatic cord within the tunica vaginalis that obstructs blood supply to the testes. Category N44.Ø lists testicular torsions by anatomic site, with an unspecified option (Ø) available. ICD-10-CM provides a unique code to classify benign cyst of testes, which is reported as an additional diagnosis. This condition is classified to a nonspecific residual subcategory code (6Ø8.89) in ICD-9-CM.

2. **N81.85   Cervical stump prolapse**
   N39.3   Stress urinary incontinence (female) (male)
   N32.81   Overactive bladder

Code N81.85 is sequenced first as the primary reason for seeking medical care. Both N39.3 and N32.81 are reported as additional diagnoses. An instructional note at code N39.3 prompts the coder to also report overactive bladder with stress urinary incontinence.

3. **I71.6** **Thoracoabdominal aortic aneurysm without rupture**
N99.Ø **Postprocedural (acute) (chronic) kidney failure**
N17.9 **Acute renal failure, unspecified**

The aortic aneurysm is listed first as the reason for the encounter/admission. An Excludes 2 notation at code block N17–N19 lists postprocedural renal failure (N99.Ø). This indicates that both the postoperative kidney failure and the specific code for the type or severity of renal failure may be reported together, since a patient may have both conditions at the same time. An instructional note at code N99.Ø states to use an additional code to report the type of kidney disease. In this scenario, code N17.9 reports the type of kidney failure as acute, not otherwise specified.

ANSWERS TO CHAPTER 15 CODING EXERCISES

1. **OØ3.4** **Incomplete spontaneous abortion without complication**

The alphabetic index lists the main term "Abortion" and subterm "with retained products of conception" with a cross-reference to "*see* Abortion, incomplete." The subterm "incomplete (spontaneous)" references code OØ3.4. Note the listed subterms for complications. Documentation of associated complication would be more appropriately classified elsewhere in category OØ3 Spontaneous abortion. Verify the code in the tabular list. The includes note at the beginning of category OØ3 confirms that incomplete abortion includes retained products of conception following spontaneous abortion.

2. **O24.41Ø** **Gestational diabetes mellitus in pregnancy, diet controlled**

The alphabetic index lists the main term "Diabetes, diabetic" and subterm "gestational, diet controlled" with reference to code O24.41Ø. The code is confirmed in the tabular list where inclusion terms verify code assignment. Note that although the diagnostic statement refers to trimesters, the fourth character represents a broader classification of "in pregnancy" (.41), "in childbirth" (.42) or "in puerperium" (.43).

3. **O2Ø.Ø** **Threatened abortion**
Z3A.19 **19 weeks gestation of pregnancy**

The alphabetic index lists the main term "Abortion" and subterm "threatened (spontaneous)" with reference to code O2Ø.Ø. Confirmation of the code in the tabular list verifies the gestational timeframe as before 20-weeks' gestation. This is a change from ICD-9-CM, where hemorrhage in early pregnancy, including threatened abortion, was classified as before 22-weeks' gestation. Furthermore, note that category O2Ø classifies hemorrhage in early pregnancy. The provider must distinguish between other hemorrhage in early pregnancy (O2Ø.8, O2Ø.9) and concern for potential (threatened) abortion (O2Ø.Ø). For hemorrhage due to abruption placentae (O45.-) or other placental condition, see category O45. Category O24 excludes pregnancy with abortive outcome (OØØ–OØ8), incomplete or complete. If the documentation is unclear, query the physician.

4.　**O47.03　False labor before 37 completed weeks of gestation, third trimester**
　　Z3A.36　36 weeks gestation of pregnancy

The alphabetic index lists the main term "Pregnancy" and subterms "threatened, labor, before 37 completed weeks of gestation" with reference to subcategory O47.0.-. Note that the subterms "premature labor" and "preterm labor, without delivery" reference code category O60 Preterm labor. The includes note at category O60 specifies inclusion of spontaneous onset of labor before 37 completed weeks of gestation. The diagnostic statement specifies 36-weeks' gestation, which upon confirmation of category O47, is included in the code descriptions as applicable to false (threatened) labor before 37 completed weeks of gestation.

5.　**O30.042　Twin pregnancy, dichorionic/diamniotic, second trimester**
　　O14.02　Mild to moderate pre-eclampsia, second trimester

In 2010, code category "Multiple Gestation Placenta Status (V91)" was added to ICD-9-CM. Likewise, ICD-10-CM was updated accordingly with combination codes that classify both the twin pregnancy and placenta/amniotic sac status in a single code. At the time of this publication, placenta and amniotic membrane status is unique to ICD-10-CM, as the current World Health Organization (WHO) ICD-10 does not include these specific codes. Note that the alphabetic index lists the main term "Pregnancy" and subterm "twin" with additional subterms to specify the number of placental and amniotic sacs. Remember to code to the highest degree of specificity as supported by the medical record documentation and query the provider if the documentation is lacking, or is otherwise unclear.

6.　**O63.1　Prolonged second stage (of labor)**
　　O70.0　First degree perineal laceration during delivery
　　Z37.0　Single live birth

The alphabetic index lists the main term "Delivery" and subterms "complicated by, prolonged labor, second stage" with reference to code O63.1. The subterms "complicated by, laceration, perineum, first degree" reference code O70.0. These codes are confirmed in the tabular list without further applicable instruction or further code specificity. As in ICD-9-CM, the official guidelines (section 1.C.15.b.5) state to code an outcome of delivery (Z37.-) on every maternal record when a delivery has occurred.

ANSWERS TO CHAPTER 15 CODING SCENARIOS

1.　**O80　Encounter for full-term uncomplicated delivery**
　　Z37.0　Single live birth
　　Z3A.39　39 weeks gestation of pregnancy

A note under the valid three-character code O80 qualifies this code as requiring minimal or no assistance, without instrumentation or manipulation. This code is intended to be used as a single diagnosis code and is not to be used with any other code from chapter 15 that would report a pregnancy-associated condition or complication affecting the management of the current pregnancy. Official guideline 1.C.15.n.2 states that code O80 may be used if the patient had a complication at some point during the pregnancy, that is resolved or not present at the time of the admission for delivery. Both the infection and cervical strain were treated and resolved prior to admission for deliver and, therefore, are not coded and reported. Code Z37.Ø is the only valid outcome of delivery code with O8Ø.

2.   **O64.1XXØ Obstructed labor due to breech presentation**
     O66.2   Obstructed labor due to unusually large fetus
     O24.429   Gestational diabetes mellitus in childbirth, unspecified control
     OØ9.523   Supervision of elderly multigravida
     Z37.Ø   Single live birth
     Z3A.38   38 weeks gestation of pregnancy

Note that malpresentation of fetus with obstructed labor (O64.-) is listed as an Excludes 1 diagnosis at category O32 Maternal care for malpresentation of fetus. Although a cesarean section was planned, the patient was admitted in active, obstructed labor. Subcategory O64 codes require a seventh character 0 for the single gestation. Fetal macrosomia is a common condition in gestational diabetics (O24.4-). A sixth character 9 should not be assigned for unspecified control without review of chart documentation. Query the physician, as appropriate. Code O66.2 is assigned for obstructed labor due to fetal macrosomia (unusually large size). The patient is G2P1, indicating multigravida status. At 38 years of age, she is classified as an elderly multigravida in ICD-10-CM. Outcome of delivery status is required on every maternal record when a delivery has occurred.

3.   **O98.43   Viral hepatitis complicating the puerperium**
     B18.1   Chronic viral hepatitis B without delta-agent
     O98.73   Human immunodeficiency virus [HIV] disease complicating the puerperium
     Z21   Asymptomatic human immunodeficiency virus [HIV] infection status

The patient is admitted within the six-week postpartum period for an activation of chronic HBV infection. Code O98.43 identifies this condition as complicated or aggravated by the puerperium state. Subcategory code O98.7 includes an instructional note to use an additional code to identify the type of HIV disease, including asymptomatic HIV and seropositive status (Z21). Similarly, an instructional note at code category Z21 states to code first HIV disease complicating pregnancy if applicable. (See official guidelines 1.C.15.f.) There is not an Excludes 1 listing to preclude reporting of both code O98.43 to report the infection complicating the puerperium, and code B18.1 to further specify the type of infection. Query the physician if an association between HIV disease and other (possibly HIV-related) illness is unclear. It is the responsibility of the provider to document an association between conditions. If such association is made, code O98.7- would be followed with code B2Ø.

ANSWERS TO CHAPTER 16 CODING EXERCISES

1.   **Z38.ØØ   Single liveborn infant, delivered vaginally**
     P12.Ø   Cephalohematoma due to birth injury

ICD-10-CM category Z38 is for use as the principal diagnosis code on the initial record of a newborn baby. It cannot be reported on subsequent admissions or by a second facility upon transfer of the infant. The alphabetic index lists the main term "Cephalematoma, Cephalhematoma," and subterm "newborn (birth injury)" with reference to code P12.Ø. Note that category

P12 Birth injury to scalp, lists several types of injury, including chignon, epicranial hemorrhage, and other bruising and injury.

2. **Z38.00   Single liveborn infant, delivered vaginally**
    P07.15   Other low birth weight newborn, 1250–1499 grams
    P07.31   Preterm newborn, gestational age 28 completed weeks

ICD-10-CM category Z38 is for use as the principal diagnosis code on the initial record of a newborn baby. It cannot be reported on subsequent admissions or by a second facility upon transfer of the infant. An instructional note at category P07 states to sequence the birth weight code before the gestational age code, when reporting both conditions.

3. **P07.15   Other low birth weight newborn, 1250–1499 grams**
    P07.31   Preterm newborn, gestational age 28 completed weeks
    P59.0   Neonatal jaundice associated with preterm delivery

A category Z38 code cannot be reported by a subsequent facility; either in readmission or transfer. An instructional note at category P07 states to sequence the birth weight code before the gestational age code, when reporting both conditions. Any subsequent conditions documented during the hospital stay would be reported as additional diagnoses. Code P59.0 is reported for the jaundice due to prematurity.

4. **P70.4   Other neonatal hypoglycemia**
    P05.9   Newborn affected by slow intrauterine growth, unspecified

The alphabetic index lists the main term "Hypoglycemia" and subterms "neonatal, transitory" with reference to code P70.4. Although the code description specifies "other" neonatal hypoglycemia, an inclusion note confirms code assignment. Code P05.9 is assigned as an additional diagnosis per official guideline (1.16.a.1), which states that chapter 16 codes may be used throughout the life of the patient if the condition is still present.

5. **P23.6   Congenital pneumonia due to other bacterial agents**
    B96.1   Klebsiella pneumoniae [k. pneumoniae] as the cause of diseases classified elsewhere

Official coding guideline 1.16.a.5 states that if a condition that may be either due to the birth process or community acquired does not indicate either as the origin of infection, the condition is coded as birth-acquired (congenital) by default. However, if, after study, the condition is determined to be community acquired in origin, the chapter 16 code would not be reported.

ANSWERS TO CHAPTER 16 CODING SCENARIOS

1. **N97.2   Female infertility of uterine origin**
    P04.8   Newborn (suspected to be) affected by other maternal noxious substances

The alphabetic index lists the main term "Infertility" and subterms "associated with, congenital anomaly, uterus" with reference to code N97.2. The code is confirmed in the tabular list where inclusion notations list female infertility associated with congenital anomaly of the uterus. The conditions are associated with exposure to DES as a fetus during her mother's pregnancy. Code P04.8 is reported as an additional diagnosis, since the intrauterine exposure resulted in adverse effects to the patient's health that persist or manifest as significant conditions into adulthood.

2. **P36.0   Sepsis of newborn due to streptococcus, group B**
   R65.20   Severe sepsis without septic shock

An instructional note at code category P36 Bacterial sepsis of newborn, prompts to use an additional code, if applicable, to identify severe sepsis (R65.2-). The fifth character 0 is assigned for "without septic shock." The patient was placed on prophylactic therapy to prevent shock, but no evidence of shock was documented or included in the diagnostic statement. The coder would also report any associated specific acute organ dysfunction, as supported by the documentation.

3. **Twin A:**
   Z38.31   Twin liveborn infant, delivered by cesarean
   P05.18   Newborn small for gestational age, 2000–2499 grams

   Twin B:
   Z38.31   Twin liveborn infant delivered by cesarean
   P24.10   Neonatal aspiration of (clear) amniotic fluid and mucus without respiratory symptoms
   P02.5   Newborn (suspected to be) affected by other compression of umbilical cord

Code Z38.31 is reported as the principal diagnosis for both infants. Code P05.18 reports the diagnosis of "small for gestational age (SGA)" with the birth weight of 2345. Twin B was not SGA, but had fetal distress in utero, which was attributed to cord compression upon delivery. Amniotic fluid aspiration was noted, but resolved with postsuctioning (P24.10).

ANSWERS TO CHAPTER 17 CODING EXERCISES

1. **Q05.7   Lumbar spina bifida without hydrocephalus**
   G82.22   Paraplegia, incomplete

The alphabetic index lists subterms for the main term "Spina bifida" by affected anatomic site. Each subterm site includes an option for classification by combination code that includes associated hydrocephalus. An instructional note at category Q05 Spina bifida, prompts the use of an additional code for any associated paraplegia. The fourth character .7 is assigned for specification of the affected spina bifida site (lumbar), and absence of documentation of hydrocephalus. The fifth character 2 is assigned for incomplete paraplegia based on the diagnostic statement.

2. **Q37.3   Cleft soft palate with unilateral cleft lip**

The alphabetic index lists the main term "Cleft" with a cross-reference to "*see also* Imperfect closure." However, the diagnostic statement can be effectively indexed by the subterms "palate, soft, with, cleft lip (unilateral)." The code is confirmed in the tabular list. Note the instruction at the beginning of code block Q35–Q37, which prompts for an additional code, if applicable, to report any associated malformation of the nose.

3. **Q21.1   Atrial septal defect**

The alphabetic index lists the main term "Foramen ovale" and nonessential modifier "(patent)" with reference to code Q21.1. Many inclusion terms are listed at code Q21.1. These diagnoses can be indexed under the main term "Defect" and subterms "ostium, secundum" or "atrial septal." Note that defects described as "atrial septal" or "atrioventricular" are more appropriately classified to code Q21.2.

4. **Q87.410   Marfan's syndrome with aortic dilation**
    Q87.43   Marfan's syndrome with skeletal manifestations

ICD-10-CM has expanded classification of Marfan's syndrome with combination codes that link the syndrome with cardiovascular, ocular, and skeletal malformations. The alphabetic index lists the main term "Syndrome" and subterm "Marfan's" with reference to codes specific to body system involvement. Since the diagnostic statement cannot be completely satisfied with only one code, two codes are assigned to report both aortic and skeletal malformations.

ANSWERS TO CHAPTER 17 CODING SCENARIOS

1. **Z38.00   Single liveborn infant, delivered vaginally**
    Q87.1   Congenital malformation syndromes predominantly associated with short stature
    Q22.1   Congenital pulmonary valve stenosis
    Q53.21   Abdominal testes, bilateral
    Q75.2   Hypertelorism
    Q17.4   Misplaced ear
    Q82.8   Other specified congenital malformations of skin

Official coding guideline 1.C.16.a.2 states that when coding the birth episode of a newborn record, the appropriate category Z38 code is listed as the principal diagnosis. The alphabetic index lists the main term "Noonan syndrome" with reference to code Q87.1. At the time of this publication, there is no subterm listing "Noonan" under the main term "Syndrome." An instructional note at category Q87 states to use additional codes to identify all associated manifestations. Code Q87.1 is assigned, along with the additional codes to describe the specific anomalies.

2. **Q85.03   Schwannomatosis**

Schwannomatosis is a rare form of neurofibromatosis that is primarily due to genetic mutation of the SMARCB1/INI1 gene. As a result, multiple tumors grow along cranial, spinal, and peripheral nerves, characterized by the exception of eighth cranial nerve involvement. Whereas ICD-9-CM classifies neurofibromatosis (237.70–237.79) as neoplasms of uncertain behavior in chapter 2, "Neoplasms," ICD-10-CM has reclassified these conditions to chapter 17. The alphabetic index lists the main term "Neurofibromatosis" with subterms according to type. Note that malignant neurofibromatosis remains classified to chapter 2, "Neoplasms." The main term "Schwannomatosis" may be directly indexed with reference to code Q85.03.

ANSWERS TO CHAPTER 18 CODING EXERCISES

1. **R11.2   Nausea with vomiting, unspecified**

   The alphabetic index lists the main term "Nausea" and subterms "with vomiting" with reference to code R11.2. The code is confirmed in the tabular list where multiple exclusions are listed at category R11. These exclusions apply to all R11 codes. An Excludes 1 notation indicates that the excluded code cannot be reported with the listed exclusions.

2. **C56.9   Malignant neoplasm of unspecified ovary**
   R18.Ø   Malignant ascites

   The alphabetic index lists the main term "Ascites" and subterm "malignant" with reference to code R18.Ø. An instructional note at code R18.Ø states to "code first the malignancy." Category C56 Malignant neoplasm of ovary, includes fourth characters that report laterality, if known.

3. **R22.31   Localized swelling, mass and lump, right upper limb**

   The alphabetic index lists the main term "Mass" and subterms "localized (skin), limb, upper" with reference to subcategory R22.3. The code is confirmed in the tabular list where an Excludes 1 notation lists multiple conditions more appropriately classified elsewhere, including edema (R6Ø-) and enlarged lymph nodes (R59-).

4. **RØ7.89   Other chest pain**

   The alphabetic index lists the main term "Pain" and subterms "chest, anterior wall" or "chest, wall (anterior)" with reference to code RØ7.89. The code is confirmed in the tabular list, where anterior chest wall pain is listed as an inclusion term. In the alphabetic index, consider the multiple subterms available under the index entry "Pain, chest."

5. **R56.9   Unspecified convulsions**

   The alphabetic index lists the main term "Convulsions" and the subterm "recurrent" with the listed code R56.9. This diagnosis is confirmed in the tabular list. In the index, note the "*see also* Seizure" cross-reference at the main term "Convulsions." A similar cross-reference is listed at the main term "Seizure" to "*see also* Convulsions." ICD-10-CM classifies the diagnosis "recurrent convusions" to code R65.9, whereas the diagnosis "recurrent seizure" is classified to epilepsy (G4Ø.9Ø9).

6. **N95.1   Menopausal and female climacteric states**
   R61   Generalized hyperhidrosis

   The alphabetic index lists the main term "Hot flashes" and subterm "menopausal" with reference to code N95.1. An instructional note at code N95.1 states to use additional codes for associated symptoms. The main term "Sweat, sweats" and subterm "night" reference code R61. The valid three-character code is confirmed in the tabular list where "night sweats" is listed as an inclusion term. The instructional note provides further sequencing instruction to "code first" menopausal and female climacteric states.

Answers to Chapter 18 Coding Scenarios

1. **R41.82**   **Altered mental status, unspecified**
   Z86.73   **Personal history of transient ischemic attack (TIA), and cerebral infarction without residual deficits**

   The alphabetic index lists the main term "Change" and subterm "mental status" with reference to code R41.82. The code is confirmed in the tabular list. An Excludes 1 note lists altered mental status due to known condition as mutually exclusive. Since the evaluation was for mental status changes, and the underlying cause is under investigation, code R41.82 is sequenced as the first-listed diagnosis. The history of TIA is listed as a secondary diagnosis. Official guideline III.A states that history codes (Z80–Z87) may be used as secondary codes if the historical condition or family history has an impact on current care or influences treatment. In this scenario, the history of TIA is documented as of significant influence in diagnosis and clinical evaluation.

2. **J96.00**   **Acute respiratory failure, unspecified whether with hypoxia or hypercapnia**
   R04.81   **Acute idiopathic pulmonary hemorrhage in infants**

   Respiratory failure is classified to category J96. Note that respiratory failure in the newborn (under 28 days old) is listed as an Excludes 1 condition. Code R04.81 classifies acute idiopathic pulmonary hemorrhage in infants (AIPHI) over 28 days old. Perinatal pulmonary hemorrhage in infants under 28 days old is excluded from R04.81, and instead classified to perinatal subcategory P26.-. Note that AIPHI cases determined to be related to von Willebrand disease, are more appropriately classified to code D68.0.

3. **R15.1**   **Fecal smearing**
   R15.2   **Fecal urgency**
   Z87.59   **Personal history of complications of pregnancy, childbirth and the puerperium**

   Codes R15.1 and R15.2 report symptoms when causation is undetermined or when the symptoms are not routinely associated with a confirmed diagnosis. In this scenario, these symptoms are under investigation pending establishment of a confirmed clinical diagnosis. Official guideline III.A states that history codes (Z80–Z87) may be used as secondary codes if the historical condition or family history has an impact on current care or influences treatment. In this scenario, the history of perineal injury during delivery is documented as being of significant influence to the current encounter. An inclusion note at subcategory Z87.5 includes conditions classifiable to code categories O00–O99.

Answers to Chapter 19 Coding Exercises

1. **S82.841A** **Displaced bimalleolar fracture of right lower leg, initial encounter**

   Official guideline I.19.c.1 states that a fracture not indicated whether displaced or not displaced should be coded to displaced. The alphabetic index lists the main term "Fracture" and subterm "bimalleolar" with a cross-reference to "see Fracture, ankle, bimalleolar." Subterms "ankle" and bimalleolar" include a parenthetical term "displaced" indicating it as the default code unless specified as nondisplaced. Code S84.84- is referenced for both subterms. Confirmation of the code in the tabular list provides fifth-character codes that further specify displaced vs. nondisplaced and laterality. A seventh character is required.

2. **S72.025G Nondisplaced fracture of epiphysis (separation) (upper) of left femur, subsequent encounter for delayed healing**

    Official guideline I.19.c.1 states that the aftercare codes should not be used for aftercare of traumatic fractures. Instead, assign the acute fracture code with the appropriate seventh character. In this case, the patient presents for delayed healing without mention of other complications, of a closed, nondisplaced fracture. In this diagnostic statement, the term "aftercare" indicates a subsequent encounter, and does not justify the use of aftercare codes, which are contraindicated by the chapter 19 guidelines. However, if the patient was evaluated and treated by a new physician for this diagnosis, seventh character A would be assigned as the initial encounter (for a new physician). See guideline I.19.c.1, paragraph 1, for further information regarding initial vs. subsequent encounters for fracture.

3. **S13.4XXA Sprain of ligaments of cervical spine, initial encounter**

    The alphabetic index lists the main term "Whiplash injury" with reference to code subcategory S13.4. The code is confirmed in the tabular list, where "whiplash injury of cervical spine" is listed as an inclusion term. A seventh character is required. However, the code is only three characters in length. When a seventh character is required, it must be submitted in the seventh-character place in order for the code to be valid. To do so, it is necessary to assign a placeholder X to fill in the empty characters.

4. **S91.349A Puncture wound with foreign body, unspecified foot, initial encounter**

    Category S91.3 includes open wound of foot with subcategories that distinguish between the types of open wound as unspecified, laceration, or puncture and indicate the presence or absence of foreign body in the wound. The sixth characters represent laterality, with an unspecified option 9. Official guideline I.B.13 states that an unspecified code is provided should the site not be identified in the medical record. An unspecified code should not be reported if the laterality information can be obtained in the record. Assign to left (2) or right (1), as appropriate, when possible. (**Note:** Code W45.0XXA would be assigned as an additional diagnosis to report the circumstances of the injury, along with place of occurrence and activity code, as supported by the medical documentation.)

5. **T39.1X2A Poisoning by 4-Aminophenol derivatives, intentional self-harm, initial encounter**
    K71.2   Toxic liver disease with acute hepatitis
    R56.9   Unspecified convulsions

    ICD-10-CM classifies poisoning (accidental or deliberate), adverse effects, and underdosing to chapter 19 by substance, with subcategories that differentiate intent. A seventh character is required to report the encounter. Unlike ICD-9-CM, no additional external cause code is required. Official guideline I.19.e provides sequencing instruction. The category T36–T65 code is listed first, followed by the codes that specify the nature of the poisoning (overdose).

6.   **T84.028D   Dislocation of other internal joint prosthesis, subsequent
            encounter**
     Z96.611   Presence of right artificial shoulder joint

The alphabetic index lists the main term "Complication" and subterms "joint prosthesis, dislocation" with reference to code subcategory T84.02-. Note that the dash (-) following a code in the alphabetic index indicates that additional characters are required. As in ICD-9-CM, do not code from the alphabetic index alone. The tabular list provides a complete listing of codes and conventions to facilitate accurate and complete code assignment. Category T84 requires a seventh character. Examination of subcategory T84.02 reveals site-specific codes. Since the shoulder prosthesis dislocation does not have a unique code available, the condition is reported with the .028 other joint prosthesis code. An instructional note prompts the use of an additional code to identify the affected joint prosthesis (Z96.6-). Subcategory Z96.61 lists the presence of an artificial shoulder joint, with sixth-character codes that specify laterality.

ANSWERS TO CHAPTER 19 CODING SCENARIOS

1.   **S61.401A   Unspecified open wound of right hand**
     L03.113   Cellulitis of right upper limb

The alphabetic index lists the main term "Wound" and subterm "hand" with reference to subcategory S61.40-. Additional subterms "bite," "laceration," and "puncture" provide cross-reference to "*see*" the main terms "Bite," "Laceration," or "Puncture," as appropriate. In this scenario, the wound is not further specified and, is therefore, coded as an unspecified open wound. Avoid reporting unspecified codes if possible. The alphabetic index lists the main term "Cellulitis" and subterm "hand" with a cross-reference to "see Cellulitis, upper limb." The "upper limb" subterm references L03.11-, if not further specified as the axilla, finger or thumb. Category L03 in the tabular list does not provide a unique code for "hand" or "palm." The diagnosis is coded to the right upper limb anatomic site. Code also the specific causal organism, if known (B95–B96). (**Note:** Code W45.8XXA would be assigned as an additional diagnosis to report the circumstances of the injury, along with place of occurrence and activity code, as supported by the medical documentation.)

2.   **T80.310A   ABO incompatibility with acute hemolytic transfusion
            reaction, initial encounter**
     D57.1   Sickle-cell disease without crisis
     Y65.0   Mismatched blood transfusion

Hemolytic transfusion reactions (HTR) are potentially serious transfusion-related complications that are often attributed to preventable medical error, such as mislabeling or other mismatch. The severity of transfusion reaction depends on the type of transfusion and nature of incompatibility. The alphabetic index lists the main term "Reaction" and subterms "incompatibility, ABO blood group" with a cross-reference to "*see* Complication(s), transfusion, incompatibility reaction, ABO." In doing so, the subterm "hemolytic transfusion reaction, acute" references code T80.310. The code is confirmed in the tabular list. An instructional note at code block T80–T88 prompts to use additional codes to identify the specified condition resulting from the complication and an additional code to identify devices and/or details of circumstances. Codes D57.1 and Y65.Ø are assigned as additional diagnoses.

3. **T2Ø.29XA** **Burn of second degree of multiple sites of head face and neck, initial encounter**
T22.291A **Burn of second degree of multiple sites of right shoulder and upper limb, except wrist and hand, initial encounter**
T22.292A **Burn of second degree of multiple sites of left shoulder and upper limb, except wrist and hand, initial encounter**
T23.291A **Burn of second degree of multiple sites of right wrist and hand, initial encounter**
T23.292A **Burn of second degree of multiple sites of left wrist and hand, initial encounter**
T31.2Ø **Burns involving 2Ø-29% of body surface with Ø% to 9% third degree burns**
F1Ø.129 **Alcohol abuse with intoxication, unspecified**
XØ3.ØXXA **Exposure to flames in controlled fire, not in building or structure, initial encounter**
Y9Ø.1 **Blood alcohol level of 2Ø-39 mg/1ØØml**
Y92.Ø17 **Garden or yard in single-family (private) house as the place of occurrence of the external cause**
Y93.G2 **Activity, grilling and smoking food**

Official guidelines I.C.19.d.1-2 state to sequence first the code that reflects the highest degree of burn. In this scenario, the patient presents with both first- and second-degree burns. Note the placeholder X is required with code T2Ø.29XA to facilitate reporting the required seventh character. The burns are reported at the highest level of severity, by site as second degree. Although the burns are reported to the highest degree, and as "multiple" due to the multiple site classification options available, the burns to the hands and wrists are classified separately from the rest of the upper extremity sites. Category T31 reports the extent of body surface involved. Subcategory T2Ø.2 lists an instructional note to use additional external cause codes to identify the source, place, and intent of the burn (XØ3.ØXXA, Y92.Ø17, Y93.G2). Note the placeholder X is required in the fifth- and sixth-character positions with code XØ3.Ø to facilitate reporting the required seventh character. Alcohol intoxication is assigned as an additional diagnosis. An includes note at category F1Ø prompts for the use of an additional code to report the blood alcohol level, if applicable (Y9Ø.1).

ANSWERS TO CHAPTER 20 CODING EXERCISES

1. **W55.Ø1XXA** **Bitten by cat**

The ICD-10-CM Index to External Causes lists the main term "Bite" and subterm "cat" with reference to code W55.Ø1. The code is confirmed in the tabular list. Note that category 55 Contact with other mammals, includes contact with the saliva, feces, or urine of mammals, which can pose serious health risks. Code W55.Ø1 requires a seventh character and placeholder X.

2. **V18.ØXXA** **Pedal cycle driver injured in noncollision transport accident in nontraffic accident**

The ICD-10-CM Index to External Causes lists the main term "Accident" and subterm "pedal cycle" with a cross-reference to "*see* Accident, transport, pedal cyclist." In doing so, the subterms "driver," "noncollision accident (traffic)," and "nontraffic" reference code V18.Ø. The code is confirmed in the tabular list where "fall or thrown from pedal cycle (without antecedent collision)" is listed as an inclusion. Code V18.Ø requires a seventh character and placeholders X.

3. **W26.ØXXA Contact with knife**
   Y92.Ø30   Kitchen in apartment as the place of occurrence of the external cause
   Y93.G1   Activity, food preparation and clean up

The ICD-10-CM Index to External Causes lists the main term "Cut, cutting" with a cross-reference to "(*see also* Contact, with, by object or machine)." The main term "Contact" and subterm "knife" references code W26.Ø. Code W26.0 requires a seventh character and placeholders X. A place of occurrence code is assigned based on the information provided under the main term "Place of occurrence" and subterms "apartment, kitchen." The activity is indexed under the main term "Activity" and subterm "food preparation and cleanup." Note that food preparation is classified separately from the grilling (Y93.G2), cooking, or baking (Y93.G3) of food.

4. **X10.2XXA Contact with fats and cooking oils**
   Y93.G3   Activity, cooking and baking
   Y92.511   Restaurant or café as the place of occurrence of the external cause
   Y99.Ø   Civilian activity done for income or pay

The ICD-10-CM Index to External Causes lists the main term "Burn" and subterms "hot, oil (cooking)" with reference to code X1Ø.2. Code X1Ø.2 requires a seventh character and placeholders X. An activity is assigned based on the information provided, by indexing the main term "Activity" and subterm "cooking and baking." A place of occurrence is indexed by the main term "Place of occurrence" and subterm "restaurant." The activity is indexed under the main term "Activity" and subterm "cooking and baking." Since this is an occupational injury, status code Y99.Ø is assigned as an additional diagnosis, based on the information provided.

Answers to Chapter 20 Coding Scenarios

1. **W55.12XA Struck by horse**
   X37.1XXA Tornado
   Y92.71   Barn as the place of occurrence of the external cause

The ICD-10-CM Index to External Causes lists the main term "Struck (accidentally) by" and subterm "animal (not being ridden)" or "mammal" with reference to code W55.89. Review of category W55 reveals mammal-specific subcategories, including W55.1 Contact with horse. This code requires a placeholder X and a seventh character. The circumstance of the tornado is significant to the injury and is reported by indexing the main term "Tornado (any injury)." Code X37.1 requires a seventh character. A place of occurrence is indexed by the main term "Place of occurrence" and subterm "barn."

2. **V47.51XA Driver of sport utility vehicle injured in collision with fixed or stationary object in traffic accident.**
    Y92.414 Local residential or business street as the place of occurrence of the external cause
    Y93.C2 Activity, hand held interactive electronic device

The ICD-10-CM Index to External Causes lists the main term "Accident" and subterms "transport, sport utility vehicle occupant, driver, collision with, stationary object (traffic)" with reference to code V47.51. A placeholder X and seventh character are required. A place of occurrence is indexed by the main term "Place of occurrence" and subterms "street or highway, local residential or business street." The activity is indexed under the main term "Activity" and subterm "cellular, communication device."

ANSWERS TO CHAPTER 21 CODING EXERCISES

1. **Z00.111 Health examination for newborn 8 to 28 days old**

The alphabetic index lists the main term "Examination" and subterm "newborn" with a cross-reference to "*see* Newborn, examination." In doing so, the subterm "examination" is further subdivided by number of days old. Code Z00.111 is referenced and confirmed in the tabular list. Note that additional codes are necessary to report any abnormal findings identified during the examination.

2. **Z38.00 Single liveborn infant, delivered vaginally**
    Z67.41 Type O blood, Rh negative

Official guideline 1.C.16.2 states that the principal diagnosis for a birth episode on a newborn record is assigned with the appropriate category Z38 code listed as the principal diagnosis. This code is assigned and reported only once on the newborn record, at the time of birth. The alphabetic index lists the main term "Type" and subterms "blood, O, Rh negative" with reference to code Z67.41. The code is confirmed in the tabular list.

3. **Z01.419 Encounter for gynecological examination (general) (routine) without abnormal findings**
    Z11.51 Encounter for screening for human papillomavirus (HPV)
    Z12.72 Encounter for screening for malignant neoplasm of vagina

The alphabetic index lists the main term "Examination" and the subterm "gynecological" (assuming normal examination), with reference to code Z01.419. Note that additional subterms differentiate between an exam with abnormal findings (Z01.411) and one performed for contraceptive maintenance (Z30.8). The code is confirmed in the tabular list where an instructional note prompts for the assignment of additional codes to report HPB screening and Pap smear, as applicable.

ANSWERS TO CHAPTER 21 CODING SCENARIOS

1. **N85.00**   **Endometrial hyperplasia, unspecified**
   Z92.23   **Personal history of estrogen therapy**

   Subcategory Z92.2 includes codes for reporting specific past drug therapies that may present hazards to health in the long term. Official guideline 1.C.21.c.4 states that history codes are acceptable on any medical record regardless of the reason for visit. These codes indicate a history of illness or other circumstance that even if no longer present, provide important information that may alter the type of treatment ordered.

2. **E89.1**   **Postprocedural hypoinsulinemia**
   E13.9   **Other specified diabetes mellitus without complications**
   Z90.411   **Acquired partial absence of pancreas**
   Z79.4   **Long term (current) use of insulin**

   Official guideline 1.C.4.a.6.b.i states that secondary diabetes due to pancreatectomy requires multiple codes in a specific sequence: code E89.1, followed by the appropriate E13 code and a code from subcategory Z90.41-. Code Z79.4 is reported as an additional diagnosis to indicate long-term insulin use. Multiple instructional notes throughout the text (E89.1, E13, Z90.41) prompt the assignment of additional codes, where appropriate.

3. **Z02.0**   **Encounter for examination for admission to educational institution**
   Z28.3   **Underimmunization status**

   The alphabetic index lists the main term "Examination" with subterms "admission to, school" with reference to code Z02.0. The code is confirmed in the tabular list. The main term "Status" and subterm "underimmunization" references code Z28.3. As a secondary diagnosis, this code supports the antibody testing procedures. In this scenario, Z02.0 reports the reason for the encounter, whereas code Z28.3 provides additional information that describes the course of treatment or testing.

Comprehensive Self-Examination

Answer each question based on the information provided. Choose the best answer for multiple choice or true/false questions. Assign the appropriate ICD-10-CM diagnosis codes for all reportable diagnoses, including external causes of morbidity (VØØ–Y99), as appropriate, according to the instructions in ICD-10-CM text and the "ICD-10-CM Draft Official Guidelines for Coding and Reporting."

Answers are listed in the next section of this book.

CHAPTER 1. CERTAIN INFECTIOUS AND PARASITIC DISEASES (AØØ–B99)

1.1 **When a patient is admitted with HIV and a related condition, sequence the related condition first, and the HIV disease as an additional diagnosis.**

☐ True

☐ False

1.2 **Category A59 lists intestinal trichomoniasis (AØ7.8) as an Excludes 2 condition. This notation should be interpreted as:**

A. "Not coded here!" Intestinal trichomoniasis (AØ7.8) cannot be reported with a code from category A59.

B. "Not included here." Code AØ7.8 is not part of the conditions classified to category A59. As such, the conditions are mutually exclusive and should never be reported together.

C. "Not coded here!" Code AØ7.8 is not classified to category A59, but may be reported with a code from category A59, as long as code AØ7.8 is sequenced first.

D. "Not included here." Intestinal trichomoniasis (AØ7.8) is excluded from category A59, and more appropriately classified elsewhere; however, it is possible for the patient to have both conditions at the same time. If so, it would be acceptable to report both AØ7.8 and a category A59 code together.

1.3 **Ciprofloxacin (fluoroquinolone)-resistant salmonella enteritis.**

_____

_____

1.4 **A patient presents with respiratory failure and shock due to severe gram negative sepsis; blood culture was positive for *Pseudomonas aeruginosa*.**

_____

_____

CHAPTER 2. NEOPLASMS (CØØ–D49)

2.1 **When an admission/encounter is for the management of an anemia associated with a malignancy, and the treatment is only for the anemia, report code D63.Ø Anemia in neoplastic disease, as the first-listed diagnosis, followed by the appropriate malignancy code.**

☐ True

☐ False

2.2 **Subcategory code C92.Ø Acute myeloblastic leukemia, list multiple inclusion terms. These terms:**

A. Represent a complete list of the various conditions included within the subcategory; any additional terms found in the alphabetic index are excluded, and instead assigned to the residual subcategory.

B. Represent a complete list of synonyms to the code title at the subcategory level, not to the codes contained therein.

C. Represent a limited listing of included conditions and synonyms to the code title. Additional terms found only in the alphabetic index may also be assigned, as appropriate.

D. Both A and B.

2.3 **Evaluation of pulmonary symptoms reveals a metastatic right upper lobe lung cancer from (existing) primary colorectal neoplasm.**

_____

_____

2.4 **A patient, status-post kidney transplant, presents for initiation of chemotherapy. The patient contracted lymphoma from malignant cells in the transplanted kidney.**

_____

_____

CHAPTER 3. DISEASES OF THE BLOOD AND BLOOD-FORMING ORGANS AND CERTAIN DISORDERS INVOLVING THE IMMUNE MECHANISM (D5∅–D89)

3.1 **Code D77 is a manifestation code identified by the phrase "in disease classified elsewhere" in the code title. These codes represent a manifestation of an underlying disease. Code D77, however, may be reported alone, when the documentation does not specify the underlying disease.**

☐ True

☐ False

3.2 **Code block D8∅–D89 Certain disorders involving the immune mechanism, includes classifications for the following conditions, except:**

A. Human immunodeficiency virus HIV disease

B. Certain immunodeficiency disorders

C. Sarcoidosis

D. Defects in the compliment system

3.3 **Iron-deficiency anemia due to chronic blood loss**

_____

_____

3.4 **A patient under treatment for tuberculous spondylitis presents with progressive weakness and shortness of breath. Laboratory tests revealed decreased hemoglobin at 47 g/L and erythrocyte count to 1.5 G/L, reticulocytes were very low (reticulocyte production index of 0.48), but bone marrow aspirate showed an accelerated erythropoiesis with ring sideroblasts. Anemia rapidly resolved after cessation of Isoniazid. Diagnosis: Isoniazid-induced sideroblastic anemia.**

_____

_____

CHAPTER 4. ENDOCRINE, NUTRITIONAL AND METABOLIC DISEASES (EØØ–E89)

4.1 Diabetes mellitus is reported with combination codes in ICD-10-CM, which report both the type of diabetes and the disease manifestation. No additional codes are required.

☐ True

☐ False

4.2 GM2, Sandhoff disease

_____

_____

4.3 A patient returns for follow-up management of glucocorticosteroid-induced Cushing's syndrome.

_____

_____

4.4 A 52-year-old male presents for evaluation of exogenous hypercholesterolemia with hypertriglyceridemia. His body mass index (BMI) has decreased to 30.9; demonstrating a 20-lb weight reduction since the last visit due to increased exercise and calorie intake modifications. Additional diagnosis: Dietary-induced borderline obesity.

_____

_____

CHAPTER 5. MENTAL AND BEHAVIORAL DISORDERS (FØ1–F99)

5.1 Interpret the following ICD-10-CM coding conventions:

F54 Psychological and behavioral factors associated with disorders or diseases classified elsewhere
Code first the associated physical disorder

A. Code F54 is a manifestation code.

B. Code F54 cannot be reported alone.

C. Code F54 is not subject to the etiology/manifestation convention.

D. Code F54 may be reported alone without documentation of etiological condition.

E. Both A. and B.

F. Both C. and D.

5.2 Bipolar disorder, manic episode with psychosis

5.3 Pathological (compulsive) gambling in a patient with obsessive compulsive personality disorder

5.4 A patient with known cocaine addiction presents to the ER with signs of intoxication. Physical exam reveals tremor and perceptual disturbance (tinnitus). The patient's severe anxiety, high blood pressure, and hyperventilation are consistent a phase I cocaine overdose.

_____

_____

CHAPTER 6. DISEASES OF THE NERVOUS SYSTEM (GØØ–G99)

6.1 Category G89 codes may be listed as the first-listed or principal diagnosis when: 1) Pain control or pain management is the reason for the admission/encounter, and 2) The encounter is for insertion of a neurostimulator for pain control.

☐ True

☐ False

6.2 Which of the following statements is *not* true? For category G81 and subcategories G83.1–G83.3, if the affected side is documented, but not specified as dominant or nondominant, and no default code is indicated:

A. Report the affected side as unspecified.

B. Report as dominant if the affected side is documented as right.

C. Report as nondominant if the affected side is documented as left.

D. Report as dominant if the patient is ambidextrous.

6.3 A patient with metastatic bone cancer, and a history of a prostate primary (previously resected), is admitted for pain control of acute neoplasm related pain.

_____

_____

6.4 A patient presents to the hospital in status migrainosus. She has a recent history of intractable migraine. Hospital course is complicated by persistent aura. Cerebrovascular imaging was negative for underlying pathology. The patient's medications were adjusted and a referral for an outpatient ophthalmology consult was provided.

_____

_____

CHAPTER 7. DISEASES OF THE EYE AND ADNEXA (H00–H59)

7.1 The Excludes note at the beginning of chapter 7 indicates that the listed conditions are classified elsewhere, and may, therefore, be interpreted as "Not coded here."

☐ True

☐ False

7.2 For conditions that are classified according to laterality, if a condition is documented as bilateral (affecting both eyes), and no bilateral code is provided within a classification, assign separate codes for both the left and right side.

☐ True

☐ False

7.3 Chronic moderate angle closure glaucoma with glaukomflecken (glaucomatous flecks) cataract, left eye

_____

_____

7.4 A patient presents with increased pain and decreased vision in his left eye over the past week. He is one month status post trabeculectomy for treatment of glaucoma. Examination reveals a purulent bleb with mild inflammation of the anterior segment. Diagnosis: stage 1 postprocedural bleb.

_____

_____

Chapter 8. Diseases of the Ear and Mastoid Process (H6Ø–H95)

8.1 Labyrinthine dysfunction, hypersensitivity, and hypofunction may all be classified to, and reported with, code H83.2.

   ☐ True

   ☐ False

8.2 Acute subperiosteal mastoiditis

   A. H71.Ø1

   B. H7Ø.Ø1

   C. H71.Ø19

   D. None of the above

8.3 Pseudomonas chondritis of pinna, right ear

_____

_____

8.4 A 7-year-old male presents with bilateral acute recurrent suppurative otitis media. Examination reveals a spontaneous attic perforated tympanic membrane, left ear.

_____

_____

CHAPTER 9. DISEASES OF THE CIRCULATORY SYSTEM (I∅∅–I99)

9.1 A causal relationship is assumed in a patient with both atherosclerosis and angina pectoris, unless the documentation indicates that angina is due to something other than the atherosclerosis.

☐ True

☐ False

9.2 When a patient requires continued care for a myocardial infarction, codes from category I21 continue to be reported for the duration of _____ (or less) from onset, regardless of the health care setting.

A. 2 weeks

B. 4 weeks

C. 8 weeks

D. 12 weeks

9.3 Coronary artery disease with crescendo angina pectoris

_____

_____

9.4 A right-handed patient with a long-standing history of hypertension presents with a sudden-onset of syncope, left-sided facial weakness, arm drift, visual field disturbances, and abnormal speech. Diagnostic imaging reveals a thrombotic infarction of the right anterior cerebral artery. Diagnosis: acute thrombotic cerebral infarction with residual left-sided hemiparesis.

_____

_____

CHAPTER 10. DISEASES OF THE RESPIRATORY SYSTEM (J00–J99)

10.1 When a respiratory condition is described as occurring in more than one site and is not specifically indexed, it should be classified to each anatomic site, as appropriate.

❑ True

❑ False

10.2 How many codes would be necessary to report an acute *Haemophillus influenza* bronchitis with an acute exacerbation of chronic obstructive pulmonary disease?

A. One: J44.0 only

B. Two: J44.0 and J44.1

C. Three: J44.0, J44.1, and J20.1

10.3 Acute recurrent streptococcal tonsillitis

_____

_____

10.4 Patient presents with progressive worsening of viral pneumonia. Viral culture was positive for respiratory syncytial virus (RSV). Diagnostic imaging reveals an abscess in the right upper lobe, which when aspirated, tested positive for methicillian-resistant *Staphylococcus aureus*. Diagnosis: RSV pneumonia complicated by MRSA bacterial pneumonia with abscess.

_____

_____

CHAPTER 11. DISEASES OF THE DIGESTIVE SYSTEM (KØØ–K94)

11.1 Conditions classifiable to categories K5Ø Crohn's disease, and K51 Ulcerative colitis, are mutually exclusive, and may never be reported together.

☐ True

☐ False

11.2 Diarrhea due to irritable bowel syndrome

A. K58.Ø

B. K58.9, R19.7

C. R19.7

D. K58.Ø, R19.7

11.3 Obstructive sliding hiatal hernia with gastroesophageal reflux esophagitis

_____

_____

11.4. A patient presents extremely ill with nausea, vomiting, fever, and severe LLQ abdominal tenderness and rectal bleeding. She has a remote history of diverticular disease diagnosed on screening colonoscopy. Upon examination, the patient's abdomen was rigid, swollen, and tender over the LLQ. Rectal examination was positive for lower GI hemorrhage. CT of the abdomen demonstrated localized peritonitis due to perforated sigmoid diverticulitis.

_____

_____

CHAPTER 12. DISEASES OF THE SKIN AND SUBCUTANEOUS TISSUE (LØØ–L99)

12.1 When coding and reporting multiple pressure ulcers, report only the highest stage (most severe) ulcer, stages 1–4.

❏ True

❏ False

12.2 If a chronic skin ulcer of the lower extremity, classified to category L97, is documented with atherosclerosis of the lower extremities, a causal relationship may be assumed and the atherosclerosis is listed first.

❏ True

❏ False

12.3 An elderly farmer with a long-standing history of sun exposure presents for treatment of skin lesions of the ears, scalp, and face. The skin biopsy obtained on the previous encounter is consistent with solar keratosis.

_____

_____

12.4 Erythema multiforme in Ritter's disease with 15 percent body surface exfoliation

_____

_____

CHAPTER 13. DISEASES OF THE MUSCULOSKELETAL SYSTEM AND CONNECTIVE TISSUE (MØØ–M99)

13.1 When coding pathological fractures, the seventh character A may be reported for the following circumstances *except*:

A. As long as the patient is receiving active treatment for the fracture

B. For surgical treatment encounters for problems associated with healing

C. Emergency department encounter

D. Evaluation and treatment by a new physician

13.2 Chapter 13 codes that represent laterality include the site of the:

A. Bone

B. Joint

C. Muscle

D. All of the above

13.3 Enteropathic arthropathy of the ankles (bilateral) associated with a long-term history of Crohn's disease

_____

_____

13.4 A 62-year-old female presents for evaluation of degenerative osteoarthritis of the lumbar spine and herniated lumbar disc. Diagnostic imaging reveals displacement of the L2–L3 intervertebral disc. Physical exam is consistent with progressive disc compression of the L2–L3 nerve root, exacerbating the sciatica symptoms. Surgical treatment options were discussed with the patient.

_____

_____

CHAPTER 14. DISEASES OF THE GENITOURINARY SYSTEM (NØØ–N99)

14.1 The sequencing of chronic kidney disease associated with other contributing conditions (e.g., hypertension, diabetes mellitus) is based on the conventions (instructions) in the tabular list.

❑ True

❑ False

14.2 A dialysis patient presents with stage 4 chronic kidney disease with end stage renal disease (ESRD).

A. N18.4, N18.6, Z99.2

B. N18.4, Z99.2

C. N18.6, Z99.2

D. N18.6

14.3 Benign prostatic hypertrophy (BPH) with reflux uropathy

_____

_____

14.4 A young immigrant woman presents with intense pelvic and vulvar pain. The physician suspects pelvic inflammatory disease or infection. Upon examination, the access to the introitus is severely compromised with external genitalia in a healed, but mutilated appearance. The patient is admitted to the hospital and scheduled for surgery. Under general anesthesia, the artificially created barrier is removed, and specimens are collected for culture and sensitivity. Pathology confirms the presence of group A streptococcus. Diagnosis: acute bacterial parametritis with pelvic cellulitis, female genital mutilation status, type III.

_____

_____

CHAPTER 15. PREGNANCY, CHILDBIRTH AND THE PUERPERIUM (O00–O9A)

15.1 Obstetric cases require codes from chapter 15. Additional codes from other chapters are excluded from maternal or obstetric reporting.

❑ True

❑ False

15.2 Which of the following statements is *not* true:

A. The final character for trimester of pregnancy should be based on the provider's documentation of trimester for the current encounter.

B. The provider's documentation of number of weeks' gestation should not be used to identify the trimester.

C. If the trimester is not a component of a code, the condition is either classified to a specific trimester, or is not applicable to the condition.

D. Not all chapter 15 codes apply to all trimesters, although certain conditions may occur in more than one trimester.

15.3 Spontaneous vaginal delivery of liveborn diamniotic/dichorionic twins at 36-weeks' gestation. Delivery complicated by third-degree perineal laceration.

_____

_____

15.4 A 39-year-old primigravida presents at 19-weeks' gestation for management of mild pre-eclampsia, mild hyperemesis gravidarum, and gestational diet-controlled diabetes mellitus.

_____

_____

CHAPTER 16. CERTAIN CONDITIONS ORIGINATING IN THE PERINATAL PERIOD (PØØ–P96)

16.1 When a condition that originates in the perinatal period continues throughout the life of the patient, the perinatal code should continue to be used to report the condition, regardless of the patient's age.

☐ True

☐ False

16.2 Which of the following statements is *not* true:

A. Codes from category PØ5 should not be assigned with codes from category PØ7.

B. Report both birth weight and gestational age codes from category PØ7, as appropriate.

C. A code for prematurity should be assigned based on the estimated gestational age of the newborn as recorded in the medical record.

D. Assignment of PØ5 and PØ7 should be based on the recorded birth weight and estimated gestational age.

16.3 A 14-day-old infant presents with agitation, crying, and poor feeding. Examination is consistent with oral thrush. Oral culture is positive for candida albicans. Diagnosis: neonatal thrush.

_____

_____

16.4 A male is born prematurely in the hospital via vaginal delivery at 35-weeks' gestation with a birth weight of 2214 grams. The mother has a history of cocaine abuse. The newborn has no manifestations or signs of withdrawal from the drug abuse; however, the infant tests positive for cocaine. During the hospitalization, the infant is treated with phototherapy for jaundice associated with prematurity.

_____

_____

CHAPTER 17. CONGENITAL MALFORMATIONS, DEFORMATIONS AND CHROMOSOMAL ABNORMALITIES (QØØ–Q99)

17.1 Codes from chapter 17 should not be reported for chromosomal anomalies identified in adulthood. Instead, the condition should be reported with the appropriate code from the affected body system chapter.

❑ True

❑ False

17.2 When no unique code is available for a malformation/deformation or chromosomal anomaly, assign additional (separate, as necessary) codes for any manifestations or associated conditions present that are not inherent components of the chapter 17 condition.

❑ True

❑ False

17.3 Aortic dilation in Marfan's syndrome

_____

_____

17.4 A 20-year-old patient with trisomy 21, mild intellectual disability (recent IQ: 62) and a history of corrected congenital heart defect, presents for treatment of congenital hypothyroidism.

_____

_____

CHAPTER 18. SYMPTOMS, SIGNS AND ABNORMAL CLINICAL AND LABORATORY FINDINGS, NOT ELSEWHERE CLASSIFIED (RØØ–R99)

18.1 **Practically all chapter 18 classification categories could be designated as "not otherwise specified," "unknown etiology," or "transient."**

☐ True

☐ False

18.2 **Chapter 18 classifications include the following, except:**

A. Signs and symptoms that point rather definitively to a given diagnosis

B. Signs or symptoms existing at the time of the initial encounter that proved to be transient

C. Provisional diagnoses in a patient who failed to return for further investigation

D. Cases in which a more precise diagnosis cannot be determined

E. Signs and symptoms that point (perhaps) equally to two or more diseases or two or more systems of the body.

18.3 **A 70-year-old female presents to her family physician's office with atypical chest pain and fatigue. She is provided with a prescription for nitroglycerin. The patient is referred for an outpatient testing and expedient consultation with a cardiologist.**

_____

_____

18.4 **A 38-year-old male presents to the outpatient radiology clinic for ultrasound of the abdomen to evaluate right upper quadrant abdominal pain. He is morbidly obese at 5'-7", 300 lbs., and a body mass index (BMI) of 46. Upon exam, the transducer was unable to capture images due to obstruction by dense fatty abdominal tissue. Multiple attempts to reposition the instrument failed to produce successful results. The patient's physician will be contacted to discuss alternate methods of imaging that will accommodate the patient's large body habitus.**

_____

_____

CHAPTER 19. INJURY, POISONING, AND CERTAIN OTHER CONSEQUENCES OF EXTERNAL CAUSES (SØØ–T88)

19.1 Codes within the T section of chapter 19 that include an external cause do not require an additional external cause code.

☐ True

☐ False

19.2 Which of the following statements regarding the coding of injuries is *not* true?

A. Assign separate codes for each injury unless a combination code is provided, in which case the combination code should be assigned.

B. The appropriate traumatic injury codes (SØØ–T14.9) should be reported for normal, healing surgical wounds and to identify complications of surgical wounds, by anatomic site.

C. The code for the most serious injury, as determined by the provider and focus of treatment, is sequenced first.

D. Code TØ7 Unspecified multiple injuries, should not be reported unless information for a more specified code is not available.

19.3 A patient presents for follow up of a closed Colles' fracture of the right wrist. Examination reveals delayed healing. Patient history is remarkable for long-term corticosteroid therapy for systemic lupus erythematosus (SLE). Diagnosis: delayed healing of Colles' fracture, SLE, corticosteroid status.

_____

_____

19.4 An elderly patient presents to the emergency department after a fall injury in the home. The patient stated that she slipped and fell in the kitchen of her private residence; falling onto her hip and shoulder, which "took the brunt of the impact," and bumping the back of her head slightly on a table, with no loss of consciousness. Examination was positive for a possible right hip fracture, and an obvious traumatic dislocation of the right shoulder. The patient's right occipital scalp was tender to palpation, with an approximate 3 cm, raised occipital contusion. Diagnostic imaging revealed no intracranial pathology; however, films were positive for a displaced, subtrochanteric fracture of the femur, and an anterior subluxation of the humerus at the glenohumeral joint. The patient was admitted and scheduled for surgery, where manual reduction of the shoulder dislocation and an open reduction with fixation of the subtrochanteric femur fracture were performed without incident.

_____

_____

CHAPTER 20. EXTERNAL CAUSES OF MORBIDITY (VØØ-Y99)

20.1 Chapter 20 codes are applicable only to injuries, poisonings, and consequences of external causes, the range of SØØ–T88.

❑ True

❑ False

20.2 A code from category Y93 Activity codes, is appropriate for use with external cause and intent codes if identifying the activity provides additional information about the event.

❑ True

❑ False

20.3 Assign the external cause codes:
A Marine officer presents for follow up of an injury sustained by friendly fire during a military operation in Afghanistan.

_____

_____

20.4 Assign the external cause codes:
A woman presents for initial treatment of an injury sustained when attempting to pet a cat, which bit her on the hand. She sustained the injury during the leisure activity of caring for her horses in a commercial self-care animal boarding facility (barn).

_____

_____

CHAPTER 21. FACTORS INFLUENCING HEALTH STATUS AND CONTACT WITH HEALTH SERVICES (ZØØ–Z99)

21.1 The use of Z codes have little practical use, and should be limited to those instances when there is no further documentation to permit more precise coding.

☐ True

☐ False

21.2 Which of the following statements regarding screening Z codes is *not* true? A screening code:

A. May be listed as a first listed code if the screening is the reason for the visit, or an additional code if the screening is done during an encounter for other health problems.

B. Is not necessary if the screening is inherent to a routine examination (e.g., Pap smear during a routine pelvic exam).

C. Is a test to rule out or confirm a suspected diagnosis due to presenting a sign or symptom.

D. Indicates that a screening exam is planned. A procedure code is required to confirm that the screening was performed.

21.3 A 57-year-old female presents to the OB/GYN clinic for follow-up vaginal Pap smear following a total abdominal hysterectomy (TAH) one year ago for cervical cancer. Radiation and chemotherapy treatments concluded approximately six months ago.

_____

_____

21.4 A patient presents with marked fatigue and vague, generalized "aches and pains." She states that her lack of energy and "aches" are interfering with her work, daily activities, and social life. She presents at this time for physical examination and laboratory testing to rule out pathology. Family history is significant for a sister who was recently diagnosed with multiple sclerosis (MS) and an aunt with systemic lupus erythematosus (SLE). Personal history is noncontributory, except for a history of mononucleosis and depression as a teenager. The patient will return to review the outpatient test results. Differential diagnosis includes latent viral infection, fibromyalgia, autoimmune disease, and depression.

_____

_____

Comprehensive Self-Examination Answers

Note: Official guidelines noted in rationale are in reference to the "ICD-10-CM Draft Official Guidelines for Coding and Reporting," 2013 version. The current version of the guidelines is available on the NCHS website at: http://www.cdc.gov/nchs/icd/icd10cm.htm#10update.

CHAPTER 1. CERTAIN INFECTIOUS AND PARASITIC DISEASES (AØØ–B99)

1.1 **False.**

Official guideline 1.C.2.a states that when a patient is admitted for an HIV related condition, the principal diagnosis should be B2Ø, followed by additional diagnosis codes for all reported HIV-related conditions.

1.2 **D. "Not included here."**

Intestinal trichomoniasis (AØ7.8) is excluded from category A59, and more appropriately classified elsewhere; however, it is possible for the patient to have both conditions at the same time. If so, it would be acceptable to report both AØ7.8 and a category A59 code together.

See the ICD-10-CM Draft Conventions in the front matter of Optum's *ICD-10-CM—The Complete Official Draft Code Set* text. In this section, the format, punctuation, abbreviations, and notations are defined to assist in complete, accurate, and consistent coding.

1.3 **AØ2.Ø** **Salmonella enteritis**
Z16.23 **Resistant to quinolones and fluoroquinolones**

The alphabetic index lists the main term "Enteritis" and subterms "Salmonella, salmonellosis" with reference to code AØ2.Ø. The code is confirmed in the tabular list, where an instructional note at the beginning of the chapter prompts the use of an additional code to identify any associated drug resistance (Z16). Category Z16 also includes an instructional note to code first (sequence first) the infection.

1.4 **A41.52** **Sepsis due to Pseudomonas**
R65.21 **Severe sepsis with septic shock**
J96.ØØ **Acute respiratory failure, unspecified whether with hypoxia or hypercapnia**

Official guidelines 1.C.1.d.1.b and 1.C.1.d.2 address the coding and sequencing of sepsis, severe sepsis, and septic shock. A minimum of two codes are required when coding sepsis and septic shock: a code for the underlying systemic infection followed by a subcategory R65.2 Severe sepsis, code. When septic shock is documented, severe sepsis is assumed. Instructional notes at subcategory R65.2 state to code first the sepsis (A41.-), and to use an additional code to identify the specific acute organ dysfunction (e.g., acute respiratory failure).

CHAPTER 2. NEOPLASMS (CØØ–D49)

2.1   **False.**

Official guideline 1.C.2.c.1 states that, in this circumstance, the malignancy is sequenced first. This is a departure from ICD-9-CM guidelines.

2.2   **C. Represent a limited listing of included conditions and synonyms to the code title. Additional terms found only in the alphabetic index may also be assigned, as appropriate.**

Official guideline 1.A.11 defines inclusion terms as noted in option C above, with the clarification that listed inclusion terms are not exhaustive. Follow the instruction in the alphabetic index and tabular list. If the alphabetic index provides additional terms in reference to a code, confirm that a code in the tabular list, and assign as appropriate.

2.3   **C78.Ø1**   **Secondary malignant neoplasm of right lung**
      C19   **Malignant neoplasm of rectosigmoid junction**

Neoplasm sequencing is dependent upon the circumstances of the admission/encounter. Sequence first the neoplasm that necessitated the encounter. If the secondary neoplasm (metastasis) is the reason for the encounter, it may be sequenced as the first-listed or principal diagnosis. The primary site would be sequenced as an additional code. The neoplasm table lists the main term "Neoplasm, neoplastic," with the subterms "colon, with rectum" with reference to code C19 in the first (Primary Malignancy) column.

It should also be noted that the terms "colorectal" and "rectosigmoid" are synonymous since the sigmoid colon and the rectum intersect.

2.4   **Z51.11**   **Encounter for antineoplastic chemotherapy**
      T86.19   **Other complication of kidney transplant**
      C8Ø.2   **Malignant neoplasm associated with transplanted organ**
      C64.9   **Malignant neoplasm of unspecified kidney, except renal pelvis**

Official guideline 1.C.2.e.2 states that admissions/encounters solely for the administration of chemotherapy are reported with the appropriate therapy code (Z51.1-) sequenced as the first-listed or principal diagnosis. Two instructional notes are listed at code C80.2. The appropriate T86 category code is to be sequenced first to report the complication of transplanted organ. An additional code is reported to identify the specific malignancy (C64.9).

Chapter 3. Diseases of the Blood and Blood-forming Organs and Certain Disorders Involving the Immune Mechanism (D5Ø–D89)

3.1 False.

The first part of this statement is true. Code D77 reports a manifestation; however, the interpretation of a manifestation code, as stated in the question, is false. A manifestation code cannot be reported as a first-listed or principal diagnosis.

3.2 A. Human immunodeficiency virus HIV disease

Although code block D8Ø–D89 Certain disorders involving the immune mechanism, includes classifications of certain immune disorders, it specifically lists human immunodeficiency virus [HIV] disease (B2Ø) as an Excludes 1 diagnosis.

3.3 D5Ø.Ø Iron deficiency anemia secondary to blood loss (chronic)

The alphabetic index lists the main term "Anemia" and subterms "deficiency, iron, secondary to blood loss (chronic)" with reference to code D5Ø.Ø. The code is confirmed in the tabular list.

3.4 D64.2 Secondary sideroblastic anemia due to drugs and toxins
T37.1X5A Adverse effect of antimycobacterial drugs, initial encounter
A18.Ø1 Tuberculosis of spine

The alphabetic index lists the main term "Anemia" and subterms "sideroblastic, secondary (due to), drugs and toxins" with reference to code D64.2. The tabular list contains and instructional note at code D64.2, which prompts to use an additional code from categories T36–T50 to report the adverse effect, with fifth or sixth character 5. Tuberculosis is assigned as an additional diagnosis.

CHAPTER 4. ENDOCRINE, NUTRITIONAL AND METABOLIC DISEASES (EØØ–E89)

4.1 False.

Although it is certainly possible to report diabetes and an associated manifestation with one combination code (e.g., E10.21 Type 1 diabetes mellitus with diabetic nephropathy), it is often necessary to assign additional codes to report a condition in its entirety. Instructional notes in the text demonstrate these circumstances. For example:

E10.22   **Type 1 diabetes mellitus with diabetic chronic kidney disease**

Use additional code to identify stage of chronic kidney disease (N18.1–N18.6)

4.2   E75.Ø1   Sandhoff disease

The alphabetic index lists the main term "Sandhoff's disease" with code E75.Ø1. The tabular list confirms subcategory E75.Ø GM2 gangliosidosis, with Sandoff disease classified to code E75.Ø1.

4.3   E24.2   Drug-induced Cushing's syndrome
T38.ØX5D Adverse effect of glucocorticoids and synthetic analogues, subsequent encounter

The alphabetic index lists the main term "Syndrome" and subterms "Cushing's, due to, drugs" with reference to code E24.2. The code is confirmed in the tabular list where an instructional note prompts to use additional code for adverse effect, if applicable, to identify drug (T36–T50 with fifth or sixth character 5). The diagnostic statement indicates this is a subsequent encounter (D).

4.4   E78.2   Mixed hyperlipidemia
E66.Ø9   Other obesity due to excess calories
Z68.3Ø   Body mass index [BMI] 3Ø.Ø–3Ø.9, adult

The alphabetic index lists the main term "Hypercholesterolemia" and subterms "with hypertriglyceridemia" with reference to code E78.2. Inclusion terms in the tabular list confirm code assignment. An instructional note at category E66 prompts for the addition of a category Z68 code to report BMI.

Chapter 5. Mental, Behavioral, and Neurodevelopmental Disorders (FØ1–F99)

5.1 E. Both A. and B.

ICD-10-CM etiology/manifestation coding conventions require the underlying condition (etiology) to be sequenced first, followed by the manifestation. Manifestation codes may not be reported alone, and may be identified by the phrase "in diseases classified elsewhere" in the code title. Follow sequencing instructions in the text and report this manifestation secondary to the underlying condition.

5.2 F31.2 Bipolar disorder, current episode manic severe with psychotic features

The alphabetic index lists the main term "Disorder" and subterms "bipolar, current episode, manic, with psychotic features" with reference to code F31.2. The code is confirmed in the tabular list. Note that bipolar disorder with single manic episode is excluded (F30-) from category F31. Review documentation carefully when coding and reporting bipolar disorder. Clarify with the provider if necessary.

5.3 F63.Ø Pathological gambling
F6Ø.5 Obsessive-compulsive personality disorder

The alphabetic index lists two subterm entries under the main term "Compulsion, compulsive." The subterm "gambling" references code F63.Ø, whereas the subterm "personality" references code F60.5. Review of the tabular list for the referenced codes lists two separate classifications. Excessive gambling by manic patients (F30, F31) and those with antisocial personality disorder (F60.2) are listed as Excludes 2 conditions. There is no notation that precludes the two codes from being reported together, and in fact, both codes are necessary to satisfy the diagnostic statement. Note that obsessive-compulsive personality disorder is classified separately from obsessive-compulsive disorder (F42). In order to code to the highest level of specificity, a code for the pathological gambling and the obsessive-compulsive disorder should be assigned. Note that if the main term "Disorder" was used to locate the obsessive-compulsive personality disorder, the encounter may not have been coded to the highest specificity. It is necessary to index the subterm "personality" to index the diagnosis of obsessive-compulsive personality disorder to code F60.5.

5.4 T4Ø.5X1A Poisoning by cocaine, accidental (unintentional), initial encounter
F14.222 Cocaine dependence with intoxication with perceptual disturbance

An overdose (accidental) is coded to "Poisoning, accidental (unintentional)." Category F14.2 Cocaine dependence, lists cocaine poisoning as an Excludes 2 condition that indicates that cocaine poisoning (overdose) is classified elsewhere, but may be reported with cocaine dependence when the two conditions coexist.

CHAPTER 6. DISEASES OF THE NERVOUS SYSTEM (GØØ–G99)

6.1 **True.**

Official guideline 1.C.6.b.1.a confirms both statements. Note, however, that if the underlying cause of the pain (necessitating pain control management) is known, it should be reported as an additional diagnosis. A category G89 code would not be sequenced first if the encounter is aimed at treated an underlying condition, and a neurostimulator is inserted for pain control during the same encounter. In that situation, the underlying condition would be listed first.

6.2 **A. Report the affected side as unspecified.**

If the affected side is documented, code to the appropriate laterality. Official guideline 1.C.6.a states that if the dominant or nondominant side status is not documented (if the patient is not documented as right or left-handed) assume dominance based on the criteria of items B–D.

6.3 **G89.3** **Neoplasm related pain (acute) (chronic)**
C79.51 **Secondary malignant neoplasm of bone**
Z85.46 **Personal history of malignant neoplasm of prostate**

Official guideline 1.C.6.5 states that code G89.3 may be sequenced as the first-listed or principal diagnosis if the reason for the encounter is pain control or pain management. The underlying neoplasms are reported as additional diagnoses.

6.4 **G43.511** **Persistent migraine aura without cerebral infarction, intractable, with status migrainosus**

The alphabetic index lists the main term "Migraine" with subterms "with aura, persistent, without cerebral infarction and intractable, intractable, with status migrainosus" with reference to G43.511. The code is confirmed in the tabular list. Notice that category G43.5 classifies migraine with aura described specifically as "persistent aura." Migraine with aura not described as persisted is classified to G43.1.

CHAPTER 7. DISEASES OF THE EYE AND ADNEXA (H00–H59)

7.1   False.

The Excludes note at the beginning of chapter 7 indicates that the listed conditions are classified elsewhere, but that they may be reported with a chapter 7 code, as appropriate, if the chapter 7 code and the excluded diagnoses coexist.

7.2   True.

Official guideline 1.B.13 supports this statement.

**7.3   H40.2222 Chronic angle closure glaucoma, left eye
         H26.232   Glaucomatous flecks (subcapsular), left eye**

The alphabetic index lists the main term "Glaucomatous flecks" with a cross-reference to "*see* Cataract, complicated." The main term "Cataract" and subterms "complicated, with, glaucomatous flecks" references subcategory H26.23-, in which the sixth character indicates laterality (2, left). An instructional note prompts to code first the underlying glaucoma (H40–H42). The type of glaucoma is specified as chronic angle closure. The index lists the main term "Glaucoma" and subterms "angle-closure, chronic" with reference to subcategory H40.22. The sixth character indicates laterality (2, left). Seventh character "2" reports disease stage.

7.4   H59.41   Inflammation (infection) of postprocedural bleb, stage 1

The alphabetic index lists the main term "Bleb" and subterms "inflamed (infected) (postprocedural), stage 1" with reference to code H59.41. The code is confirmed in the tabular list.

CHAPTER 8. DISEASES OF THE EAR AND MASTOID PROCESS (H6Ø–H95)

8.1   **False.**

While these conditions are included in subcategory H83.2, it would be invalid to report these conditions without the required sixth character. Subcategory H83.2 is further subdivided into a fifth-character subclassification that requires an additional sixth character laterality designation. Official guideline 1.A.3 states that for reporting purposes, only codes are permissible not categories (three characters) or subcategories (three to six characters). A code is invalid if it is not assigned the full number of characters required (1.B.2).

8.2   **C. Subperiosteal abscess of mastoid, unspecified ear**

The alphabetic index lists the main term "Mastoiditis" and subterms "acute, subacute, periosteal" with reference to code H7Ø.Ø1-. The dash (-) indicates that the code is further subdivided. Upon confirmation in the tabular list, six-character codes are listed within subcategory H7Ø.Ø1 in which laterality must be reported, if known. The laterality is not stated and, therefore, cannot be assumed. Code H7Ø.Ø19 reports unspecified laterality (unspecified ear).

8.3   **H61.Ø31**   **Chondritis of right external ear**
        B96.5   **Pseudomonas (aeruginosa) (mallei) (pseudomallei) as the cause of diseases classified elsewhere**

Official guideline 1.C.1.b states to assign the appropriate code from categories B95–B97 to report infectious agents as the cause of diseases classified elsewhere. Although the condition (chondritis) and laterality (right) may be reported with code H61.Ø31, an additional code is necessary to report the causal infectious organism (pseudomonas).

8.4   **H66.ØØ4**   **Acute suppurative otitis media without spontaneous rupture of ear drum, recurrent, right ear**
        H66.Ø15   **Acute suppurative otitis media with spontaneous rupture of ear drum, recurrent, left ear**
        H72.12   **Attic perforation of tympanic membrane, left ear**

Instructional notes at code categories H66 and H72 prompt for multiple coding in the event of otitis media with associated perforated tympanic membrane. Subcategory H66.Ø is further divided by associated rupture (H66.Ø1). Since only the left ear has an associated perforation, it is separately reported from the right, even though both conditions are classified as acute, suppurative, and recurrent.

CHAPTER 9. DISEASES OF THE CIRCULATORY SYSTEM (I00–I99)

9.1   True.

This statement is supported by official guideline 1.C.9.b.

9.2   B. 4 weeks

Official guideline I.C.9.e.1 supports this statement. This is a departure from ICD-9-CM coding practices in which the episode of care concept required the reporting of a subsequent episode (fifth character 2) designation for subsequent encounters for further treatment of an acute MI within eight weeks following the initial episode. The episode of care concept has been eliminated in ICD-10-CM. Instead, ICD-10-CM classifies AMI into two categories, initial AMI or subsequent AMI, regardless of the episode of care.

9.3   I25.110   Atherosclerotic heart disease of native coronary artery with unstable angina pectoris

The alphabetic index provides a cross-reference at the main term "Disease" and subterms "artery, coronary" to "*see* Arteriosclerosis, coronary (artery)." Subcategory I25.1 includes coronary artery disease (CAD). Note that native coronary artery disease is assumed unless there is a documented history of coronary artery bypass. In that situation, the coder would determine whether the native or bypass vessels were affected, and code accordingly or to "unspecified" if specific information is not available. The main term "Angina" lists subterm "crescendo" with a cross-reference to "*see* Angina, unstable." As such, the crescendo angina pectoris is classified as unstable.

9.4   I63.321   Cerebral infarction due to thrombosis of right anterior cerebral artery
**   G81.94   Hemiplegia, unspecified, affecting left nondominant side**
**   I10   Essential (primary) hypertension**

Code I63.321 identifies the cerebral infarction by type (thrombosis) and site (right anterior cerebral artery). Code G81.94 identifies the residual hemiplegia. A note at category G81 clarifies that the category is for use in multiple coding to identify hemiplegia, by type resulting from any cause. The hemiplegia, unspecified to type is specified to laterality, as affecting the left (nondominant) side in a right-handed patient. Hypertension is reported as an additional diagnosis.

CHAPTER 10. DISEASES OF THE RESPIRATORY SYSTEM (JØØ–J99)

10.1 False.

The note at the beginning of chapter 10 instructs to classify the condition to the lower anatomic site. Specifically, the note states: "When a respiratory condition is described as occurring in more than one site and is not specifically indexed, it should be classified to the lower anatomic site (e.g., tracheobronchitis to bronchitis in J40)."

10.2 C. Three, J44.Ø, J44.1 and J2Ø.1

The instructional note at code J44.Ø prompts to use an additional code to identify the infection. An Excludes 2 note at the beginning of code block J2Ø–J22 indicates that codes from that block may be reported with code J44.Ø. Similarly, the Excludes 2 note at code J44.1 indicates that both J44.Ø and J44.1 may be reported together when both conditions coexist.

10.3 J03.01   Acute recurrent streptococcal tonsillitis

The alphabetic index lists the main term "Tonsillitis" and subterms "streptococcal, recurrent" with reference to code J03.01. Note that subcategory J03.0 includes the organism within the code description. As such, no additional code is required to identify the infectious agent.

10.4 J15.212   Pneumonia due to methicillin resistant Staphylococcus aureus
J85.1   Abscess of lung with pneumonia
J12.1   Respiratory syncytial virus pneumonia

Three codes are required to satisfy the diagnostic statement. Instructional notes at categories J15 and J12 prompt to code also associated abscess, if applicable (J85.1).

Chapter 11. Diseases of the Digestive System (KØØ–K94)

11.1 True.

This statement is an example of the correct interpretation of Excludes 1 notations.

11.2 A. K58.Ø

Code K58.Ø Irritable bowel syndrome with diarrhea, is a combination code that identifies a condition and an associated complication or secondary process (manifestation). Official guideline 1.B.9 states to assign only the combination code when it identifies the diagnostic conditions involved. Multiple coding should not be used when the classification provides a combination code that clearly satisfies the diagnostic statement.

11.3 K44.Ø   Diaphragmatic hernia with obstruction, without gangrene
K21.Ø   Gastro-esophageal reflux disease with esophagitis

The alphabetic index lists the main term "Hernia, hernial" and subterms "hiatal, with, obstruction" with reference to code K44.Ø. Category K44 Diaphragmatic hernia, includes hiatus hernia (sliding). Gastroesophageal reflux disease (GERD) is classified to category K21, with fourth-character codes that differentiate between GERD with or without reflux. Note that code block K20–K31 lists hiatus hernia as an Excludes 2 condition. Both codes may be reported, as appropriate when they coexist.

11.4 K57.21   Diverticulitis of large intestine with perforation and abscess with bleeding

The alphabetic index lists the main term "Diverticulitis" with subterms "intestine, large, with abscess, perforation or peritonitis, with bleeding" with reference to code K57.21. The combination code is confirmed in the tabular list. No additional codes are required, as the combination code satisfies the diagnostic statement.

CHAPTER 12. DISEASES OF THE SKIN AND SUBCUTANEOUS TISSUE (LØØ–L99)

12.1 False.

Category L89 is composed of combination codes that identify the site and severity of pressure ulcer. Official guideline 1.C.12.1. states to assign as many codes from category L89 as needed to identify all the pressure ulcers (by site) that the patient has.

12.2 True.

The note at category L97 supports this statement. If any of the conditions listed in the "code first any associated condition" notation at category L97 is documented, with a lower extremity ulcer, a causal condition should be assumed. Multiple coding and sequencing practices are reinforced by instructional notes at the listed I7Ø subcategories, which prompt the coder to use an additional code to identify the severity of the (lower extremity) ulcer with the appropriate fifth character.

12.3 L57.Ø   Actinic keratosis
X32.XXXD Exposure to sunlight, subsequent encounter

The alphabetic index lists the main term "Keratosis" and subterm "solar" with reference to L57.0. Solar keratosis is listed as an inclusion term in the tabular list. An instructional note at category L57 prompts to use an additional code to identify the source of the ultraviolet radiation. Category X32 reports the exposure to sunlight. A seventh character D is required to report the subsequent encounter for the condition resulting from the exposure. Placeholders (X) are required to fill the vacant character positions.

12.4 LØØ   Staphylococcal scalded skin syndrome
L49.3   Exfoliation due to erythematous condition involving 3Ø–39 percent of body surface

The Excludes 1 notation at category L51 precludes the use of a category L51 code with Ritter's disease (LØØ). Only Ritter's disease (staphylococcal scalded skin syndrome) is reported, followed by code L49.3 to report the extent of body surface involved.

CHAPTER 13. DISEASES OF THE MUSCULOSKELETAL SYSTEM AND CONNECTIVE TISSUE (MØØ–M99)

13.1 **B. For surgical treatment encounters for problems associated with healing**

Official guidelines for coding 1.C.13.c states that the seventh character A is for use as long as the patient is receiving active treatment for the fracture. Examples of active treatment include surgical treatment, emergency department encounters, and evaluation and treatment by a new physician. However, after the patient has completed active treatment and presents for subsequent encounters associated with complications of healing (e.g., malunion, nonunion, and sequelae) an other appropriate seventh characters should be reported, as appropriate (e.g., D, G, K, P, S) to the subcategory.

13.2 **D. All of the above**

Official guideline 1.C.13.a supports the application of site to either the bone, joint, or muscle involved, as appropriate.

13.3 **M07.671** **Enteropathic arthropathies, right ankle and foot**
 M07.672 **Enteropathic arthropathies, left ankle and foot**
 K5Ø.918 **Crohn's disease, unspecified with other complication**

Official guideline 1.B.13 states that for a condition which affects bilateral sites, but no bilateral code is provided, separate codes should be assigned for both the left and the right side.

Code K5Ø.9Ø reports Crohn's disease, NOS. However, since the disease has progressed outside the gastrointestinal system with the development of associated arthropathy, one may question whether code K5Ø.918 would be a more appropriate code. In lieu of official advice whether the designation of a "complication" extends beyond the gastrointestinal disease process, code K5Ø.9Ø is reported by default.

13.4 **M51.16** **Intervertebral disc disorders with radiculopathy, lumbar region**
 M47.816 **Spondylosis without myelopathy or radiculopathy, lumbar region**

The alphabetic index lists the main term "Osteoarthritis" and subterm "spine" with a cross-reference to "*see* Spondylosis." The main term "Spondylosis" lists the subterms "without myelopathy or radiculopathy, lumbar region" with reference to M47.816. The code is confirmed in the tabular list. The scenario attributes the progression of symptoms with sciatica due to the disc displacement. The main term "Displacement" and subterms "intervertebral disc, lumbar region, with neuritis, radiculitis, radiculopathy or sciatica" references code M51.16. The code is also confirmed in the tabular list.

Chapter 14. Diseases of the Genitourinary System (NØØ–N99)

14.1 True.

Official guideline 1.C.14.a.3 supports this statement. The conventions (instructions) in the tabular list include those as specified in the instructional notes, includes and excludes notations.

14.2 C. N18.6, Z99.2

Official guideline 1.C.14.1 states that if both a stage of CKD and ESRD are documented, assign code N18.6 only. The diagnostic statement is not completely satisfied, however, without the addition of code Z99.2 to report dialysis status. The addition of this status code is supported by an instructional note at code N18.6, which prompts to use an additional code to identify dialysis status (N99.2).

14.3 N4Ø.1 Enlarged prostate with lower urinary tract symptoms [LUTS]
N13.8 Other obstructive and reflux uropathy

The alphabetic index lists the main term "Hypertrophy" and subterms "prostate" with a cross-reference to "*see* Enlargement, enlarged, prostate." In doing so, the subterms "prostate, with lower urinary tract symptoms (LUTS)" references code N40.1. The code is confirmed in the tabular list where an instructional note prompts to use additional codes to report associated symptoms, when specified. The main term "Uropathy" and subterms "reflux, specified NEC" references code N13.8. An instructional note provides sequencing instruction to code, if applicable, any causal condition first, such as enlarged prostate (N4Ø.1). Note that fourth character .1 is indicated, since lower urinary tract symptoms (reflux uropathy) are present.

14.4 N73.Ø Acute parametritis and pelvic cellulitis
B95.Ø Streptococcus, group A, as the cause of diseases classified elsewhere
N9Ø.813 Female genital mutilation Type III status

The main term "Parametritis" and subterm "acute" references code N73.0. A cross-reference is provided to "see also Disease, pelvis, inflammatory." In the tabular list, an instructional note at category N73 prompts to use an additional code (B95–B97) to identify the infectious agent. Code B95.0 is assigned as an additional diagnosis. The alphabetic index lists the main term "Female genital mutilation status (FGM)" and subterms "type III" with reference to code N90.813.

Chapter 15. Pregnancy, Childbirth and the Puerperium (O00–O9A)

15.1 False.

Although obstetric cases require codes from chapter 15, which take sequencing priority, additional codes from other chapters may be used in conjunction with chapter 15 codes to further specify condition (official guideline 1.C.15.a.1).

15.2 B. The provider's documentation of number of weeks' gestation should not be used to identify the trimester.

Official guideline 1.C.15.a.3 states that the provider's documentation of number of weeks gestation may be used to identify the trimester. Assignment of the final character designating trimester should be based on the provider's documentation, whether it is specified as a specific trimester or documented in number of weeks' gestation. This applies to the assignment of trimester for pre-existing conditions as well as those that develop during or are due to the pregnancy.

15.3 O30.043 **Twin pregnancy, dichorionic/diamniotic, third trimester**
O70.2 **Third degree perineal laceration during delivery**
Z37.2 **Outcome of delivery, twins both liveborn**
Z3A.36 **36 weeks gestation**

Code O3.04 requires the sixth character 3 to specify trimester of pregnancy at the time of the encounter. The perineal laceration is assigned as an additional diagnosis, and does not require a trimester character, since the code description identifies the occurrence as "during delivery." An outcome of delivery status is required as an additional code on the mother's record (excluding stillbirth P95).

15.4 O14.02 **Mild to moderate pre-eclampsia, second trimester**
O21.0 **Mild hyperemesis gravidarum**
O24.410 **Gestational diabetes mellitus in pregnancy, diet controlled**
O09.512 **Supervision of elderly primigravida, second trimester**
Z3A.19 **19 weeks gestation**

The alphabetic index lists conditions pre-eclampsia and hyperemesis gravidarum under the main term "Pregnancy" and subterm "complicated by." Cross-references are provided for hyperemesis gravidarum and gestational diabetes to index these conditions under alternate terms. Trimester designations are assigned as second trimester based on the gestational weeks provided. Code O09.512 is assigned to report the patient as elderly primigravida; as 35 years and older at expected date of delivery.

CHAPTER 16. CERTAIN CONDITIONS ORIGINATING IN THE PERINATAL PERIOD (P00–P96)

16.1 True.

Official guideline 1.C.16.4 supports this statement.

16.2 C. A code for prematurity should be assigned based on the estimated gestational age of the newborn as recorded in the medical record.

Providers use different criteria in determining prematurity. As such, a code for prematurity should not be assigned unless prematurity is documented by the provider (official guideline 1.C.16.d).

16.3 P37.5 Neonatal candidiasis

Oral thrush in a newborn can be indexed in a number of ways, including via the main term "Thrush" and subterm "newborn" or "Candidiasis," and subterm "neonatal." The code is confirmed in the tabular list.

16.4 Z38.00 Single liveborn infant, delivered vaginally
P07.18 Other low birth weight newborn, 2000–2499 grams
P07.38 Preterm newborn, gestational age 35 completed weeks
P04.41 Newborn (suspected to be) affected by maternal use of cocaine
P59.0 Neonatal jaundice, preterm

Category code Z38 Liveborn infant, is listed as the principal diagnosis for the birth record (official guideline 1.C.16.a.2). The diagnosis of prematurity is assigned as documented. The birth weight is sequenced before the gestational age (1.C.16.d). The alphabetic index lists the main term "Newborn" and subterms "affected by, cocaine" with reference to code P04.41. The main term "Newborn" and subterm "jaundice, of prematurity" references code P59.0. The codes are confirmed in the tabular list.

CHAPTER 17. CONGENITAL MALFORMATIONS, DEFORMATIONS AND CHROMOSOMAL ABNORMALITIES (QØØ–Q99)

17.1 False.

Chapter 17 codes may be assigned and reported, as appropriate, throughout the life of the patient. Official guideline 1.C.17. states that although present at birth, a malformation, deformation, or chromosomal abnormality may not be identified until later in life. Whenever the condition is diagnosed by the physician, it is appropriate to assign a chapter 17 code.

17.2 True.

Official guideline 1.C.17 supports this statement. Assign additional codes to report any manifestations or associated conditions present, as necessary, which are not inherent components of the chapter 17 condition.

17.3 Q87.41Ø   Marfan's syndrome with aortic dilation

Chapter 17 classifications include many combination codes similar to Q87.41Ø that facilitate the reporting of a condition and certain associated symptoms or manifestations with a single code. Otherwise, when the code description specifically identifies the malformation/deformation/anomaly, manifestations that are an *inherent* part of the anomaly should not be coded separately.

17.4 EØ3.1   Congenital hypothyroidism without goiter
     Q90.9   Down syndrome, unspecified
     F7Ø   Mild intellectual disabilities
     Z87.74   Personal history of (corrected) congenital malformations of heart and circulatory system

Although Down syndrome has a unique code assignment, congenital hypothyroidism is a commonly associated condition that is not an inherent part of the syndrome. As such, the hypothyroidism is reported separately and listed first as the reason for the encounter.

Instructional notes at category E9Ø and code block F7Ø–F79 prompt for multiple coding, where applicable, and provide sequencing guidance. The alphabetic index lists the main term "History" and subterms "personal (of), congenital malformation (corrected), heart (corrected)" with reference to code Z87.74. The code is confirmed in the tabular list.

Chapter 18. Symptoms, Signs and Abnormal Clinical and Laboratory Findings, Not Elsewhere Classified (R00–R99)

18.1 True.

The notation at the beginning of chapter 18 supports this statement.

18.2 A. Signs and symptoms that point rather definitively to a given diagnosis

The note at the beginning of chapter 18 defines the chapter contents. It is noted that signs and symptoms that point rather definitively to a given diagnosis have been assigned to a category in other chapters of the classification (official guideline 1.C.18).

18.3 R07.89 Other chest pain
R53.83 Other fatigue

The alphabetic index lists the main term "Pain" and subterms "atypical" with reference to code R07.89. Similarly, the main term "Fatigue" references code R53.83. The codes are confirmed in the tabular list. Symptom codes are reported when a related definitive diagnosis has not been established (confirmed) by the provider (official guideline 1.C.18.a).

18.4 R10.11 Right upper quadrant pain
R93.9 Diagnostic imaging inconclusive to excess body fat of patient
E66.01 Morbid (severe) obesity due to excessive calories
Z68.42 Body mass index (BMI) 45.0–49.9, adult

The right upper quadrant abdominal pain is sequenced as the first listed diagnosis as the reason for the encounter. The alphabetic index lists the main term "Findings, abnormal, inconclusive, without diagnosis" with the subterms "radiologic (x-ray), inconclusive due to excess body fat of patient" with reference to code R93.9. The code is confirmed in the tabular list. Morbid obesity and BMI status are reported as additional diagnoses.

CHAPTER 19. INJURY, POISONING, AND CERTAIN OTHER CONSEQUENCES OF EXTERNAL CAUSES (SØØ–T88)

19.1 True.

An instructional note at the beginning of chapter 19 supports this statement. Chapter 19 includes two initial alpha characters: S and T. The T section classifies injuries to unspecified body regions, poisonings, and other certain consequences of external causes.

19.2 B. The appropriate traumatic injury codes (SØØ–T14.9) should be reported for normal, healing surgical wounds and to identify complications of surgical wounds, by anatomic site.

This statement is not true. Official guideline 1.C.19.b states the contrary; that traumatic injury codes (SØØ–T14.9) should *not* be reported for normal, healing surgical wounds and to identify complications of surgical wounds. Normal, healing surgical wounds are not reported as traumatic injuries. Instead, index the terms "Aftercare" or "Complication," as appropriate, to report the specific circumstance or condition.

19.3 S52.531G Colles' fracture of right radius, subsequent encounter for closed fracture with delayed healing
M32.9   Systemic lupus erythematosus, unspecified
Z79.52   Long term (current) use of systemic steroids

The alphabetic index lists the main term "Fracture" and subterm "Colles'" with a cross-reference to "*see* Colles' fracture." In doing so, code S53.51- is referenced. A sixth character is required (1, right). The seventh character G indicates delayed healing of the closed fracture. The lupus and long-term steroid status are reported as additional diagnoses.

19.4 S72.21XA Displaced subtrochanteric fracture of right femur, initial encounter
S43.Ø11A Anterior subluxation of right humerus, initial encounter
SØØ.Ø3XA Contusion of scalp, initial encounter
WØ1.19ØA Fall on same level from slipping, tripping and stumbling with subsequent striking against furniture, initial encounter
Y92.Ø1Ø   Kitchen of single-family non-institutional (private) house as the place of occurrence of the external cause

The displaced hip fracture is sequenced first, as the most serious injury (official guideline 1.C.19.b). Separate codes for each injury are assigned (fracture, dislocation, contusion). If a more serious injury, such as an intracranial injury or concussion were determined to be present, the contusion would not have been separately assigned (1.C19.b.1). In this scenario, intracranial injury was ruled out, and the contusion was reported by anatomic site (scalp). The external cause is identified by indexing the main term "Fall" in the ICD-10-CM Index to External Causes. Similarly, the main terms "Place of occurrence" reference the appropriate Y92 category code. The activity is not stated, so Y93.9 Unspecified activity, is not assigned (1.C.2Ø.c). If the external cause status were stated, the appropriate Y99 code would be assigned. All codes, except for the place of occurrence (Y92.Ø1Ø), require seventh characters.

CHAPTER 20. EXTERNAL CAUSES OF MORBIDITY (VØØ–Y99)

20.1 False.

External cause codes may be assigned and reported with any code in the range of AØØ–T88.9, and ZØØ–Z99 that is a health condition due to an external cause. These codes are valid for reporting any infection, health condition, or injury due to an external source or cause. Note, however, that no additional external cause is required for poisonings, toxic effects, adverse effects, and underdosing codes (T36–T65) (official guideline 1.C.19.e).

20.2 True.

Official guideline 1.C.20.c supports this statement.

20.3 Y37.92XD Military operations involving friendly fire, subsequent encounter

The ICD-10-CM Index to External Causes lists the main terms "Military operations" and subterms "friendly fire" with reference to code Y37.92. A seventh character is required. A placeholder "X" fills the sixth-character position. Note that a place of occurrence code (Y92), an activity code (Y93), and an external cause status code (Y99) are used only once, at the initial encounter for treatment (A) (official guideline 1.C.20.b.c.k).

20.4 W55.Ø1XA Bitten by cat, initial encounter
Y93.K9   Activity, other involving animal care
Y92.71   Barn as the place of occurrence of the external cause
Y99.8   Other external cause status

The Index to External Causes lists the main term "Bite" and subterm "cat" with reference to code W55.Ø1. A placeholder "X" fills the sixth character position for the required seventh character (A, initial encounter). The main term "Activity" and subterms "animal care NEC" reference code Y93.K9. The code is confirmed as a valid five-character code in the tabular list. The main terms "Place of occurrence" lists the subterm "barn" with reference to code Y92.71. There is no classification distinction between a private or commercial barn. The external cause status is specified as leisure activity (Y99.8).

CHAPTER 21. FACTORS INFLUENCING HEALTH STATUS AND CONTACT WITH HEALTH SERVICES (ZØØ–Z99)

21.1 False.

This statement partially applies only to nonspecific Z codes (typically with a .9 last character). As for the remainder of the chapter 21 classifications, Z codes are intended for use in any health care setting (official guideline 1.C.21.a). The note at the beginning of chapter 21 defines the chapter contents to include reasons for encounters, and describe circumstances other than "disease" or "injury" that are recorded as "diagnoses" or "problems."

21.2 C. Is a testing to rule out or confirm a suspected diagnosis due to presenting a sign or symptom.

Official guideline 1.C.21.5 contradicts this statement. A screening exam is not synonymous with a testing to rule out or confirm a suspected diagnosis due to the presence of some sign or symptom. Such is a diagnostic examination, not a screening. Diagnostic examinations are reported with a code that indicates the presenting sign or symptom as the reason for the encounter.

21.3 ZØ8   **Encounter for follow-up examination after completed treatment for malignant neoplasm**

Z85.41   **Personal history of malignant neoplasm of cervix uteri**

Z9Ø.71Ø   **Acquired absence of both cervix and uterus**

Z92.21   **Personal history of antineoplastic chemotherapy**

Z92.3   **Personal history of irradiation**

Code ZØ8 is assigned as the first-listed diagnosis to explain the continuing surveillance following treatment of malignant neoplasm. Follow up codes are reported only when the condition has been fully treated and no longer exists. This code is reported in conjunction with history codes to provide the full picture of the healed condition and its course of treatment (official guideline 1.C.21.8). Instructional notes at code ZØ8 prompt for the use of additional codes to identify acquired absence of organs (Z9Ø-) and personal history of malignant neoplasm (Z85-). However, if a condition is found to recur during a follow up visit, then the diagnosis code would be assigned in place of the follow-up code.

21.4 R52   **Pain, unspecified**

R53.83   **Other fatigue**

Z86.59   **Personal history of other mental and behavioral disorders**

Z86.19   **Personal history of other infectious and parasitic diseases**

Z82.Ø   **Family history of epilepsy and other disease of the nervous system**

Z82.69   **Family history of other diseases of the musculoskeletal system and connective tissue**

In lieu of an established diagnosis, the patient's symptoms are listed as the reason for the encounter and diagnostic testing (official guideline 1.C.18.a).

Official guideline 1.C.21.4 defines the use of history codes. Personal history codes for the patient's past depression and mononucleosis are assigned, as they have potential for recurrence, or influencing the monitoring and treatment. Similarly, the family history codes are assigned to report the history of diseases that place the patient at increased risk. These codes may be used regardless of the reason for the visit, and provide important information that may explain or alter the type of treatment ordered.

Appendix A: ICD-10-CM Draft Official Guidelines for Coding and Reporting 2013

Narrative changes appear in bold text

Items <u>underlined</u> have been moved within the guidelines since the 2012 version

***Italics* are used to indicate revisions to heading changes**

The Centers for Medicare and Medicaid Services (CMS) and the National Center for Health Statistics (NCHS), two departments within the U.S. Federal Government's Department of Health and Human Services (DHHS) provide the following guidelines for coding and reporting using the International Classification of Diseases, 10th Revision, Clinical Modification (ICD-10-CM). These guidelines should be used as a companion document to the official version of the ICD-10-CM as published on the NCHS website. The ICD-10-CM is a morbidity classification published by the United States for classifying diagnoses and reason for visits in all health care settings. The ICD-10-CM is based on the ICD-10, the statistical classification of disease published by the World Health Organization (WHO).

These guidelines have been approved by the four organizations that make up the Cooperating Parties for the ICD-10-CM: the American Hospital Association (AHA), the American Health Information Management Association (AHIMA), CMS, and NCHS.

These guidelines are a set of rules that have been developed to accompany and complement the official conventions and instructions provided within the ICD-10-CM itself. The instructions and conventions of the classification take precedence over guidelines. These guidelines are based on the coding and sequencing instructions in the Tabular List and Alphabetic Index of ICD-10-CM, but provide additional instruction. Adherence to these guidelines when assigning ICD-10-CM diagnosis codes is required under the Health Insurance Portability and Accountability Act (HIPAA). The diagnosis codes (Tabular List and Alphabetic Index) have been adopted under HIPAA for all healthcare settings. A joint effort between the healthcare provider and the coder is essential to achieve complete and accurate documentation, code assignment, and reporting of diagnoses and procedures. These guidelines have been developed to assist both the healthcare provider and the coder in identifying those diagnoses and procedures that are to be reported. The importance of consistent, complete documentation in the medical record cannot be overemphasized. Without such documentation accurate coding cannot be achieved. The entire record should be reviewed to determine the specific reason for the encounter and the conditions treated.

The term encounter is used for all settings, including hospital admissions. In the context of these guidelines, the term provider is used throughout the guidelines to mean physician or any qualified health care practitioner who is legally accountable for establishing the patient's diagnosis. Only this set of guidelines, approved by the Cooperating Parties, is official.

The guidelines are organized into sections. Section I includes the structure and conventions of the classification and general guidelines that apply to the entire classification, and chapter-specific guidelines that correspond to the chapters as they are arranged in the classification. Section II includes guidelines for selection of principal diagnosis for non-outpatient settings. Section III includes guidelines for reporting additional diagnoses in non-outpatient settings. Section IV is for outpatient coding and reporting. It is necessary to review all sections of the guidelines to fully understand all of the rules and instructions needed to code properly.

Section I. Conventions, general coding guidelines and chapter specific guidelines

The conventions, general guidelines and chapter-specific guidelines are applicable to all health care settings unless otherwise indicated. The conventions and instructions of the classification take precedence over guidelines.

A. Conventions for the ICD-10-CM

The conventions for the ICD-10-CM are the general rules for use of the classification independent of the guidelines. These conventions are incorporated within the Alphabetic Index and Tabular List of the ICD-10-CM as instructional notes.

1. **The Alphabetic Index and Tabular List**

   The ICD-10-CM is divided into the Alphabetic Index, an alphabetical list of terms and their corresponding code, and the Tabular List, a structured chronological list of codes divided into chapters based on body system or condition. The Alphabetic Index consists of the following parts: the Index of Diseases and Injury, the Index of External Causes of Injury, the Table of Neoplasms and the Table of Drugs and Chemicals.

   See Section I.C2. General guidelines

   See Section I.C.19. Adverse effects, poisoning, underdosing and toxic effects

2. **Format and Structure:**

   The ICD-10-CM Tabular List contains categories, subcategories and codes. Characters for categories, subcategories and codes may be either a letter or a number. All categories are 3 characters. A three-character category that has no further subdivision is equivalent to a code. Subcategories are either 4 or 5 characters. Codes may be 3, 4, 5, 6 or 7 characters. That is, each level of subdivision after a category is a subcategory. The final level of subdivision is a code. Codes that have applicable 7th characters are still referred to as codes, not subcategories. A code that has an applicable 7th character is considered invalid without the 7th character.

   The ICD-10-CM uses an indented format for ease in reference.

3. **Use of codes for reporting purposes**

   For reporting purposes only codes are permissible, not categories or subcategories, and any applicable 7th character is required.

4. **Placeholder character**

   The ICD-10-CM utilizes a placeholder character "x". The "x" is used as a placeholder at certain codes to allow for future expansion. An example of this is at the poisoning, adverse effect and underdosing codes, categories T36-T50.

   Where a placeholder exists, the x must be used in order for the code to be considered a valid code.

5. **7th Characters**

   Certain ICD-10-CM categories have applicable 7th characters. The applicable 7th character is required for all codes within the category, or as the notes in the Tabular List instruct. The 7th character must always be the 7th character in the data field. If a code that requires a 7th character is not 6 characters, a placeholder X must be used to fill in the empty characters.

6. **Abbreviations**
   a. **Alphabetic Index abbreviations**

   NEC   "Not elsewhere classifiable"
   This abbreviation in the Alphabetic Index represents "other specified". When a specific code is not available for a condition, the Alphabetic Index directs the coder to the "other specified" code in the Tabular List.

   NOS   "Not otherwise specified"
   This abbreviation is the equivalent of unspecified.

   b. **Tabular List abbreviations**

   NEC   "Not elsewhere classifiable"
   This abbreviation in the Tabular List represents "other specified". When a specific code is not available for a condition the Tabular List includes an NEC entry under a code to identify the code as the "other specified" code.

   NOS   "Not otherwise specified"
   This abbreviation is the equivalent of unspecified.

7. **Punctuation**

   [ ]   Brackets are used in the Tabular List to enclose synonyms, alternative wording or explanatory phrases. Brackets are used in the Alphabetic Index to identify manifestation codes.

   ( )   Parentheses are used in both the Alphabetic Index and Tabular List to enclose supplementary words that may be present or absent in the statement of a disease or procedure without affecting the code number to which it is assigned. The terms within the parentheses are referred to as nonessential modifiers.

   :   Colons are used in the Tabular List after an incomplete term which needs one or more of the modifiers following the colon to make it assignable to a given category.

8. **Use of "and"**
   See Section I.A.14. Use of the term "And"

9. **Other and Unspecified codes**
   a. **"Other" codes**
   Codes titled "other" or "other specified" are for use when the information in the medical record provides detail for which a specific code does not exist. Alphabetic Index entries with NEC in the line designate "other" codes in the Tabular List. These Alphabetic Index entries represent specific disease entities for which no specific code exists so the term is included within an "other" code.

   b. **"Unspecified" codes**
   Codes titled "unspecified" are for use when the information in the medical record is insufficient to assign a more specific code. For those categories for which an unspecified code is not provided, the "other specified" code may represent both other and unspecified.

10. **Includes Notes**
    This note appears immediately under a three character code title to further define, or give examples of, the content of the category.

11. **Inclusion Terms**
    List of terms is included under some codes. These terms are the conditions for which that code is to be used. The terms may be synonyms of the code title, or, in the case of "other specified" codes, the terms are a list of the various conditions assigned to that code. The inclusion terms are not necessarily exhaustive. Additional terms found only in the Alphabetic Index may also be assigned to a code.

12. **Excludes Notes**
    The ICD-10-CM has two types of excludes notes. Each type of note has a different definition for use but they are all similar in

that they indicate that codes excluded from each other are independent of each other.

   a. **Excludes1**
   A type 1 Excludes note is a pure excludes note. It means "NOT CODED HERE!" An Excludes1 note indicates that the code excluded should never be used at the same time as the code above the Excludes1 note. An Excludes1 is used when two conditions cannot occur together, such as a congenital form versus an acquired form of the same condition.

   b. **Excludes2**
   A type 2 Excludes note represents "Not included here". An excludes2 note indicates that the condition excluded is not part of the condition represented by the code, but a patient may have both conditions at the same time. When an Excludes2 note appears under a code, it is acceptable to use both the code and the excluded code together, when appropriate.

13. **Etiology/manifestation convention ("code first", "use additional code" and "in diseases classified elsewhere" notes)**
    Certain conditions have both an underlying etiology and multiple body system manifestations due to the underlying etiology. For such conditions, the ICD-10-CM has a coding convention that requires the underlying condition be sequenced first followed by the manifestation. Wherever such a combination exists, there is a "use additional code" note at the etiology code, and a "code first" note at the manifestation code. These instructional notes indicate the proper sequencing order of the codes, etiology followed by manifestation.

    In most cases the manifestation codes will have in the code title, "in diseases classified elsewhere." Codes with this title are a component of the etiology/ manifestation convention. The code title indicates that it is a manifestation code. "In diseases classified elsewhere" codes are never permitted to be used as first-listed or principal diagnosis codes. They must be used in conjunction with an underlying condition code and they must be listed following the underlying condition. See category F02, Dementia in other diseases classified elsewhere, for an example of this convention.

    There are manifestation codes that do not have "in diseases classified elsewhere" in the title. For such codes, **there is a "use additional code" note at the etiology code and a "code first" note at the manifestation code and the rules for sequencing apply.**

    In addition to the notes in the Tabular List, these conditions also have a specific Alphabetic Index entry structure. In the Alphabetic Index both conditions are listed together with the etiology code first followed by the manifestation codes in brackets. The code in brackets is always to be sequenced second.

    An example of the etiology/manifestation convention is dementia in Parkinson's disease. In the Alphabetic Index, code G20 is listed first, followed by code F02.80 or F02.81 in brackets. Code G20 represents the underlying etiology, Parkinson's disease, and must be sequenced first, whereas codes F02.80 and F02.81 represent the manifestation of dementia in diseases classified elsewhere, with or without behavioral disturbance.

    "Code first" and "Use additional code" notes are also used as sequencing rules in the classification for certain codes that are not part of an etiology/ manifestation combination.

    See Section I.B.7. Multiple coding for a single condition.

14. **"And"**
    The word "and" should be interpreted to mean either "and" or "or" when it appears in a title.

    For example, cases of "tuberculosis of bones", "tuberculosis of joints" and "tuberculosis of bones and joints" are

classified to subcategory A18.0, Tuberculosis of bones and joints.

15. "With"

The word "with" should be interpreted to mean "associated with" or "due to" when it appears in a code title, the Alphabetic Index, or an instructional note in the Tabular List.

The word "with" in the Alphabetic Index is sequenced immediately following the main term, not in alphabetical order.

16. "See" and "See Also"

The "see" instruction following a main term in the Alphabetic Index indicates that another term should be referenced. It is necessary to go to the main term referenced with the "see" note to locate the correct code.

A "see also" instruction following a main term in the Alphabetic Index instructs that there is another main term that may also be referenced that may provide additional Alphabetic Index entries that may be useful. It is not necessary to follow the "see also" note when the original main term provides the necessary code.

17. "Code also note"

A "code also" note instructs that two codes may be required to fully describe a condition, but this note does not provide sequencing direction.

18. Default codes

A code listed next to a main term in the ICD-10-CM Alphabetic Index is referred to as a default code. The default code represents that condition that is most commonly associated with the main term, or is the unspecified code for the condition. If a condition is documented in a medical record (for example, appendicitis) without any additional information, such as acute or chronic, the default code should be assigned.

B. General Coding Guidelines

1. Locating a code in the ICD-10-CM

To select a code in the classification that corresponds to a diagnosis or reason for visit documented in a medical record, first locate the term in the Alphabetic Index, and then verify the code in the Tabular List. Read and be guided by instructional notations that appear in both the Alphabetic Index and the Tabular List.

It is essential to use both the Alphabetic Index and Tabular List when locating and assigning a code. The Alphabetic Index does not always provide the full code. Selection of the full code, including laterality and any applicable 7th character can only be done in the Tabular List. A dash (-) at the end of an Alphabetic Index entry indicates that additional characters are required. Even if a dash is not included at the Alphabetic Index entry, it is necessary to refer to the Tabular List to verify that no 7th character is required.

2. Level of Detail in Coding

Diagnosis codes are to be used and reported at their highest number of characters available.

ICD-10-CM diagnosis codes are composed of codes with 3, 4, 5, 6 or 7 characters. Codes with three characters are included in ICD-10-CM as the heading of a category of codes that may be further subdivided by the use of fourth and/or fifth characters and/or sixth characters, which provide greater detail.

A three-character code is to be used only if it is not further subdivided. A code is invalid if it has not been coded to the full number of characters required for that code, including the 7th character, if applicable.

3. Code or codes from A00.0 through T88.9, Z00-Z99.8

The appropriate code or codes from A00.0 through T88.9, Z00-Z99.8 must be used to identify diagnoses, symptoms, conditions, problems, complaints or other reason(s) for the encounter/visit.

4. Signs and symptoms

Codes that describe symptoms and signs, as opposed to diagnoses, are acceptable for reporting purposes when a related definitive diagnosis has not been established (confirmed) by the provider. Chapter 18 of ICD-10-CM, Symptoms, Signs, and Abnormal Clinical and Laboratory Findings, Not Elsewhere Classified (codes R00.0 - R99) contains many, but not all codes for symptoms.

5. Conditions that are an integral part of a disease process

Signs and symptoms that are associated routinely with a disease process should not be assigned as additional codes, unless otherwise instructed by the classification.

6. Conditions that are not an integral part of a disease process

Additional signs and symptoms that may not be associated routinely with a disease process should be coded when present.

7. Multiple coding for a single condition

In addition to the etiology/manifestation convention that requires two codes to fully describe a single condition that affects multiple body systems, there are other single conditions that also require more than one code. "Use additional code" notes are found in the Tabular List at codes that are not part of an etiology/manifestation pair where a secondary code is useful to fully describe a condition. The sequencing rule is the same as the etiology/manifestation pair, "use additional code" indicates that a secondary code should be added.

For example, for bacterial infections that are not included in chapter 1, a secondary code from category B95, Streptococcus, Staphylococcus, and Enterococcus, as the cause of diseases classified elsewhere, or B96, Other bacterial agents as the cause of diseases classified elsewhere, may be required to identify the bacterial organism causing the infection. A "use additional code" note will normally be found at the infectious disease code, indicating a need for the organism code to be added as a secondary code.

"Code first" notes are also under certain codes that are not specifically manifestation codes but may be due to an underlying cause. When there is a "code first" note and an underlying condition is present, the underlying condition should be sequenced first.

"Code, if applicable, any causal condition first", notes indicate that this code may be assigned as a principal diagnosis when the causal condition is unknown or not applicable. If a causal condition is known, then the code for that condition should be sequenced as the principal or first-listed diagnosis.

Multiple codes may be needed for sequela, complication codes and obstetric codes to more fully describe a condition. See the specific guidelines for these conditions for further instruction.

8. Acute and Chronic Conditions

If the same condition is described as both acute (subacute) and chronic, and separate subentries exist in the Alphabetic Index at the same indentation level, code both and sequence the acute (subacute) code first.

9. Combination Code

A combination code is a single code used to classify:

Two diagnoses, or

> A diagnosis with an associated secondary process (manifestation)

> A diagnosis with an associated complication

Combination codes are identified by referring to subterm entries in the Alphabetic Index and by reading the inclusion and exclusion notes in the Tabular List.

Assign only the combination code when that code fully identifies the diagnostic conditions involved or when the Alphabetic Index so directs. Multiple coding should not be used when the

---

classification provides a combination code that clearly identifies all of the elements documented in the diagnosis. When the combination code lacks necessary specificity in describing the manifestation or complication, an additional code should be used as a secondary code.

10. Sequela (Late Effects)

A sequela is the residual effect (condition produced) after the acute phase of an illness or injury has terminated. There is no time limit on when a sequela code can be used. The residual may be apparent early, such as in cerebral infarction, or it may occur months or years later, such as that due to a previous injury. Coding of sequela generally requires two codes sequenced in the following order: The condition or nature of the sequela is sequenced first. The sequela code is sequenced second.

An exception to the above guidelines are those instances where the code for the sequela is followed by a manifestation code identified in the Tabular List and title, or the sequela code has been expanded (at the fourth, fifth or sixth character levels) to include the manifestation(s). The code for the acute phase of an illness or injury that led to the sequela is never used with a code for the late effect.

See Section I.C.9. Sequelae of cerebrovascular disease

See Section I.C.15. Sequelae of complication of pregnancy, childbirth and the puerperium

See Section I.C.19. Application of 7th characters for Chapter 19

11. Impending or Threatened Condition

Code any condition described at the time of discharge as "impending" or "threatened" as follows:

If it did occur, code as confirmed diagnosis.

If it did not occur, reference the Alphabetic Index to determine if the condition has a subentry term for "impending" or "threatened" and also reference main term entries for "Impending" and for "Threatened."

If the subterms are listed, assign the given code.

If the subterms are not listed, code the existing underlying condition(s) and not the condition described as impending or threatened.

12. Reporting Same Diagnosis Code More than Once

Each unique ICD-10-CM diagnosis code may be reported only once for an encounter. This applies to bilateral conditions when there are no distinct codes identifying laterality or two different conditions classified to the same ICD-10-CM diagnosis code.

13. Laterality

Some ICD-10-CM codes indicate laterality, **specifying whether the condition occurs on the left, right or is bilateral.** If no bilateral code is provided and the condition is bilateral, assign separate codes for both the left and right side. **If the side is not identified in the medical record, assign the code for the unspecified side.**

14. Documentation for BMI and Pressure Ulcer Stages

For the Body Mass Index (BMI)**, depth of non-pressure chronic ulcers** and pressure ulcer stage codes, code assignment may be based on medical record documentation from clinicians who are not the patient's provider (i.e., physician or other qualified healthcare practitioner legally accountable for establishing the patient's diagnosis), since this information is typically documented by other clinicians involved in the care of the patient (e.g., a dietitian often documents the BMI and nurses often documents the pressure ulcer stages). However, the associated diagnosis (such as overweight, obesity, or pressure ulcer) must be documented by the patient's provider. If there is conflicting medical record documentation, either from the same clinician or different clinicians, the patient's attending provider should be queried for clarification.

The BMI codes should only be reported as secondary diagnoses. As with all other secondary diagnosis codes, the BMI codes should only be assigned when they meet the definition of a reportable additional diagnosis (see Section III, Reporting Additional Diagnoses).

15. Syndromes

Follow the Alphabetic Index guidance when coding syndromes. In the absence of Alphabetic Index guidance, assign codes for the documented manifestations of the syndrome.

Additional codes for manifestations that are not an integral part of the disease process may also be assigned when the condition does not have a unique code.

16. Documentation of Complications of Care

Code assignment is based on the provider's documentation of the relationship between the condition and the care or procedure. The guideline extends to any complications of care, regardless of the chapter the code is located in. It is important to note that not all conditions that occur during or following medical care or surgery are classified as complications. There must be a cause-and-effect relationship between the care provided and the condition, and an indication in the documentation that it is a complication. Query the provider for clarification, if the complication is not clearly documented.

17. Borderline Diagnosis

If the provider documents a "borderline" diagnosis at the time of discharge, the diagnosis is coded as confirmed, unless the classification provides a specific entry (e.g., borderline diabetes). If a borderline condition has a specific index entry in ICD-10-CM, it should be coded as such. Since borderline conditions are not uncertain diagnoses, no distinction is made between the care setting (inpatient versus outpatient). Whenever the documentation is unclear regarding a borderline condition, coders are encouraged to query for clarification.

C. Chapter-Specific Coding Guidelines

In addition to general coding guidelines, there are guidelines for specific diagnoses and/or conditions in the classification. Unless otherwise indicated, these guidelines apply to all health care settings. Please refer to Section II for guidelines on the selection of principal diagnosis.

1. Chapter 1: Certain Infectious and Parasitic Diseases (A00-B99)

a. Human immunodeficiency virus (HIV) infections

1) Code only confirmed cases

Code only confirmed cases of HIV infection/illness. This is an exception to the hospital inpatient guideline Section II, H.

In this context, "confirmation" does not require documentation of positive serology or culture for HIV; the provider's diagnostic statement that the patient is HIV positive, or has an HIV-related illness is sufficient.

2) Selection and sequencing of HIV codes

(a) Patient admitted for HIV-related condition

If a patient is admitted for an HIV-related condition, the principal diagnosis should be B20, **Human immunodeficiency virus [HIV] disease** followed by additional diagnosis codes for all reported HIV-related conditions.

(b) Patient with HIV disease admitted for unrelated condition

If a patient with HIV disease is admitted for an unrelated condition (such as a traumatic injury), the code for the unrelated condition (e.g., the nature of injury code) should be the principal diagnosis.

Other diagnoses would be B20 followed by additional diagnosis codes for all reported HIV-related conditions.

(c) Whether the patient is newly diagnosed

Whether the patient is newly diagnosed or has had previous admissions/encounters for HIV conditions is irrelevant to the sequencing decision.

(d) Asymptomatic human immunodeficiency virus

Z21, Asymptomatic human immunodeficiency virus [HIV] infection status, is to be applied when the patient without any documentation of symptoms is listed as being "HIV positive," "known HIV," "HIV test positive," or similar terminology. Do not use this code if the term "AIDS" is used or if the patient is treated for any HIV-related illness or is described as having any condition(s) resulting from his/her HIV positive status; use B20 in these cases.

(e) Patients with inconclusive HIV serology

Patients with inconclusive HIV serology, but no definitive diagnosis or manifestations of the illness, may be assigned code R75, Inconclusive laboratory evidence of human immunodeficiency virus [HIV].

(f) Previously diagnosed HIV-related illness

Patients with any known prior diagnosis of an HIV-related illness should be coded to B20. Once a patient has developed an HIV-related illness, the patient should always be assigned code B20 on every subsequent admission/encounter. Patients previously diagnosed with any HIV illness (B20) should never be assigned to R75 or Z21, Asymptomatic human immunodeficiency virus [HIV] infection status.

(g) HIV infection in pregnancy, childbirth and the puerperium

During pregnancy, childbirth or the puerperium, a patient admitted (or presenting for a health care encounter) because of an HIV-related illness should receive a principal diagnosis code of O98.7-, Human immunodeficiency [HIV] disease complicating pregnancy, childbirth and the puerperium, followed by B20 and the code(s) for the HIV-related illness(es). Codes from Chapter 15 always take sequencing priority.

Patients with asymptomatic HIV infection status admitted (or presenting for a health care encounter) during pregnancy, childbirth, or the puerperium should receive codes of O98.7- and Z21.

(h) Encounters for testing for HIV

If a patient is being seen to determine his/her HIV status, use code Z11.4, Encounter for screening for human immunodeficiency virus [HIV]. Use additional codes for any associated high risk behavior.

If a patient with signs or symptoms is being seen for HIV testing, code the signs and symptoms. An additional counseling code Z71.7, Human immunodeficiency virus [HIV] counseling, may be used if counseling is provided during the encounter for the test.

When a patient returns to be informed of his/her HIV test results and the test result is negative, use code Z71.7, Human immunodeficiency virus [HIV] counseling.

If the results are positive, see previous guidelines and assign codes as appropriate.

b. Infectious agents as the cause of diseases classified to other chapters

Certain infections are classified in chapters other than Chapter 1 and no organism is identified as part of the infection code. In these instances, it is necessary to use an additional code from Chapter 1 to identify the organism. A code from category B95, Streptococcus, Staphylococcus, and Enterococcus as the cause of diseases classified to other chapters, B96, Other bacterial agents as the cause of diseases classified to other chapters, or B97, Viral agents as the cause of diseases classified to other chapters, is to be used as an additional code to identify the organism. An instructional note will be found at the infection code advising that an additional organism code is required.

c. Infections resistant to antibiotics

Many bacterial infections are resistant to current antibiotics. It is necessary to identify all infections documented as antibiotic resistant. Assign a code from category Z16, Resistance to antimicrobial drugs, following the infection code only if the infection code does not identify drug resistance.

d. Sepsis, severe sepsis, and septic shock

1) Coding of sepsis and severe sepsis

(a) Sepsis

For a diagnosis of sepsis, assign the appropriate code for the underlying systemic infection. If the type of infection or causal organism is not further specified, assign code A41.9, Sepsis, unspecified organism.

A code from subcategory R65.2, Severe sepsis, should not be assigned unless severe sepsis or an associated acute organ dysfunction is documented.

(i) Negative or inconclusive blood cultures and sepsis

Negative or inconclusive blood cultures do not preclude a diagnosis of sepsis in patients with clinical evidence of the condition, however, the provider should be queried.

(ii) Urosepsis

The term urosepsis is a nonspecific term. It is not to be considered synonymous with sepsis. It has no default code in the Alphabetic Index. Should a provider use this term, he/she must be queried for clarification.

(iii) Sepsis with organ dysfunction

If a patient has sepsis and associated acute organ dysfunction or multiple organ dysfunction (MOD), follow the instructions for coding severe sepsis.

(iv) Acute organ dysfunction that is not clearly associated with the sepsis

If a patient has sepsis and an acute organ dysfunction, but the medical record documentation indicates that the acute organ dysfunction is related to a medical condition other than the sepsis, do not assign a code from subcategory R65.2, Severe sepsis. An acute organ dysfunction must be associated with the sepsis in order to assign the severe sepsis code. If the documentation is not clear as to whether an acute organ dysfunction is related to the sepsis or another medical condition, query the provider.

(b) Severe sepsis

The coding of severe sepsis requires a minimum of 2 codes: first a code for the underlying systemic infection, followed by a code from subcategory

---

R65.2, Severe sepsis. If the causal organism is not documented, assign code A41.9, Sepsis, unspecified organism, for the infection. Additional code(s) for the associated acute organ dysfunction are also required.

Due to the complex nature of severe sepsis, some cases may require querying the provider prior to assignment of the codes.

2) Septic shock

(a) Septic shock generally refers to circulatory failure associated with severe sepsis, and therefore, it represents a type of acute organ dysfunction. For all cases of septic shock, the code for the underlying systemic infection should be sequenced first, followed by code R65.21, Severe sepsis with septic shock. Any additional codes for the other acute organ dysfunctions should also be assigned. For cases of septic shock, the code for the systemic infection should be sequenced first, followed by code R65.21, Severe sepsis with septic shock or code T81.12, Postprocedural septic shock. Any additional codes for the other acute organ dysfunctions should also be assigned. As noted in the sequencing instructions in the Tabular List, the code for septic shock cannot be assigned as a principal diagnosis.

3) Sequencing of severe sepsis

If severe sepsis is present on admission, and meets the definition of principal diagnosis, the underlying systemic infection should be assigned as principal diagnosis followed by the appropriate code from subcategory R65.2 as required by the sequencing rules in the Tabular List. A code from subcategory R65.2 can never be assigned as a principal diagnosis.

When severe sepsis develops during an encounter (it was not present on admission) the underlying systemic infection and the appropriate code from subcategory R65.2 should be assigned as secondary diagnoses.

Severe sepsis may be present on admission but the diagnosis may not be confirmed until sometime after admission. If the documentation is not clear whether severe sepsis was present on admission, the provider should be queried.

4) Sepsis and severe sepsis with a localized infection

If the reason for admission is both sepsis or severe sepsis and a localized infection, such as pneumonia or cellulitis, a code(s) for the underlying systemic infection should be assigned first and the code for the localized infection should be assigned as a secondary diagnosis. If the patient has severe sepsis, a code from subcategory R65.2 should also be assigned as a secondary diagnosis. If the patient is admitted with a localized infection, such as pneumonia, and sepsis/severe sepsis doesn't develop until after admission, the localized infection should be assigned first, followed by the appropriate sepsis/severe sepsis codes.

5) Sepsis due to a postprocedural infection

(a) Documentation of causal relationship

As with all postprocedural complications, code assignment is based on the provider's documentation of the relationship between the infection and the procedure.

(b) Sepsis due to a postprocedural infection

For such cases, the postprocedural infection code, such as, T80.2, Infections following infusion, transfusion, and therapeutic injection, T81.4, Infection following a procedure, T88.0, Infection following immunization, or O86.0, Infection of obstetric surgical wound, should be coded first, followed by the code for the specific infection. If the patient has severe sepsis the appropriate code from subcategory R65.2 should also be assigned with the additional code(s) for any acute organ dysfunction.

(c) Postprocedural infection and postprocedural septic shock

In cases where a postprocedural infection has occurred and has resulted in severe sepsis and postprocedural septic shock, the code for the precipitating complication such as code T81.4, Infection following a procedure, or O86.0, Infection of obstetrical surgical wound should be coded first followed by code R65.21, Severe sepsis with septic shock and a code for the systemic infection.

6) Sepsis and severe sepsis associated with a noninfectious process (condition)

In some cases a noninfectious process (condition), such as trauma, may lead to an infection which can result in sepsis or severe sepsis. If sepsis or severe sepsis is documented as associated with a noninfectious condition, such as a burn or serious injury, and this condition meets the definition for principal diagnosis, the code for the noninfectious condition should be sequenced first, followed by the code for the resulting infection. If severe sepsis, is present a code from subcategory R65.2 should also be assigned with any associated organ dysfunction(s) codes. It is not necessary to assign a code from subcategory R65.1, Systemic inflammatory response syndrome (SIRS) of non-infectious origin, for these cases.

If the infection meets the definition of principal diagnosis it should be sequenced before the non-infectious condition. When both the associated non-infectious condition and the infection meet the definition of principal diagnosis either may be assigned as principal diagnosis.

Only one code from category R65, Symptoms and signs specifically associated with systemic inflammation and infection, should be assigned. Therefore, when a non-infectious condition leads to an infection resulting in severe sepsis, assign the appropriate code from subcategory R65.2, Severe sepsis. Do not additionally assign a code from subcategory R65.1, Systemic inflammatory response syndrome (SIRS) of non-infectious origin.

See Section I.C.18. SIRS due to non-infectious process

7) Sepsis and septic shock complicating abortion, pregnancy, childbirth, and the puerperium
See Section I.C.15. Sepsis and septic shock complicating abortion, pregnancy, childbirth and the puerperium

8) Newborn sepsis
See Section I.C.16. f. Bacterial sepsis of Newborn

e. Methicillin resistant *Staphylococcus aureus* (MRSA) conditions

1) Selection and sequencing of MRSA codes

(a) Combination codes for MRSA infection

When a patient is diagnosed with an infection that is due to methicillin resistant *Staphylococcus aureus* (MRSA), and that infection has a combination code that includes the causal organism (e.g., sepsis, pneumonia) assign the appropriate combination code for the condition (e.g., code A41.02, Sepsis due to Methicillin resistant *Staphylococcus aureus* or code J15.212, Pneumonia due to Methicillin resistant *Staphylococcus aureus*). Do not assign code B95.62,

Methicillin resistant *Staphylococcus aureus* infection as the cause of diseases classified elsewhere, as an additional code because the combination code includes the type of infection and the MRSA organism. Do not assign a code from subcategory Z16.11, Resistance to penicillins, as an additional diagnosis.

See Section C.1. for instructions on coding and sequencing of sepsis and severe sepsis.

(b) Other codes for MRSA infection

When there is documentation of a current infection (e.g., wound infection, stitch abscess, urinary tract infection) due to MRSA, and that infection does not have a combination code that includes the causal organism, assign the appropriate code to identify the condition along with code B95.62, Methicillin resistant *Staphylococcus aureus* infection as the cause of diseases classified elsewhere for the MRSA infection. Do not assign a code from subcategory Z16.11, Resistance to penicillins.

(c) Methicillin susceptible *Staphylococcus aureus* (MSSA) and MRSA colonization

The condition or state of being colonized or carrying MSSA or MRSA is called colonization or carriage, while an individual person is described as being colonized or being a carrier. Colonization means that MSSA or MSRA is present on or in the body without necessarily causing illness. A positive MRSA colonization test might be documented by the provider as "MRSA screen positive" or "MRSA nasal swab positive".

Assign code Z22.322, Carrier or suspected carrier of Methicillin resistant *Staphylococcus aureus*, for patients documented as having MRSA colonization. Assign code Z22.321, Carrier or suspected carrier of Methicillin susceptible *Staphylococcus aureus*, for patient documented as having MSSA colonization. Colonization is not necessarily indicative of a disease process or as the cause of a specific condition the patient may have unless documented as such by the provider.

(d) MRSA colonization and infection

If a patient is documented as having both MRSA colonization and infection during a hospital admission, code Z22.322, Carrier or suspected carrier of Methicillin resistant *Staphylococcus aureus*, and a code for the MRSA infection may both be assigned.

2. Chapter 2: Neoplasms (C00-D49)

General guidelines

Chapter 2 of the ICD-10-CM contains the codes for most benign and all malignant neoplasms. Certain benign neoplasms, such as prostatic adenomas, may be found in the specific body system chapters. To properly code a neoplasm it is necessary to determine from the record if the neoplasm is benign, in-situ, malignant, or of uncertain histologic behavior. If malignant, any secondary (metastatic) sites should also be determined.

Primary malignant neoplasms overlapping site boundaries

A primary malignant neoplasm that overlaps two or more contiguous (next to each other) sites should be classified to the subcategory/code .8 ('overlapping lesion'), unless the combination is specifically indexed elsewhere. For multiple neoplasms of the same site that are not contiguous such as tumors in different quadrants of the same breast, codes for each site should be assigned.

Malignant neoplasm of ectopic tissue

Malignant neoplasms of ectopic tissue are to be coded to the site **of origin** mentioned, e.g., ectopic pancreatic malignant neoplasms **involving the stomach** are coded to pancreas, unspecified (C25.9).

The neoplasm table in the Alphabetic Index should be referenced first. However, if the histological term is documented, that term should be referenced first, rather than going immediately to the Neoplasm Table, in order to determine which column in the Neoplasm Table is appropriate. For example, if the documentation indicates "adenoma," refer to the term in the Alphabetic Index to review the entries under this term and the instructional note to "see also neoplasm, by site, benign." The table provides the proper code based on the type of neoplasm and the site. It is important to select the proper column in the table that corresponds to the type of neoplasm. The Tabular List should then be referenced to verify that the correct code has been selected from the table and that a more specific site code does not exist.

See Section I.C.21. Factors influencing health status and contact with health services, Status, for information regarding Z15.0, codes for genetic susceptibility to cancer.

a. Treatment directed at the malignancy

If the treatment is directed at the malignancy, designate the malignancy as the principal diagnosis.

The only exception to this guideline is if a patient admission/encounter is solely for the administration of chemotherapy, immunotherapy or radiation therapy, assign the appropriate Z51.-- code as the first-listed or principal diagnosis, and the diagnosis or problem for which the service is being performed as a secondary diagnosis.

b. Treatment of secondary site

When a patient is admitted because of a primary neoplasm with metastasis and treatment is directed toward the secondary site only, the secondary neoplasm is designated as the principal diagnosis even though the primary malignancy is still present.

c. Coding and sequencing of complications

Coding and sequencing of complications associated with the malignancies or with the therapy thereof are subject to the following guidelines:

1) Anemia associated with malignancy

When admission/encounter is for management of an anemia associated with the malignancy, and the treatment is only for anemia, the appropriate code for the malignancy is sequenced as the principal or first-listed diagnosis followed by the appropriate code for the anemia (such as code D63.0, Anemia in neoplastic disease).

2) Anemia associated with chemotherapy, immunotherapy and radiation therapy

When the admission/encounter is for management of an anemia associated with an adverse effect of the administration of chemotherapy or immunotherapy and the only treatment is for the anemia, the anemia code is sequenced first followed by the appropriate codes for the neoplasm and the adverse effect (T45.1X5, Adverse effect of antineoplastic and immunosuppressive drugs).

When the admission/encounter is for management of an anemia associated with an adverse effect of radiotherapy, the anemia code should be sequenced first, followed by the appropriate neoplasm code and code Y84.2, Radiological procedure and radiotherapy as the cause of abnormal reaction of the patient, or of later complication, without mention of misadventure at the time of the procedure.

3) Management of dehydration due to the malignancy

When the admission/encounter is for management of dehydration due to the malignancy and only the dehydration is being treated (intravenous rehydration), the dehydration is sequenced first, followed by the code(s) for the malignancy.

4) Treatment of a complication resulting from a surgical procedure

When the admission/encounter is for treatment of a complication resulting from a surgical procedure, designate the complication as the principal or first-listed diagnosis if treatment is directed at resolving the complication.

d. Primary malignancy previously excised

When a primary malignancy has been previously excised or eradicated from its site and there is no further treatment directed to that site and there is no evidence of any existing primary malignancy, a code from category Z85, Personal history of malignant neoplasm, should be used to indicate the former site of the malignancy. Any mention of extension, invasion, or metastasis to another site is coded as a secondary malignant neoplasm to that site. The secondary site may be the principal or first-listed with the Z85 code used as a secondary code.

e. Admissions/Encounters involving chemotherapy, immunotherapy and radiation therapy

1) Episode of care involves surgical removal of neoplasm

When an episode of care involves the surgical removal of a neoplasm, primary or secondary site, followed by adjunct chemotherapy or radiation treatment during the same episode of care, the code for the neoplasm should be assigned as principal or first-listed diagnosis.

2) Patient admission/encounter solely for administration of chemotherapy, immunotherapy and radiation therapy

If a patient admission/encounter is solely for the administration of chemotherapy, immunotherapy or radiation therapy assign code Z51.0, Encounter for antineoplastic radiation therapy, or Z51.11, Encounter for antineoplastic chemotherapy, or Z51.12, Encounter for antineoplastic immunotherapy as the first-listed or principal diagnosis. If a patient receives more than one of these therapies during the same admission more than one of these codes may be assigned, in any sequence.

The malignancy for which the therapy is being administered should be assigned as a secondary diagnosis.

3) Patient admitted for radiation therapy, chemotherapy or immunotherapy and develops complications

When a patient is admitted for the purpose of radiotherapy, immunotherapy or chemotherapy and develops complications such as uncontrolled nausea and vomiting or dehydration, the principal or first-listed diagnosis is Z51.0, Encounter for antineoplastic radiation therapy, or Z51.11, Encounter for antineoplastic chemotherapy, or Z51.12, Encounter for antineoplastic immunotherapy followed by any codes for the complications.

f. Admission/encounter to determine extent of malignancy

When the reason for admission/encounter is to determine the extent of the malignancy, or for a procedure such as paracentesis or thoracentesis, the primary malignancy or appropriate metastatic site is designated as the principal or first-listed diagnosis, even though chemotherapy or radiotherapy is administered.

g. Symptoms, signs, and abnormal findings listed in Chapter 18 associated with neoplasms

Symptoms, signs, and ill-defined conditions listed in Chapter 18 characteristic of, or associated with, an existing primary or secondary site malignancy cannot be used to replace the malignancy as principal or first-listed diagnosis, regardless of the number of admissions or encounters for treatment and care of the neoplasm.

See section I.C.21. Factors influencing health status and contact with health services, Encounter for prophylactic organ removal.

h. Admission/encounter for pain control/management

See Section I.C.6. for information on coding admission/encounter for pain control/management.

i. Malignancy in two or more noncontiguous sites

A patient may have more than one malignant tumor in the same organ. These tumors may represent different primaries or metastatic disease, depending on the site. Should the documentation be unclear, the provider should be queried as to the status of each tumor so that the correct codes can be assigned.

j. Disseminated malignant neoplasm, unspecified

Code C80.0, Disseminated malignant neoplasm, unspecified, is for use only in those cases where the patient has advanced metastatic disease and no known primary or secondary sites are specified. It should not be used in place of assigning codes for the primary site and all known secondary sites.

k. Malignant neoplasm without specification of site

Code C80.1, Malignant (primary) neoplasm, unspecified, equates to Cancer, unspecified. This code should only be used when no determination can be made as to the primary site of a malignancy. This code should rarely be used in the inpatient setting.

l. Sequencing of neoplasm codes

1) Encounter for treatment of primary malignancy

If the reason for the encounter is for treatment of a primary malignancy, assign the malignancy as the principal/first-listed diagnosis. The primary site is to be sequenced first, followed by any metastatic sites.

2) Encounter for treatment of secondary malignancy

When an encounter is for a primary malignancy with metastasis and treatment is directed toward the metastatic (secondary) site(s) only, the metastatic site(s) is designated as the principal/first-listed diagnosis. The primary malignancy is coded as an additional code.

3) Malignant neoplasm in a pregnant patient

When a pregnant woman has a malignant neoplasm, a code from subcategory O9A.1-, Malignant neoplasm complicating pregnancy, childbirth, and the puerperium, should be sequenced first, followed by the appropriate code from Chapter 2 to indicate the type of neoplasm.

4) Encounter for complication associated with a neoplasm

When an encounter is for management of a complication associated with a neoplasm, such as dehydration, and the treatment is only for the complication, the complication is coded first, followed by the appropriate code(s) for the neoplasm.

The exception to this guideline is anemia. When the admission/encounter is for management of an anemia associated with the malignancy, and the treatment is only for anemia, the appropriate code for the malignancy is sequenced as the principal or first-listed diagnosis followed by code D63.0, Anemia in neoplastic disease.

5) Complication from surgical procedure for treatment of a neoplasm

When an encounter is for treatment of a complication resulting from a surgical procedure performed for the treatment of the neoplasm, designate the complication as the principal/first-listed diagnosis. See guideline regarding the coding of a current malignancy versus personal history to determine if the code for the neoplasm should also be assigned.

6) Pathologic fracture due to a neoplasm

When an encounter is for a pathological fracture due to a neoplasm, and the focus of treatment is the fracture, a code from subcategory M84.5, Pathological fracture in neoplastic disease, should be sequenced first, followed by the code for the neoplasm.

If the focus of treatment is the neoplasm with an associated pathological fracture, the neoplasm code should be sequenced first, followed by a code from M84.5 for the pathological fracture.

m. Current malignancy versus personal history of malignancy

When a primary malignancy has been excised but further treatment, such as an additional surgery for the malignancy, radiation therapy or chemotherapy is directed to that site, the primary malignancy code should be used until treatment is completed.

When a primary malignancy has been previously excised or eradicated from its site, there is no further treatment (of the malignancy) directed to that site, and there is no evidence of any existing primary malignancy, a code from category Z85, Personal history of malignant neoplasm, should be used to indicate the former site of the malignancy.

See Section I.C.21. Factors influencing health status and contact with health services, History (of)

n. Leukemia, multiple myeloma, and malignant plasma cell neoplasms in remission versus personal history

The categories for leukemia, and category C90, Multiple myeloma and malignant plasma cell neoplasms, have codes indicating whether or not the leukemia has achieved remission. There are also codes Z85.6, Personal history of leukemia, and Z85.79, Personal history of other malignant neoplasms of lymphoid, hematopoietic and related tissues. If the documentation is unclear, as to whether the leukemia has achieved remission, the provider should be queried.

See Section I.C.21. Factors influencing health status and contact with health services, History (of)

o. Aftercare following surgery for neoplasm

See Section I.C.21. Factors influencing health status and contact with health services, Aftercare

p. Follow-up care for completed treatment of a malignancy

See Section I.C.21. Factors influencing health status and contact with health services, Follow-up

q. Prophylactic organ removal for prevention of malignancy

See Section I.C. 21, Factors influencing health status and contact with health services, Prophylactic organ removal

r. Malignant neoplasm associated with transplanted organ

A malignant neoplasm of a transplanted organ should be coded as a transplant complication. Assign first the appropriate code from category T86.-, Complications of transplanted organs and tissue, followed by code C80.2, Malignant neoplasm associated with transplanted organ. Use an additional code for the specific malignancy.

3. Chapter 3: Disease of the Blood and Blood-forming Organs and Certain Disorders Involving the Immune Mechanism (D50-D89)

Reserved for future guideline expansion

4. Chapter 4: Endocrine, Nutritional, and Metabolic Diseases (E00-E89)

a. Diabetes mellitus

The diabetes mellitus codes are combination codes that include the type of diabetes mellitus, the body system affected, and the complications affecting that body system. As many codes within a particular category as are necessary to describe all of the complications of the disease may be used. They should be sequenced based on the reason for a particular encounter. Assign as many codes from categories E08 – E13 as needed to identify all of the associated conditions that the patient has.

1) Type of diabetes

The age of a patient is not the sole determining factor, though most type 1 diabetics develop the condition before reaching puberty. For this reason type 1 diabetes mellitus is also referred to as juvenile diabetes.

2) Type of diabetes mellitus not documented

If the type of diabetes mellitus is not documented in the medical record the default is E11.-, Type 2 diabetes mellitus.

3) Diabetes mellitus and the use of insulin

If the documentation in a medical record does not indicate the type of diabetes but does indicate that the patient uses insulin, code E11, Type 2 diabetes mellitus, should be assigned. Code Z79.4, Long-term (current) use of insulin, should also be assigned to indicate that the patient uses insulin. Code Z79.4 should not be assigned if insulin is given temporarily to bring a type 2 patient's blood sugar under control during an encounter.

4) Diabetes mellitus in pregnancy and gestational diabetes

See Section I.C.15. Diabetes mellitus in pregnancy.

See Section I.C.15. Gestational (pregnancy induced) diabetes

5) Complications due to insulin pump malfunction

(a) Underdose of insulin due to insulin pump failure

An underdose of insulin due to an insulin pump failure should be assigned to a code from subcategory T85.6, Mechanical complication of other specified internal and external prosthetic devices, implants and grafts, that specifies the type of pump malfunction, as the principal or first-listed code, followed by code T38.3x6-, Underdosing of insulin and oral hypoglycemic [antidiabetic] drugs. Additional codes for the type of diabetes mellitus and any associated complications due to the underdosing should also be assigned.

(b) Overdose of insulin due to insulin pump failure

The principal or first-listed code for an encounter due to an insulin pump malfunction resulting in an overdose of insulin, should also be T85.6-, Mechanical complication of other specified internal and external prosthetic devices, implants and grafts, followed by code T38.3X1-, Poisoning by insulin and oral hypoglycemic [antidiabetic] drugs, accidental (unintentional).

6) Secondary diabetes mellitus

Codes under categories E08, Diabetes mellitus due to underlying condition, E09, Drug or chemical induced diabetes mellitus, **and E13, Other specified diabetes mellitus,** identify complications/manifestations associated with secondary diabetes mellitus. Secondary diabetes is always caused by another condition or event (e.g., cystic fibrosis, malignant neoplasm of pancreas, pancreatectomy, adverse effect of drug, or poisoning).

(a) Secondary diabetes mellitus and the use of insulin

For patients who routinely use insulin, code Z79.4, Long-term (current) use of insulin, should also be assigned. Code Z79.4 should not be assigned if insulin is given temporarily to bring a patient's blood sugar under control during an encounter.

(b) Assigning and sequencing secondary diabetes codes and its causes

The sequencing of the secondary diabetes codes in relationship to codes for the cause of the diabetes is based on the Tabular List instructions for categories E08, E09 and E13.

(i) Secondary diabetes mellitus due to pancreatectomy

For postpancreatectomy diabetes mellitus (lack of insulin due to the surgical removal of all or part of the pancreas), assign code E89.1, Postprocedural hypoinsulinemia. Assign a code from category E13 and a code from subcategory Z90.41-, Acquired absence of pancreas, as additional codes.

(ii) Secondary diabetes due to drugs

Secondary diabetes may be caused by an adverse effect of correctly administered medications, poisoning or sequela of poisoning.

See section I.C.19.e for coding of adverse effects and poisoning, and section I.C.20 for external cause code reporting.

5. **Chapter 5: Mental and behavioral disorders (F01 – F99)**

   a. **Pain disorders related to psychological factors**

   Assign code F45.41, for pain that is exclusively related to psychological disorders. As indicated by the Excludes 1 note under category G89, a code from category G89 should not be assigned with code F45.41

   Code F45.42, Pain disorders with related psychological factors, should be used with a code from category G89, Pain, not elsewhere classified, if there is documentation of a psychological component for a patient with acute or chronic pain.

   See Section I.C.6. Pain

   b. **Mental and behavioral disorders due to psychoactive substance use**

   1) **In remission**

   Selection of codes for "in remission" for categories F10-F19, Mental and behavioral disorders due to psychoactive substance use (categories F10-F19 with -.21) requires the provider's clinical judgment. The appropriate codes for "in remission" are assigned only on the basis of provider documentation (as defined in the Official Guidelines for Coding and Reporting).

   2) **Psychoactive substance use, abuse and dependence**

   When the provider documentation refers to use, abuse and dependence of the same substance (e.g. alcohol, opioid, cannabis, etc.), only one code should be assigned to identify the pattern of use based on the following hierarchy:

- If both use and abuse are documented, assign only the code for abuse
- If both abuse and dependence are documented, assign only the code for dependence
- If use, abuse and dependence are all documented, assign only the code for dependence
- If both use and dependence are documented, assign only the code for dependence.

   3) **Psychoactive substance use**

   As with all other diagnoses, the codes for psychoactive substance use (F10.9-, F11.9-, F12.9-, F13.9-, F14.9-, F15.9-, F16.9-) should only be assigned based on provider documentation and when they meet the definition of a reportable diagnosis (see Section III, Reporting Additional Diagnoses). The codes are to be used only when the psychoactive substance use is associated with a mental or behavioral disorder, and such a relationship is documented by the provider.

6. **Chapter 6: Diseases of Nervous System (G00-G99)**

   a. **Dominant/nondominant side**

   Codes from category G81, Hemiplegia and hemiparesis, and subcategories, G83.1, Monoplegia of lower limb, G83.2, Monoplegia of upper limb, and G83.3, Monoplegia, unspecified, identify whether the dominant or nondominant side is affected. Should the affected side be documented, but not specified as dominant or nondominant, and the classification system does not indicate a default, code selection is as follows:

- For ambidextrous patients, the default should be dominant.
- If the left side is affected, the default is non-dominant.
- If the right side is affected, the default is dominant.

   b. **Pain - Category G89**

   1) **General coding information**

   Codes in category G89, Pain, not elsewhere classified, may be used in conjunction with codes from other categories and chapters to provide more detail about acute or chronic pain and neoplasm-related pain, unless otherwise indicated below.

   If the pain is not specified as acute or chronic, post-thoracotomy, postprocedural, or neoplasm-related, do not assign codes from category G89.

   A code from category G89 should not be assigned if the underlying (definitive) diagnosis is known, unless the reason for the encounter is pain control/ management and not management of the underlying condition.

   When an admission or encounter is for a procedure aimed at treating the underlying condition (e.g., spinal fusion, kyphoplasty), a code for the underlying condition (e.g., vertebral fracture, spinal stenosis) should be assigned as the principal diagnosis. No code from category G89 should be assigned.

   (a) Category G89 codes as principal or first-listed diagnosis

   Category G89 codes are acceptable as principal diagnosis or the first-listed code:

- When pain control or pain management is the reason for the admission/encounter (e.g., a patient with displaced intervertebral disc, nerve impingement and severe back pain presents for injection of steroid into the spinal canal). The underlying cause of the pain should be reported as an additional diagnosis, if known.

- When a patient is admitted for the insertion of a neurostimulator for pain control, assign the appropriate pain code as the principal or first-listed diagnosis. When an admission or encounter is for a procedure aimed at treating the underlying condition and a neurostimulator is inserted for pain control during the same admission/encounter, a code for the underlying condition should be assigned as the principal diagnosis and the appropriate pain code should be assigned as a secondary diagnosis.

(b) Use of category G89 codes in conjunction with site specific pain codes

(i) Assigning category G89 and site-specific pain codes

Codes from category G89 may be used in conjunction with codes that identify the site of pain (including codes from chapter 18) if the category G89 code provides additional information. For example, if the code describes the site of the pain, but does not fully describe whether the pain is acute or chronic, then both codes should be assigned.

(ii) Sequencing of category G89 codes with site-specific pain codes

The sequencing of category G89 codes with site-specific pain codes (including chapter 18 codes), is dependent on the circumstances of the encounter/admission as follows:

- If the encounter is for pain control or pain management, assign the code from category G89 followed by the code identifying the specific site of pain (e.g., encounter for pain management for acute neck pain from trauma is assigned code G89.11, Acute pain due to trauma, followed by code M54.2, Cervicalgia, to identify the site of pain).
- If the encounter is for any other reason except pain control or pain management, and a related definitive diagnosis has not been established (confirmed) by the provider, assign the code for the specific site of pain first, followed by the appropriate code from category G89.

2) Pain due to devices, implants and grafts

See Section I.C.19. Pain due to medical devices

3) Postoperative pain

The provider's documentation should be used to guide the coding of postoperative pain, as well as *Section III. Reporting Additional Diagnoses* and *Section IV. Diagnostic Coding and Reporting in the Outpatient Setting.*

The default for post-thoracotomy and other postoperative pain not specified as acute or chronic is the code for the acute form.

Routine or expected postoperative pain immediately after surgery should not be coded.

(a) Postoperative pain not associated with specific postoperative complication

Postoperative pain not associated with a specific postoperative complication is assigned to the appropriate postoperative pain code in category G89.

(b) Postoperative pain associated with specific postoperative complication

Postoperative pain associated with a specific postoperative complication (such as painful wire sutures) is assigned to the appropriate code(s) found in Chapter 19, Injury, poisoning, and certain other consequences of external causes. If appropriate, use additional code(s) from category G89 to identify acute or chronic pain (G89.18 or G89.28).

4) Chronic pain

Chronic pain is classified to subcategory G89.2. There is no time frame defining when pain becomes chronic pain. The provider's documentation should be used to guide use of these codes.

5) Neoplasm related pain

Code G89.3 is assigned to pain documented as being related, associated or due to cancer, primary or secondary malignancy, or tumor. This code is assigned regardless of whether the pain is acute or chronic.

This code may be assigned as the principal or first-listed code when the stated reason for the admission/encounter is documented as pain control/pain management. The underlying neoplasm should be reported as an additional diagnosis.

When the reason for the admission/encounter is management of the neoplasm and the pain associated with the neoplasm is also documented, code G89.3 may be assigned as an additional diagnosis. It is not necessary to assign an additional code for the site of the pain.

See Section I.C.2 for instructions on the sequencing of neoplasms for all other stated reasons for the admission/encounter (except for pain control/pain management).

6) Chronic pain syndrome

Central pain syndrome (G89.Ø) and chronic pain syndrome (G89.4) are different than the term "chronic pain," and therefore codes should only be used when the provider has specifically documented this condition.

See Section I.C.5. Pain disorders related to psychological factors

7. Chapter 7: Diseases of Eye and Adnexa (HØØ-H59)

a. Glaucoma

1) Assigning glaucoma codes

Assign as many codes from category H4Ø, Glaucoma, as needed to identify the type of glaucoma, the affected eye, and the glaucoma stage.

2) Bilateral glaucoma with same type and stage

When a patient has bilateral glaucoma and both eyes are documented as being the same type and stage, and there is a code for bilateral glaucoma, report only the code for the type of glaucoma, bilateral, with the seventh character for the stage.

When a patient has bilateral glaucoma and both eyes are documented as being the same type and stage, and the classification does not provide a code for bilateral glaucoma (i.e. subcategories H4Ø.1Ø, H4Ø.11 and H4Ø.2Ø) report only one code for the type of glaucoma with the appropriate seventh character for the stage.

3) Bilateral glaucoma stage with different types or stages

When a patient has bilateral glaucoma and each eye is documented as having a different type or stage, and the classification distinguishes laterality, assign the appropriate code for each eye rather than the code for bilateral glaucoma.

When a patient has bilateral glaucoma and each eye is documented as having a different type, and the classification does not distinguish laterality (i.e. subcategories H40.10, H40.11 and H40.20), assign one code for each type of glaucoma with the appropriate seventh character for the stage.

When a patient has bilateral glaucoma and each eye is documented as having the same type, but different stage, and the classification does not distinguish laterality (i.e. subcategories H40.10, H40.11 and H40.20), assign a code for the type of glaucoma for each eye with the seventh character for the specific glaucoma stage documented for each eye.

4) **Patient admitted with glaucoma and stage evolves during the admission**
If a patient is admitted with glaucoma and the stage progresses during the admission, assign the code for highest stage documented.

5) **Indeterminate stage glaucoma**
Assignment of the seventh character "4" for "indeterminate stage" should be based on the clinical documentation. The seventh character "4" is used for glaucomas whose stage cannot be clinically determined. This seventh character should not be confused with the seventh character "0", unspecified, which should be assigned when there is no documentation regarding the stage of the glaucoma.

8. **Chapter 8: Diseases of Ear and Mastoid Process (H60-H95)**
Reserved for future guideline expansion

9. **Chapter 9: Diseases of Circulatory System (I00-I99)**
   a. **Hypertension**
   1) **Hypertension with heart disease**
   Heart conditions classified to I50.- or I51.4-I51.9, are assigned to, a code from category I11, Hypertensive heart disease, when a causal relationship is stated (due to hypertension) or implied (hypertensive). Use an additional code from category I50, Heart failure, to identify the type of heart failure in those patients with heart failure.

   The same heart conditions (I50.-, I51.4-I51.9) with hypertension, but without a stated causal relationship, are coded separately. Sequence according to the circumstances of the admission/encounter.

   2) **Hypertensive chronic kidney disease**
   Assign codes from category I12, Hypertensive chronic kidney disease, when both hypertension and a condition classifiable to category N18, Chronic kidney disease (CKD), are present. Unlike hypertension with heart disease, ICD-10-CM presumes a cause-and-effect relationship and classifies chronic kidney disease with hypertension as hypertensive chronic kidney disease.

   The appropriate code from category N18 should be used as a secondary code with a code from category I12 to identify the stage of chronic kidney disease.

   See Section I.C.14. Chronic kidney disease.

   If a patient has hypertensive chronic kidney disease and acute renal failure, an additional code for the acute renal failure is required.

   3) **Hypertensive heart and chronic kidney disease**
   Assign codes from combination category I13, Hypertensive heart and chronic kidney disease, when both hypertensive kidney disease and hypertensive heart disease are stated in the diagnosis. Assume a

relationship between the hypertension and the chronic kidney disease, whether or not the condition is so designated. If heart failure is present, assign an additional code from category I50 to identify the type of heart failure.

The appropriate code from category N18, Chronic kidney disease, should be used as a secondary code with a code from category I13 to identify the stage of chronic kidney disease.

See Section I.C.14. Chronic kidney disease.

The codes in category I13, Hypertensive heart and chronic kidney disease, are combination codes that include hypertension, heart disease and chronic kidney disease. The Includes note at I13 specifies that the conditions included at I11 and I12 are included together in I13. If a patient has hypertension, heart disease and chronic kidney disease then a code from I13 should be used, not individual codes for hypertension, heart disease and chronic kidney disease, or codes from I11 or I12.

For patients with both acute renal failure and chronic kidney disease an additional code for acute renal failure is required.

4) **Hypertensive cerebrovascular disease**
For hypertensive cerebrovascular disease, first assign the appropriate code from categories I60-I69, followed by the appropriate hypertension code.

5) **Hypertensive retinopathy**
Subcategory H35.0, Background retinopathy and retinal vascular changes, should be used with a code from category I10 – I15, Hypertensive disease to include the systemic hypertension. The sequencing is based on the reason for the encounter.

6) **Hypertension, secondary**
Secondary hypertension is due to an underlying condition. Two codes are required: one to identify the underlying etiology and one from category I15 to identify the hypertension. Sequencing of codes is determined by the reason for admission/encounter.

7) **Hypertension, transient**
Assign code R03.0, Elevated blood pressure reading without diagnosis of hypertension, unless patient has an established diagnosis of hypertension. Assign code O13.-, Gestational [pregnancy-induced] hypertension without significant proteinuria, or O14.-, Pre-eclampsia, for transient hypertension of pregnancy.

8) **Hypertension, controlled**
This diagnostic statement usually refers to an existing state of hypertension under control by therapy. Assign the appropriate code from categories I10-I15, Hypertensive diseases.

9) **Hypertension, uncontrolled**
Uncontrolled hypertension may refer to untreated hypertension or hypertension not responding to current therapeutic regimen. In either case, assign the appropriate code from categories I10-I15, Hypertensive diseases.

b. **Atherosclerotic coronary artery disease and angina**
ICD-10-CM has combination codes for atherosclerotic heart disease with angina pectoris. The subcategories for these codes are I25.11, Atherosclerotic heart disease of native coronary artery with angina pectoris and I25.7, Atherosclerosis of coronary artery bypass graft(s) and coronary artery of transplanted heart with angina pectoris.

When using one of these combination codes it is not necessary to use an additional code for angina pectoris. A causal relationship can be assumed in a patient with both atherosclerosis and angina pectoris, unless the documentation indicates the angina is due to something other than the atherosclerosis.

If a patient with coronary artery disease is admitted due to an acute myocardial infarction (AMI), the AMI should be sequenced before the coronary artery disease.

See Section I.C.9. Acute myocardial infarction (AMI)

c. Intraoperative and postprocedural cerebrovascular accident

Medical record documentation should clearly specify the cause- and-effect relationship between the medical intervention and the cerebrovascular accident in order to assign a code for intraoperative or postprocedural cerebrovascular accident.

Proper code assignment depends on whether it was an infarction or hemorrhage and whether it occurred intraoperatively or postoperatively. If it was a cerebral hemorrhage, code assignment depends on the type of procedure performed.

d. Sequelae of cerebrovascular disease

1) Category I69, sequelae of cerebrovascular disease

Category I69 is used to indicate conditions classifiable to categories I60-I67 as the causes of sequela (neurologic deficits), themselves classified elsewhere. These "late effects" include neurologic deficits that persist after initial onset of conditions classifiable to categories I60-I67. The neurologic deficits caused by cerebrovascular disease may be present from the onset or may arise at any time after the onset of the condition classifiable to categories I60-I67.

Codes from category I69, Sequelae of cerebrovascular disease, that specify hemiplegia, hemiparesis and monoplegia identify whether the dominant or nondominant side is affected. Should the affected side be documented, but not specified as dominant or nondominant, and the classification system does not indicate a default, code selection is as follows:

-   **For ambidextrous patients, the default should be dominant.**
-   **If the left side is affected, the default is non-dominant.**
-   **If the right side is affected, the default is dominant.**

2) Codes from category I69 with codes from I60-I67

Codes from category I69 may be assigned on a health care record with codes from I60-I67, if the patient has a current cerebrovascular disease and deficits from an old cerebrovascular disease.

3) Codes from category I69 *and Personal history of transient ischemic attack (TIA) and cerebral infarction (Z86.73)*

Codes from category I69 should not be assigned if the patient does not have neurologic deficits.

See Section I.C.21. 4. History (of) for use of personal history codes

e. Acute myocardial infarction (AMI)

1) ST elevation myocardial infarction (STEMI) and non ST elevation myocardial infarction (NSTEMI)

The ICD-10-CM codes for acute myocardial infarction (AMI) identify the site, such as anterolateral wall or true posterior wall. Subcategories I21.0-I21.2 and code I21.3

are used for ST elevation myocardial infarction (STEMI). Code I21.4, Non-ST elevation (NSTEMI) myocardial infarction, is used for non ST elevation myocardial infarction (NSTEMI) and nontransmural MIs.

If NSTEMI evolves to STEMI, assign the STEMI code. If STEMI converts to NSTEMI due to thrombolytic therapy, it is still coded as STEMI.

For encounters occurring while the myocardial infarction is equal to, or less than, four weeks old, including transfers to another acute setting or a postacute setting, and the patient requires continued care for the myocardial infarction, codes from category I21 may continue to be reported. For encounters after the 4 week time frame and the patient is still receiving care related to the myocardial infarction, the appropriate aftercare code should be assigned, rather than a code from category I21. For old or healed myocardial infarctions not requiring further care, code I25.2, Old myocardial infarction, may be assigned.

2) Acute myocardial infarction, unspecified

Code I21.3, ST elevation (STEMI) myocardial infarction of unspecified site, is the default for the unspecified term acute myocardial infarction. If only STEMI or transmural MI without the site is documented, query the provider as to the site, or assign code I21.3.

3) AMI documented as nontransmural or subendocardial but site provided

If an AMI is documented as nontransmural or subendocardial, but the site is provided, it is still coded as a subendocardial AMI.

See Section I.C.21.3 for information on coding status post administration of tPA in a different facility within the last 24 hrs.

4) Subsequent acute myocardial infarction

A code from category I22, Subsequent ST elevation (STEMI) and non ST elevation (NSTEMI) myocardial infarction, is to be used when a patient who has suffered an AMI has a new AMI within the 4 week time frame of the initial AMI. A code from category I22 must be used in conjunction with a code from category I21. The sequencing of the I22 and I21 codes depends on the circumstances of the encounter.

10. Chapter 10: Diseases of *the* Respiratory System (J00-J99)

a. Chronic Obstructive Pulmonary Disease [COPD] and Asthma

1) Acute exacerbation of chronic obstructive bronchitis and asthma

The codes in categories J44 and J45 distinguish between uncomplicated cases and those in acute exacerbation. An acute exacerbation is a worsening or a decompensation of a chronic condition. An acute exacerbation is not equivalent to an infection superimposed on a chronic condition, though an exacerbation may be triggered by an infection.

b. Acute Respiratory Failure

1) Acute respiratory failure as principal diagnosis

A code from subcategory J96.0, Acute respiratory failure, or subcategory J96.2, Acute and chronic respiratory failure, may be assigned as a principal diagnosis when it is the condition established after study to be chiefly responsible for occasioning the admission to the hospital, and the selection is supported by the Alphabetic Index and Tabular List. However, chapter-specific coding guidelines (such as obstetrics, poisoning, HIV, newborn) that provide sequencing direction take precedence.

2) **Acute respiratory failure as secondary diagnosis**
Respiratory failure may be listed as a secondary diagnosis if it occurs after admission, or if it is present on admission, but does not meet the definition of principal diagnosis.

3) **Sequencing of acute respiratory failure and another acute condition**
When a patient is admitted with respiratory failure and another acute condition, (e.g., myocardial infarction, cerebrovascular accident, aspiration pneumonia), the principal diagnosis will not be the same in every situation. This applies whether the other acute condition is a respiratory or nonrespiratory condition. Selection of the principal diagnosis will be dependent on the circumstances of admission. If both the respiratory failure and the other acute condition are equally responsible for occasioning the admission to the hospital, and there are no chapter-specific sequencing rules, the guideline regarding two or more diagnoses that equally meet the definition for principal diagnosis (Section II, C.) may be applied in these situations.

If the documentation is not clear as to whether acute respiratory failure and another condition are equally responsible for occasioning the admission, query the provider for clarification.

c. **Influenza due to certain identified influenza viruses**
Code only confirmed cases of influenza due to certain identified influenza viruses (category J09), **and due to other identified influenza virus (category J10)**. This is an exception to the hospital inpatient guideline Section II, H. (Uncertain Diagnosis).

In this context, "confirmation" does not require documentation of positive laboratory testing specific for avian or other novel influenza A **or other identified influenza virus**. However, coding should be based on the provider's diagnostic statement that the patient has avian influenza, or other novel influenza A, **for category J09, or has another particular identified strain of influenza, such as H1N1 or H3N2, but not identified as novel or variant, for category J10.**

If the provider records "suspected" or "possible" or "probable" avian influenza, **or novel influenza, or other identified influenza, then** the appropriate influenza code from category J11, Influenza due to unidentified influenza virus, should be assigned. A code from category J09, Influenza due to certain identified influenza viruses, should not be assigned **nor should a code from category J10, Influenza due to other identified influenza virus.**

d. **Ventilator associated pneumonia**
1) **Documentation of ventilator associated pneumonia**
As with all procedural or postprocedural complications, code assignment is based on the provider's documentation of the relationship between the condition and the procedure.

Code J95.851, Ventilator associated pneumonia, should be assigned only when the provider has documented ventilator associated pneumonia (VAP). An additional code to identify the organism (e.g., Pseudomonas aeruginosa, code B96.5) should also be assigned. Do not assign an additional code from categories J12-J18 to identify the type of pneumonia.

Code J95.851 should not be assigned for cases where the patient has pneumonia and is on a mechanical ventilator and the provider has not specifically stated that the pneumonia is ventilator-associated pneumonia. If the documentation is unclear as to whether the

patient has a pneumonia that is a complication attributable to the mechanical ventilator, query the provider.

2) **Ventilator associated pneumonia develops after admission**
A patient may be admitted with one type of pneumonia (e.g., code J13, Pneumonia due to Streptococcus pneumonia) and subsequently develop VAP. In this instance, the principal diagnosis would be the appro- priate code from categories J12-J18 for the pneumonia diagnosed at the time of admission. Code J95.851, Ventilator associated pneumonia, would be assigned as an additional diagnosis when the provider has also documented the presence of ventilator associated pneumonia.

11. **Chapter 11: Diseases of *the* Digestive System (K00-K95)**
Reserved for future guideline expansion

12. **Chapter 12: Diseases of *the* Skin and Subcutaneous Tissue (L00-L99)**
a. **Pressure ulcer stage codes**
1) **Pressure ulcer stages**
Codes from category L89, Pressure ulcer, are combination codes that identify the site of the pressure ulcer as well as the stage of the ulcer.

The ICD-10-CM classifies pressure ulcer stages based on severity, which is designated by stages 1-4, unspecified stage and unstageable.

Assign as many codes from category L89 as needed to identify all the pressure ulcers the patient has, if applicable.

2) **Unstageable pressure ulcers**
Assignment of the code for unstageable pressure ulcer (L89.--0) should be based on the clinical documentation. These codes are used for pressure ulcers whose stage cannot be clinically determined (e.g., the ulcer is covered by eschar or has been treated with a skin or muscle graft) and pressure ulcers that are documented as deep tissue injury but not documented as due to trauma. This code should not be confused with the codes for unspecified stage (L89.--9). When there is no documentation regarding the stage of the pressure ulcer, assign the appropriate code for unspecified stage (L89.--9).

3) **Documented pressure ulcer stage**
Assignment of the pressure ulcer stage code should be guided by clinical documentation of the stage or documentation of the terms found in the Alphabetic Index. For clinical terms describing the stage that are not found in the Alphabetic Index, and there is no documentation of the stage, the provider should be queried.

4) **Patients admitted with pressure ulcers documented as healed**
No code is assigned if the documentation states that the pressure ulcer is completely healed.

5) **Patients admitted with pressure ulcers documented as healing**
Pressure ulcers described as healing should be assigned the appropriate pressure ulcer stage code based on the documentation in the medical record. If the documentation does not provide information about the stage of the healing pressure ulcer, assign the appropriate code for unspecified stage.

If the documentation is unclear as to whether the patient has a current (new) pressure ulcer or if the patient is being treated for a healing pressure ulcer, query the provider.

6) Patient admitted with pressure ulcer evolving into another stage during the admission

If a patient is admitted with a pressure ulcer at one stage and it progresses to a higher stage, assign the code for the highest stage reported for that site.

13. Chapter 13: Diseases of the Musculoskeletal System and Connective Tissue (M00-M99)

a. Site and laterality

Most of the codes within Chapter 13 have site and laterality designations. The site represents the bone, joint or the muscle involved. For some conditions where more than one bone, joint or muscle is usually involved, such as osteoarthritis, there is a "multiple sites" code available. For categories where no multiple site code is provided and more than one bone, joint or muscle is involved, multiple codes should be used to indicate the different sites involved.

1) Bone versus joint

For certain conditions, the bone may be affected at the upper or lower end, (e.g., avascular necrosis of bone, M87, Osteoporosis, M80, M81). Though the portion of the bone affected may be at the joint, the site designation will be the bone, not the joint.

b. Acute traumatic versus chronic or recurrent musculoskeletal conditions

Many musculoskeletal conditions are a result of previous injury or trauma to a site, or are recurrent conditions. Bone, joint or muscle conditions that are the result of a healed injury are usually found in chapter 13. Recurrent bone, joint or muscle conditions are also usually found in chapter 13. Any current, acute injury should be coded to the appropriate injury code from chapter 19. Chronic or recurrent conditions should generally be coded with a code from chapter 13. If it is difficult to determine from the documentation in the record which code is best to describe a condition, query the provider.

c. Coding of Pathologic Fractures

7th character A is for use as long as the patient is receiving active treatment for the fracture. Examples of active treatment are: surgical treatment, emergency department encounter, evaluation and treatment by a new physician. 7th character, D is to be used for encounters after the patient has completed active treatment. The other 7th characters, listed under each subcategory in the Tabular List, are to be used for subsequent encounters for treatment of problems associated with the healing, such as malunions, nonunions, and sequelae.

Care for complications of surgical treatment for fracture repairs during the healing or recovery phase should be coded with the appropriate complication codes.

See Section I.C.19. Coding of traumatic fractures.

d. Osteoporosis

Osteoporosis is a systemic condition, meaning that all bones of the musculoskeletal system are affected. Therefore, site is not a component of the codes under category M81, Osteoporosis without current pathological fracture. The site codes under category M80, Osteoporosis with current pathological fracture, identify the site of the fracture, not the osteoporosis.

1) Osteoporosis without pathological fracture

Category M81, Osteoporosis without current pathological fracture, is for use for patients with osteoporosis who do not currently have a pathologic fracture due to the osteoporosis, even if they have had a fracture in the past. For patients with a history of

osteoporosis fractures, status code Z87.310, Personal history of (healed) osteoporosis fracture, should follow the code from M81.

2) Osteoporosis with current pathological fracture

Category M80, Osteoporosis with current pathological fracture, is for patients who have a current pathologic fracture at the time of an encounter. The codes under M80 identify the site of the fracture. A code from category M80, not a traumatic fracture code, should be used for any patient with known osteoporosis who suffers a fracture, even if the patient had a minor fall or trauma, if that fall or trauma would not usually break a normal, healthy bone.

14. Chapter 14: Diseases of Genitourinary System (N00-N99)

a. Chronic kidney disease

1) Stages of chronic kidney disease (CKD)

The ICD-10-CM classifies CKD based on severity. The severity of CKD is designated by stages 1-5. Stage 2, code N18.2, equates to mild CKD; stage 3, code N18.3, equates to moderate CKD; and stage 4, code N18.4, equates to severe CKD. Code N18.6, End stage renal disease (ESRD), is assigned when the provider has documented end-stage-renal disease (ESRD).

If both a stage of CKD and ESRD are documented, assign code N18.6 only.

2) Chronic kidney disease and kidney transplant status

Patients who have undergone kidney transplant may still have some form of chronic kidney disease (CKD) because the kidney transplant may not fully restore kidney function. Therefore, the presence of CKD alone does not constitute a transplant complication. Assign the appropriate N18 code for the patient's stage of CKD and code Z94.0, Kidney transplant status. If a transplant complication such as failure or rejection or other transplant complication is documented, see section I.C.19.g for information on coding complications of a kidney transplant. If the documentation is unclear as to whether the patient has a complication of the transplant, query the provider.

3) Chronic kidney disease with other conditions

Patients with CKD may also suffer from other serious conditions, most commonly diabetes mellitus and hypertension. The sequencing of the CKD code in relationship to codes for other contributing conditions is based on the conventions in the Tabular List.

See I.C.9. Hypertensive chronic kidney disease.

See I.C.19. Chronic kidney disease and kidney transplant complications.

15. Chapter 15: Pregnancy, Childbirth, and the Puerperium (O00-O9A)

a. General Rules for Obstetric Cases

1) Codes from chapter 15 and sequencing priority

Obstetric cases require codes from chapter 15, codes in the range O00-O9A, Pregnancy, Childbirth, and the Puerperium. Chapter 15 codes have sequencing priority over codes from other chapters. Additional codes from other chapters may be used in conjunction with chapter 15 codes to further specify conditions. Should the provider document that the pregnancy is incidental to the encounter, then code Z33.1, Pregnant state, incidental, should be used in place of any chapter 15 codes. It is the provider's responsibility to state that the condition being treated is not affecting the pregnancy.

2) Chapter 15 codes used only on the maternal record

Chapter 15 codes are to be used only on the maternal record, never on the record of the newborn.

3) Final character for trimester

The majority of codes in Chapter 15 have a final character indicating the trimester of pregnancy. The timeframes for the trimesters are indicated at the beginning of the chapter. If trimester is not a component of a code it is because the condition always occurs in a specific trimester, or the concept of trimester of pregnancy is not applicable. Certain codes have characters for only certain trimesters because the condition does not occur in all trimesters, but it may occur in more than just one.

Assignment of the final character for trimester should be based on the provider's documentation of the trimester (or number of weeks) for the current admission/encounter. This applies to the assignment of trimester for pre-existing conditions as well as those that develop during or are due to the pregnancy. The provider's documentation of the number of weeks may be used to assign the appropriate code identifying the trimester.

Whenever delivery occurs during the current admission, and there is an "in childbirth" option for the obstetric complication being coded, the "in childbirth" code should be assigned.

4) Selection of trimester for inpatient admissions that encompass more than one trimesters

In instances when a patient is admitted to a hospital for complications of pregnancy during one trimester and remains in the hospital into a subsequent trimester, the trimester character for the antepartum complication code should be assigned on the basis of the trimester when the complication developed, not the trimester of the discharge. If the condition developed prior to the current admission/encounter or represents a pre-existing condition, the trimester character for the trimester at the time of the admission/encounter should be assigned.

5) Unspecified trimester

Each category that includes codes for trimester has a code for "unspecified trimester." The "unspecified trimester" code should rarely be used, such as when the documentation in the record is insufficient to determine the trimester and it is not possible to obtain clarification.

6) 7th character for fetus identification

Where applicable, a 7th character is to be assigned for certain categories (O31, O32, O33.3 - O33.6, O35, O36, O40, O41, O60.1, O60.2, O64, and O69) to identify the fetus for which the complication code applies.

Assign 7th character "∅":

- For single gestations
- When the documentation in the record is insufficient to determine the fetus affected and it is not possible to obtain clarification.
- When it is not possible to clinically determine which fetus is affected.

b. Selection of OB principal or first-listed diagnosis

1) Routine outpatient prenatal visits

For routine outpatient prenatal visits when no complications are present, a code from category Z34, Encounter for supervision of normal pregnancy, should be used as the first-listed diagnosis. These codes should not be used in conjunction with chapter 15 codes.

2) Prenatal outpatient visits for high-risk patients

For routine prenatal outpatient visits for patients with high-risk pregnancies, a code from category O09, Supervision of high-risk pregnancy, should be used as the first-listed diagnosis. Secondary chapter 15 codes may be used in conjunction with these codes if appropriate.

3) Episodes when no delivery occurs

In episodes when no delivery occurs, the principal diagnosis should correspond to the principal complication of the pregnancy which necessitated the encounter. Should more than one complication exist, all of which are treated or monitored, any of the complications codes may be sequenced first.

4) When a delivery occurs

When a delivery occurs, the principal diagnosis should correspond to the main circumstances or complication of the delivery. In cases of cesarean delivery, the selection of the principal diagnosis should be the condition established after study that was responsible for the patient's admission. If the patient was admitted with a condition that resulted in the performance of a cesarean procedure, that condition should be selected as the principal diagnosis. If the reason for the admission/encounter was unrelated to the condition resulting in the cesarean delivery, the condition related to the reason for the admission/encounter should be selected as the principal diagnosis.

5) Outcome of delivery

A code from category Z37, Outcome of delivery, should be included on every maternal record when a delivery has occurred. These codes are not to be used on subsequent records or on the newborn record.

c. Pre-existing conditions versus conditions due to the pregnancy

Certain categories in Chapter 15 distinguish between conditions of the mother that existed prior to pregnancy (pre-existing) and those that are a direct result of pregnancy. When assigning codes from Chapter 15, it is important to assess if a condition was pre-existing prior to pregnancy or developed during or due to the pregnancy in order to assign the correct code.

Categories that do not distinguish between pre-existing and pregnancy-related conditions may be used for either. It is acceptable to use codes specifically for the puerperium with codes complicating pregnancy and childbirth if a condition arises postpartum during the delivery encounter.

d. Pre-existing hypertension in pregnancy

Category O10, Pre-existing hypertension complicating pregnancy, childbirth and the puerperium, includes codes for hypertensive heart and hypertensive chronic kidney disease. When assigning one of the O10 codes that includes hypertensive heart disease or hypertensive chronic kidney disease, it is necessary to add a secondary code from the appropriate hypertension category to specify the type of heart failure or chronic kidney disease.

See Section I.C.9. Hypertension.

e. Fetal conditions affecting the management of the mother

1) Codes from categories O35 and O36

Codes from categories O35, Maternal care for known or suspected fetal abnormality and damage, and O36, Maternal care for other fetal problems, are assigned only when the fetal condition is actually responsible for modifying the management of the mother, i.e., by requiring diagnostic studies, additional observation, special care, or termination of pregnancy. The fact that the fetal condition exists does not justify assigning a code from this series to the mother's record.

2) In utero surgery

In cases when surgery is performed on the fetus, a diagnosis code from category O35, Maternal care for known or suspected fetal abnormality and damage, should be assigned identifying the fetal condition. Assign the appropriate procedure code for the procedure performed.

No code from Chapter 16, the perinatal codes, should be used on the mother's record to identify fetal conditions. Surgery performed in utero on a fetus is still to be coded as an obstetric encounter.

f. HIV Infection in pregnancy, childbirth and the puerperium

During pregnancy, childbirth or the puerperium, a patient admitted because of an HIV-related illness should receive a principal diagnosis from subcategory O98.7-, Human immunodeficiency [HIV] disease complicating pregnancy, childbirth and the puerperium, followed by the code(s) for the HIV-related illness(es).

Patients with asymptomatic HIV infection status admitted during pregnancy, childbirth, or the puerperium should receive codes of O98.7- and Z21, Asymptomatic human immunodeficiency virus [HIV] infection status.

g. Diabetes mellitus in pregnancy

Diabetes mellitus is a significant complicating factor in pregnancy. Pregnant women who are diabetic should be assigned a code from category O24, Diabetes mellitus in pregnancy, childbirth, and the puerperium, first, followed by the appropriate diabetes code(s) (E08-E13) from Chapter 4.

h. Long term use of insulin

Code Z79.4, Long-term (current) use of insulin, should also be assigned if the diabetes mellitus is being treated with insulin.

i. Gestational (pregnancy induced) diabetes

Gestational (pregnancy induced) diabetes can occur during the second and third trimester of pregnancy in women who were not diabetic prior to pregnancy. Gestational diabetes can cause complications in the pregnancy similar to those of pre-existing diabetes mellitus. It also puts the woman at greater risk of developing diabetes after the pregnancy. Codes for gestational diabetes are in subcategory O24.4, Gestational diabetes mellitus. No other code from category O24, Diabetes mellitus in pregnancy, childbirth, and the puerperium, should be used with a code from O24.4.

The codes under subcategory O24.4 include diet controlled and insulin controlled. If a patient with gestational diabetes is treated with both diet and insulin, only the code for insulin-controlled is required.

Code Z79.4, Long-term (current) use of insulin, should not be assigned with codes from subcategory O24.4.

An abnormal glucose tolerance in pregnancy is assigned a code from subcategory O99.81, Abnormal glucose complicating pregnancy, childbirth, and the puerperium.

j. Sepsis and septic shock complicating abortion, pregnancy, childbirth and the puerperium

When assigning a chapter 15 code for sepsis complicating abortion, pregnancy, childbirth, and the puerperium, a code for the specific type of infection should be assigned as an additional diagnosis. If severe sepsis is present, a code from subcategory R65.2, Severe sepsis, and code(s) for associated organ dysfunction(s) should also be assigned as additional diagnoses.

k. Puerperal sepsis

Code O85, Puerperal sepsis, should be assigned with a secondary code to identify the causal organism (e.g., for a bacterial infection, assign a code from category B95-B96, Bacterial infections in conditions classified elsewhere). A code from category A40, Streptococcal sepsis, or A41, Other sepsis, should not be used for puerperal sepsis. If applicable, use additional codes to identify severe sepsis (R65.2-) and any associated acute organ dysfunction.

l. Alcohol and tobacco use during pregnancy, childbirth and the puerperium

1) Alcohol use during pregnancy, childbirth and the puerperium

Codes under subcategory O99.31, Alcohol use complicating pregnancy, childbirth, and the puerperium, should be assigned for any pregnancy case when a mother uses alcohol during the pregnancy or postpartum. A secondary code from category F10, Alcohol related disorders, should also be assigned to identify manifestations of the alcohol use.

2) Tobacco use during pregnancy, childbirth and the puerperium

Codes under subcategory O99.33, Smoking (tobacco) complicating pregnancy, childbirth, and the puerperium, should be assigned for any pregnancy case when a mother uses any type of tobacco product during the pregnancy or postpartum. A secondary code from category F17, Nicotine dependence, or code Z72.0, Tobacco use, should also be assigned to identify the type of nicotine dependence.

m. Poisoning, toxic effects, adverse effects and underdosing in a pregnant patient

A code from subcategory O9A.2, Injury, poisoning and certain other consequences of external causes complicating pregnancy, childbirth, and the puerperium, should be sequenced first, followed by the appropriate injury, poisoning, toxic effect, adverse effect or underdosing code, and then the additional code(s) that specifies the condition caused by the poisoning, toxic effect, adverse effect or underdosing.

See Section I.C.19. Adverse effects, poisoning, underdosing and toxic effects.

n. Normal delivery, code O80

1) Encounter for full term uncomplicated delivery

Code O80 should be assigned when a woman is admitted for a full-term normal delivery and delivers a single, healthy infant without any complications antepartum, during the delivery, or postpartum during the delivery episode. Code O80 is always a principal diagnosis. It is not to be used if any other code from chapter 15 is needed to describe a current complication of the antenatal, delivery, or perinatal period. Additional codes from other chapters may be used with code O80 if they are not related to or are in any way complicating the pregnancy.

2) Uncomplicated delivery with resolved antepartum complication

Code O80 may be used if the patient had a complication at some point during the pregnancy, but the complication is not present at the time of the admission for delivery.

3) Outcome of delivery for O80

Z37.0, Single live birth, is the only outcome of delivery code appropriate for use with O80.

o. **The peripartum and postpartum periods**

1) **Peripartum and postpartum periods**

The postpartum period begins immediately after delivery and continues for six weeks following delivery. The peripartum period is defined as the last month of pregnancy to five months postpartum.

2) **Peripartum and postpartum complication**

A postpartum complication is any complication occurring within the six-week period.

3) **Pregnancy-related complications after 6 week period**

Chapter 15 codes may also be used to describe pregnancy-related complications after the peripartum or postpartum period if the provider documents that a condition is pregnancy related.

4) **Admission for routine postpartum care following delivery outside hospital**

When the mother delivers outside the hospital prior to admission and is admitted for routine postpartum care and no complications are noted, code Z39.0, Encounter for care and examination of mother immediately after delivery, should be assigned as the principal diagnosis.

5) **Pregnancy associated cardiomyopathy**

Pregnancy associated cardiomyopathy, code O90.3, is unique in that it may be diagnosed in the third trimester of pregnancy but may continue to progress months after delivery. For this reason, it is referred to as peripartum cardiomyopathy. Code O90.3 is only for use when the cardiomyopathy develops as a result of pregnancy in a woman who did not have pre-existing heart disease.

p. **Code O94, Sequelae of complication of pregnancy, childbirth, and the puerperium**

1) **Code O94**

Code O94, Sequelae of complication of pregnancy, childbirth, and the puerperium, is for use in those cases when an initial complication of a pregnancy develops a sequelae requiring care or treatment at a future date.

2) **After the initial postpartum period**

This code may be used at any time after the initial postpartum period.

3) **Sequencing of code O94**

This code, like all late effect codes, is to be sequenced following the code describing the sequelae of the complication.

q. *Termination of Pregnancy and Spontaneous Abortions*

1) **Abortion with liveborn fetus**

When an attempted termination of pregnancy results in a liveborn fetus, assign code **Z33.2, Encounter for elective termination of pregnancy** and a code from category Z37, Outcome of Delivery.

2) **Retained products of conception following an abortion**

Subsequent encounters for retained products of conception following a spontaneous abortion or elective termination of pregnancy are assigned the appropriate code from category O03, Spontaneous abortion, or codes O07.4, Failed attempted termination of pregnancy without complication and Z33.2, Encounter for elective termination of pregnancy. This advice is appropriate even when the patient was discharged previously with a discharge diagnosis of complete abortion.

3) **Complications leading to abortion**

Codes from Chapter 15 may be used as additional codes to identify any documented complications of the pregnancy in conjunction with codes in categories in O07 and O08.

r. **Abuse in a pregnant patient**

For suspected or confirmed cases of abuse of a pregnant patient, a code(s) from subcategories O9A.3, Physical abuse complicating pregnancy, childbirth, and the puerperium, O9A.4, Sexual abuse complicating pregnancy, childbirth, and the puerperium, and O9A.5, Psychological abuse complicating pregnancy, childbirth, and the puerperium, should be sequenced first, followed by the appropriate codes (if applicable) to identify any associated current injury due to physical abuse, sexual abuse, and the perpetrator of abuse.

See Section I.C.19.f. Adult and child abuse, neglect and other maltreatment.

16. **Chapter 16: Certain Conditions Origination in the Perinatal Period (P00-P96)**

For coding and reporting purposes the perinatal period is defined as before birth through the 28th day following birth. The following guidelines are provided for reporting purposes

a. **General Perinatal Rules**

1) **Use of Chapter 16 codes**

Codes in this chapter are <u>never</u> for use on the maternal record. Codes from Chapter 15, the obstetric chapter, are never permitted on the newborn record. Chapter 16 codes may be used throughout the life of the patient if the condition is still present.

2) **Principal diagnosis for birth record**

When coding the birth episode in a newborn record, assign a code from category Z38, Liveborn infants according to place of birth and type of delivery, as the principal diagnosis. A code from category Z38 is assigned only once, to a newborn at the time of birth. If a newborn is transferred to another institution, a code from category Z38 should not be used at the receiving hospital.

A code from category Z38 is used only on the newborn record, not on the mother's record.

3) **Use of codes from other chapters with codes from Chapter 16**

Codes from other chapters may be used with codes from chapter 16 if the codes from the other chapters provide more specific detail. Codes for signs and symptoms may be assigned when a definitive diagnosis has not been established. If the reason for the encounter is a perinatal condition, the code from chapter 16 should be sequenced first.

4) **Use of Chapter 16 codes after the perinatal period**

Should a condition originate in the perinatal period, and continue throughout the life of the patient, the perinatal code should continue to be used regardless of the patient's age.

5) **Birth process or community acquired conditions**

If a newborn has a condition that may be either due to the birth process or community acquired and the documentation does not indicate which it is, the default is due to the birth process and the code from Chapter 16 should be used. If the condition is community-acquired, a code from Chapter 16 should not be assigned.

6) **Code all clinically significant conditions**

All clinically significant conditions noted on routine newborn examination should be coded. A condition is clinically significant if it requires:

- clinical evaluation; or
- therapeutic treatment; or
- diagnostic procedures; or
- extended length of hospital stay; or
- increased nursing care and/or monitoring; or
- has implications for future health care needs

Note: The perinatal guidelines listed above are the same as the general coding guidelines for "additional diagnoses", except for the final point regarding implications for future health care needs. Codes should be assigned for conditions that have been specified by the provider as having implications for future health care needs.

b. **Observation and evaluation of newborns for suspected conditions not found**

Reserved for future expansion

c. **Coding Additional Perinatal Diagnoses**

1) **Assigning codes for conditions that require treatment**

Assign codes for conditions that require treatment or further investigation, prolong the length of stay, or require resource utilization.

2) **Codes for conditions specified as having implications for future health care needs**

Assign codes for conditions that have been specified by the provider as having implications for future health care needs.

Note: This guideline should not be used for adult patients.

d. **Prematurity and fetal growth retardation**

Providers utilize different criteria in determining prematurity. A code for prematurity should not be assigned unless it is documented. Assignment of codes in categories P05, Disorders of newborn related to slow fetal growth and fetal malnutrition, and P07, Disorders of newborn related to short gestation and low birth weight, not elsewhere classified, should be based on the recorded birth weight and estimated gestational age. Codes from category P05 should not be assigned with codes from category P07.

When both birth weight and gestational age are available, two codes from category P07 should be assigned, with the code for birth weight sequenced before the code for gestational age.

A code from P05 and codes from P07.2 and P07.3 may be used to specify weeks of gestation as documented by the provider in the record.

e. **Low birth weight and immaturity status**

Codes from category P07, Disorders of newborn related to short gestation and low birth weight, not elsewhere classified, are for use for a child or adult who was premature or had a low birth weight as a newborn and this is affecting the patient's current health status.

See Section I.C.21. Factors influencing health status and contact with health services, Status.

f. **Bacterial sepsis of newborn**

Category P36, Bacterial sepsis of newborn, includes congenital sepsis. If a perinate is documented as having sepsis without documentation of congenital or community acquired, the default is congenital and a code from category P36 should be assigned. If the P36 code includes the causal

organism, an additional code from category B95, Streptococcus, Staphylococcus, and Enterococcus as the cause of diseases classified elsewhere, or B96, Other bacterial agents as the cause of diseases classified elsewhere, should not be assigned. If the P36 code does not include the causal organism, assign an additional code from category B96. If applicable, use additional codes to identify severe sepsis (R65.2-) and any associated acute organ dysfunction.

g. **Stillbirth**

Code P95, Stillbirth, is only for use in institutions that maintain separate records for stillbirths. No other code should be used with P95. Code P95 should not be used on the mother's record.

17. **Chapter 17: Congenital Malformations, Deformations, and Chromosomal Abnormalities (Q00-Q99)**

Assign an appropriate code(s) from categories Q00-Q99, Congenital malformations, deformations, and chromosomal abnormalities when a malformation/deformation or chromosomal abnormality is documented. A malformation/deformation/or chromosomal abnormality may be the principal/first-listed diagnosis on a record or a secondary diagnosis.

When a malformation/deformation/or chromosomal abnormality does not have a unique code assignment, assign additional code(s) for any manifestations that may be present.

When the code assignment specifically identifies the malformation/deformation/or chromosomal abnormality, manifestations that are an inherent component of the anomaly should not be coded separately. Additional codes should be assigned for manifestations that are not an inherent component.

Codes from Chapter 17 may be used throughout the life of the patient. If a congenital malformation or deformity has been corrected, a personal history code should be used to identify the history of the malformation or deformity. Although present at birth, malformation/deformation/or chromosomal abnormality may not be identified until later in life. Whenever the condition is diagnosed by the physician, it is appropriate to assign a code from codes Q00-Q99.

For the birth admission, the appropriate code from category Z38, Liveborn infants, according to place of birth and type of delivery, should be sequenced as the principal diagnosis, followed by any congenital anomaly codes, Q00- Q99.

18. **Chapter 18: Symptoms, Signs, and Abnormal Clinical and Laboratory Findings, Not Elsewhere Classified (R00-R99)**

Chapter 18 includes symptoms, signs, abnormal results of clinical or other investigative procedures, and ill-defined conditions regarding which no diagnosis classifiable elsewhere is recorded. Signs and symptoms that point to a specific diagnosis have been assigned to a category in other chapters of the classification.

a. **Use of symptom codes**

Codes that describe symptoms and signs are acceptable for reporting purposes when a related definitive diagnosis has not been established (confirmed) by the provider.

b. **Use of a symptom code with a definitive diagnosis code**

Codes for signs and symptoms may be reported in addition to a related definitive diagnosis when the sign or symptom is not routinely associated with that diagnosis, such as the various signs and symptoms associated with complex syndromes. The definitive diagnosis code should be sequenced before the symptom code.

Signs or symptoms that are associated routinely with a disease process should not be assigned as additional codes, unless otherwise instructed by the classification.

c. **Combination codes that include symptoms**

ICD-10-CM contains a number of combination codes that identify both the definitive diagnosis and common symptoms of that diagnosis. When using one of these combination codes, an additional code should not be assigned for the symptom.

d. **Repeated falls**

Code R29.6, Repeated falls, is for use for encounters when a patient has recently fallen and the reason for the fall is being investigated.

Code Z91.81, History of falling, is for use when a patient has fallen in the past and is at risk for future falls. When appropriate, both codes R29.6 and Z91.81 may be assigned together.

e. *Coma* **scale**

The coma scale codes (R40.2-) can be used in conjunction with traumatic brain injury codes, acute cerebrovascular disease or sequelae of cerebrovascular disease codes. These codes are primarily for use by trauma registries, but they may be used in any setting where this information is collected. The coma scale codes should be sequenced after the diagnosis code(s).

These codes, one from each subcategory, are needed to complete the scale. The 7th character indicates when the scale was recorded. The 7th character should match for all three codes.

At a minimum, report the initial score documented on presentation at your facility. This may be a score from the emergency medicine technician (EMT) or in the emergency department. If desired, a facility may choose to capture multiple Glasgow coma scale scores.

Assign code R40.24, Glasgow coma scale, total score, when only the total score is documented in the medical record and not the individual score(s).

f. **Functional quadriplegia**

Functional quadriplegia (code R53.2) is the lack of ability to use one's limbs or to ambulate due to extreme debility. It is not associated with neurologic deficit or injury, and code R53.2 should not be used for cases of neurologic quadriplegia. It should only be assigned if functional quadriplegia is specifically documented in the medical record.

g. **SIRS due to non-infectious process**

The systemic inflammatory response syndrome (SIRS) can develop as a result of certain non-infectious disease processes, such as trauma, malignant neoplasm, or pancreatitis. When SIRS is documented with a noninfectious condition, and no subsequent infection is documented, the code for the underlying condition, such as an injury, should be assigned, followed by code R65.10, Systemic inflammatory response syndrome (SIRS) of non-infectious origin without acute organ dysfunction, or code R65.11, Systemic inflammatory response syndrome (SIRS) of non-infectious origin with acute organ dysfunction. If an associated acute organ dysfunction is documented, the appropriate code(s) for the specific type of organ dysfunction(s) should be assigned in addition to code R65.11. If acute organ dysfunction is documented, but it cannot be determined if the acute organ dysfunction is associated with SIRS or due to another condition (e.g., directly due to the trauma), the provider should be queried.

h. **Death NOS**

Code R99, Ill-defined and unknown cause of mortality, is only for use in the very limited circumstance when a patient who has already died is brought into an emergency department or other healthcare facility and is pronounced dead upon arrival. It does not represent the discharge disposition of death.

19. **Chapter 19: Injury, Poisoning, and Certain Other Consequences of External Causes (S00-T88)**

a. **Application of 7th Characters in Chapter 19**

Most categories in chapter 19 have a 7th character requirement for each applicable code. Most categories in this chapter have three 7th character values (with the exception of fractures): A, initial encounter, D, subsequent encounter and S, sequela. Categories for traumatic fractures have additional 7th character values.

7th character "A", initial encounter is used while the patient is receiving active treatment for the condition. Examples of active treatment are: surgical treatment, emergency department encounter, and evaluation and treatment by a new physician.

7th character "D" subsequent encounter is used for encounters after the patient has received active treatment of the condition and is receiving routine care for the condition during the healing or recovery phase. Examples of subsequent care are: cast change or removal, removal of external or internal fixation device, medication adjustment, other aftercare and follow up visits following treatment of the injury or condition.

The aftercare Z codes should not be used for aftercare for conditions such as injuries or poisonings, where 7th characters are provided to identify subsequent care. For example, for aftercare of an injury, assign the acute injury code with the 7th character "D" (subsequent encounter).

7th character "S", sequela, is for use for complications or conditions that arise as a direct result of a condition, such as scar formation after a burn. The scars are sequelae of the burn. When using 7th character "S", it is necessary to use both the injury code that precipitated the sequela and the code for the sequela itself. The "S" is added only to the injury code, not the sequela code. The 7th character "S" identifies the injury responsible for the sequela. The specific type of sequela (e.g. scar) is sequenced first, followed by the injury code.

b. **Coding of injuries**

When coding injuries, assign separate codes for each injury unless a combination code is provided, in which case the combination code is assigned. Code T07, Unspecified multiple injuries should not be assigned in the inpatient setting unless information for a more specific code is not available. Traumatic injury codes (S00-T14.9) are not to be used for normal, healing surgical wounds or to identify complications of surgical wounds.

The code for the most serious injury, as determined by the provider and the focus of treatment, is sequenced first.

1) **Superficial injuries**

Superficial injuries such as abrasions or contusions are not coded when associated with more severe injuries of the same site.

2) **Primary injury with damage to nerves/blood vessels**

When a primary injury results in minor damage to peripheral nerves or blood vessels, the primary injury is sequenced first with additional code(s) for injuries to nerves and spinal cord (such as category S04), and/or injury to blood vessels (such as category S15). When the primary injury is to the blood vessels or nerves, that injury should be sequenced first.

c. **Coding of traumatic fractures**

The principles of multiple coding of injuries should be followed in coding fractures. Fractures of specified sites are coded individually by site in accordance with both the provisions within categories S02, S12, S22, S32, S42, S49, S52, S59, S62, S72, S79, S82, S89, S92 and the level of detail furnished by medical record content.

A fracture not indicated as open or closed should be coded to closed. A fracture not indicated whether displaced or not displaced should be coded to displaced.

More specific guidelines are as follows:

1) **Initial vs. subsequent encounter for fractures**

   Traumatic fractures are coded using the appropriate 7th character extension for initial encounter (A, B, C) while the patient is receiving active treatment for the fracture. Examples of active treatment are: surgical treatment, emergency department encounter, and evaluation and treatment by a new physician. The appropriate 7th character for initial encounter should also be assigned for a patient who delayed seeking treatment for the fracture or nonunion.

   Fractures are coded using the appropriate 7th character extension for subsequent care for encounters after the patient has completed active treatment of the fracture and is receiving routine care for the fracture during the healing or recovery phase. Examples of fracture aftercare are: cast change or removal, removal of external or internal fixation device, medication adjustment, and follow-up visits following fracture treatment.

   Care for complications of surgical treatment for fracture repairs during the healing or recovery phase should be coded with the appropriate complication codes.

   Care of complications of fractures, such as malunion and nonunion, should be reported with the appropriate 7th character extensions for subsequent care with nonunion (K, M, N,) or subsequent care with malunion (P, Q, R).

   A code from category M80, not a traumatic fracture code, should be used for any patient with known osteoporosis who suffers a fracture, even if the patient had a minor fall or trauma, if that fall or trauma would not usually break a normal, healthy bone.

   See Section I.C.13. Osteoporosis.

   The aftercare Z codes should not be used for aftercare for traumatic fractures. For aftercare of a traumatic fracture, assign the acute fracture code with the appropriate 7th character.

2) **Multiple fractures sequencing**

   Multiple fractures are sequenced in accordance with the severity of the fracture.

d. Coding of burns and corrosions

The ICD-10-CM makes a distinction between burns and corrosions. The burn codes are for thermal burns, except sunburns, that come from a heat source, such as a fire or hot appliance. The burn codes are also for burns resulting from electricity and radiation. Corrosions are burns due to chemicals. The guidelines are the same for burns and corrosions.

Current burns (T20-T25) are classified by depth, extent and by agent (X code). Burns are classified by depth as first degree (erythema), second degree (blistering), and third degree (full-thickness involvement). Burns of the eye and internal organs (T26-T28) are classified by site, but not by degree.

1) **Sequencing of burn and related condition codes**

   Sequence first the code that reflects the highest degree of burn when more than one burn is present.

   a. When the reason for the admission or encounter is for treatment of external multiple burns, sequence first the code that reflects the burn of the highest degree.

   b. When a patient has both internal and external burns, the circumstances of admission govern the selection of the principal diagnosis or first-listed diagnosis.

   c. When a patient is admitted for burn injuries and other related conditions such as smoke inhalation and/or respiratory failure, the circumstances of admission govern the selection of the principal or first-listed diagnosis.

2) **Burns of the same local site**

   Classify burns of the same local site (three-character category level, T20-T28) but of different degrees to the subcategory identifying the highest degree recorded in the diagnosis.

3) **Non-healing burns**

   Non-healing burns are coded as acute burns.

   Necrosis of burned skin should be coded as a non-healed burn.

4) **Infected burn**

   For any documented infected burn site, use an additional code for the infection.

5) **Assign separate codes for each burn site**

   When coding burns, assign separate codes for each burn site. Category T30, Burn and corrosion, body region unspecified is extremely vague and should rarely be used.

6) **Burns and corrosions classified according to extent of body surface involved**

   Assign codes from category T31, Burns classified according to extent of body surface involved, or T32, Corrosions classified according to extent of body surface involved, when the site of the burn is not specified or when there is a need for additional data. It is advisable to use category T31 as additional coding when needed to provide data for evaluating burn mortality, such as that needed by burn units. It is also advisable to use category T31 as an additional code for reporting purposes when there is mention of a third-degree burn involving 20 percent or more of the body surface.

   Categories T31 and T32 are based on the classic "rule of nines" in estimating body surface involved: head and neck are assigned nine percent, each arm nine percent, each leg 18 percent, the anterior trunk 18 percent, posterior trunk 18 percent, and genitalia one percent. Providers may change these percentage assignments where necessary to accommodate infants and children who have proportionately larger heads than adults, and patients who have large buttocks, thighs, or abdomen that involve burns.

7) **Encounters for treatment of *sequela* of burns**

   Encounters for the treatment of the late effects of burns or corrosions (i.e., scars or joint contractures) should be coded with a burn or corrosion code with the 7th character "S" for sequela.

8) **Sequelae with a late effect code and current burn**

   When appropriate, both a code for a current burn or corrosion with 7th character "A" or "D" and a burn or corrosion code with 7th character "S" may be assigned on the same record (when both a current burn and sequelae of an old burn exist). Burns and corrosions do not heal at the same rate and a current healing wound may still exist with sequela of a healed burn or corrosion.

9) Use of an external cause code with burns and corrosions

An external cause code should be used with burns and corrosions to identify the source and intent of the burn, as well as the place where it occurred.

e. Adverse effects, poisoning, underdosing and toxic effects

Codes in categories T36-T65 are combination codes that include the substance that was taken as well as the intent. No additional external cause code is required for poisonings, toxic effects, adverse effects and underdosing codes.

1) Do not code directly from the Table of Drugs

Do not code directly from the Table of Drugs and Chemicals. Always refer back to the Tabular List.

2) Use as many codes as necessary to describe

Use as many codes as necessary to describe completely all drugs, medicinal or biological substances.

3) If the same code would describe the causative agent

If the same code would describe the causative agent for more than one adverse reaction, poisoning, toxic effect or underdosing, assign the code only once.

4) If two or more drugs, medicinal or biological substances

If two or more drugs, medicinal or biological substances are reported, code each individually unless a combination code is listed in the Table of Drugs and Chemicals.

5) The occurrence of drug toxicity is classified in ICD-1Ø-CM as follows:

(a) Adverse effect

When coding an adverse effect of a drug that has been correctly prescribed and properly administered, assign the appropriate code for the nature of the adverse effect followed by the appropriate code for the adverse effect of the drug (T36-T5Ø). The code for the drug should have a 5th or 6th character "5" (for example T36.ØX5-) Examples of the nature of an adverse effect are tachycardia, delirium, gastrointestinal hemorrhaging, vomiting, hypokalemia, hepatitis, renal failure, or respiratory failure.

(b) Poisoning

When coding a poisoning or reaction to the improper use of a medication (e.g., overdose, wrong substance given or taken in error, wrong route of administration), first assign the appropriate code from categories T36-T5Ø. The poisoning codes have an associated intent as their 5th or 6th character (accidental, intentional self-harm, assault and undetermined. Use additional code(s) for all manifestations of poisonings.

If there is also a diagnosis of abuse or dependence of the substance, the abuse or dependence is assigned as an additional code.

Examples of poisoning include:

(i) Error was made in drug prescription

Errors made in drug prescription or in the administration of the drug by provider, nurse, patient, or other person.

(ii) Overdose of a drug intentionally taken

If an overdose of a drug was intentionally taken or administered and resulted in drug toxicity, it would be coded as a poisoning.

(iii) Nonprescribed drug taken with correctly prescribed and properly administered drug

If a nonprescribed drug or medicinal agent was taken in combination with a correctly prescribed and properly administered drug, any drug toxicity or other reaction resulting from the interaction of the two drugs would be classified as a poisoning.

(iv) Interaction of drug(s) and alcohol

When a reaction results from the interaction of a drug(s) and alcohol, this would be classified as poisoning.

See Section I.C.4. if poisoning is the result of insulin pump malfunctions.

(c) Underdosing

Underdosing refers to taking less of a medication than is prescribed by a provider or a manufacturer's instruction. For underdosing, assign the code from categories T36-T5Ø (fifth or sixth character "6").

Codes for underdosing should never be assigned as principal or first-listed codes. If a patient has a relapse or exacerbation of the medical condition for which the drug is prescribed because of the reduction in dose, then the medical condition itself should be coded.

Noncompliance (Z91.12-, Z91.13-) or complication of care (Y63.61, Y63.8-Y63.9) codes are to be used with an underdosing code to indicate intent, if known.

(d) Toxic effects

When a harmful substance is ingested or comes in contact with a person, this is classified as a toxic effect. The toxic effect codes are in categories T51-T65.

Toxic effect codes have an associated intent: accidental, intentional self-harm, assault and undetermined.

f. Adult and child abuse, neglect and other maltreatment

Sequence first the appropriate code from categories T74.- (Adult and child abuse, neglect and other maltreatment, confirmed) or T76.- (Adult and child abuse, neglect and other maltreatment, suspected) for abuse, neglect and other maltreatment, followed by any accompanying mental health or injury code(s).

If the documentation in the medical record states abuse or neglect it is coded as confirmed (T74.-). It is coded as suspected if it is documented as suspected (T76.-).

For cases of confirmed abuse or neglect an external cause code from the assault section (X92-YØ8) should be added to identify the cause of any physical injuries. A perpetrator code (YØ7) should be added when the perpetrator of the abuse is known. For suspected cases of abuse or neglect, do not report external cause or perpetrator code.

If a suspected case of abuse, neglect or mistreatment is ruled out during an encounter code ZØ4.71, Encounter for examination and observation following alleged physical adult abuse, ruled out, or code ZØ4.72, Encounter for examination and observation following alleged child physical abuse, ruled out, should be used, not a code from T76.

If a suspected case of alleged rape or sexual abuse is ruled out during an encounter code ZØ4.41, Encounter for examination and observation following alleged physical adult abuse, ruled out, or code Z04.42, Encounter for examination and observation following alleged rape or sexual abuse, ruled out, should be used, not a code from T76.

See Section I.C.15. Abuse in a pregnant patient.

g. **Complications of care**

1) General guidelines for **complications of care**

   (a) **Documentation of complications of care**

   See Section I.B.16. for information on documentation of complications of care.

2) **Pain due to medical devices**

   Pain associated with devices, implants or grafts left in a surgical site (for example painful hip prosthesis) is assigned to the appropriate code(s) found in Chapter 19, Injury, poisoning, and certain other consequences of external causes. Specific codes for pain due to medical devices are found in the T code section of the ICD-10-CM. Use additional code(s) from category G89 to identify acute or chronic pain due to presence of the device, implant or graft (G89.18 or G89.28).

3) **Transplant complications**

   (a) **Transplant complications other than kidney**

   Codes under category T86, Complications of transplanted organs and tissues, are for use for both complications and rejection of transplanted organs. A transplant complication code is only assigned if the complication affects the function of the transplanted organ. Two codes are required to fully describe a transplant complication: the appropriate code from category T86 and a secondary code that identifies the complication.

   Pre-existing conditions or conditions that develop after the transplant are not coded as complications unless they affect the function of the transplanted organs.

   See I.C.21. for transplant organ removal status

   See I.C.2. for malignant neoplasm associated with transplanted organ.

   (b) *Kidney transplant complications*

   Patients who have undergone kidney transplant may still have some form of chronic kidney disease (CKD) because the kidney transplant may not fully restore kidney function. Code T86.1- should be assigned for documented complications of a kidney transplant, such as transplant failure or rejection or other transplant complication. Code T86.1- should not be assigned for post kidney transplant patients who have chronic kidney (CKD) unless a transplant complication such as transplant failure or rejection is documented. If the documentation is unclear as to whether the patient has a complication of the transplant, query the provider.

   Conditions that affect the function of the transplanted kidney, other than CKD, should be assigned a code from subcategory T86.1, Complications of transplanted organ, Kidney, and a secondary code that identifies the complication.

   For patients with CKD following a kidney transplant, but who do not have a complication such as failure or rejection, *see section I.C.14. Chronic kidney disease and kidney transplant status.*

4) **Complication codes that include the external cause**

   As with certain other T codes, some of the complications of care codes have the external cause included in the code. The code includes the nature of the complication as well as the type of procedure that caused the complication. No external cause code indicating the type of procedure is necessary for these codes.

5) **Complications of care codes within the body system chapters**

   Intraoperative and postprocedural complication codes are found within the body system chapters with codes specific to the organs and structures of that body system. These codes should be sequenced first, followed by a code(s) for the specific complication, if applicable.

20. **Chapter 20: External Causes of Morbidity (V01-Y99)**

Introduction: These guidelines are provided for the reporting of external causes of morbidity codes in order that there will be standardization in the process. These codes are secondary codes for use in any health care setting.

External cause codes are intended to provide data for injury research and evaluation of injury prevention strategies. These codes capture how the injury or health condition happened (cause), the intent (unintentional or accidental; or intentional, such as suicide or assault), the place where the event occurred the activity of the patient at the time of the event, and the person's status (e.g., civilian, military).

a. **General external cause coding guidelines**

1) **Used with any code in the range of A00.0-T88.9, Z00-Z99**

   An external cause code may be used with any code in the range of A00.0-T88.9, Z00-Z99, classification that is a health condition due to an external cause. Though they are most applicable to injuries, they are also valid for use with such things as infections or diseases due to an external source, and other health conditions, such as a heart attack that occurs during strenuous physical activity.

2) **External cause code used for length of treatment**

   Assign the external cause code, with the appropriate 7th character (initial encounter, subsequent encounter or sequela) for each encounter for which the injury or condition is being treated.

3) **Use the full range of external cause codes**

   Use the full range of external cause codes to completely describe the cause, the intent, the place of occurrence, and if applicable, the activity of the patient at the time of the event, and the patient's status, for all injuries, and other health conditions due to an external cause.

4) **Assign as many external cause codes as necessary**

   Assign as many external cause codes as necessary to fully explain each cause. If only one external code can be recorded, assign the code most related to the principal diagnosis.

5) **The selection of the appropriate external cause code**

   The selection of the appropriate external cause code is guided by the Alphabetic Index of External Causes and by Inclusion and Exclusion notes in the Tabular List.

6) **External cause code can never be a principal diagnosis**

   An external cause code can never be a principal (first-listed) diagnosis.

7) **Combination external cause codes**

   Certain of the external cause codes are combination codes that identify sequential events that result in an injury, such as a fall which results in striking against an object. The injury may be due to either event or both. The combination external cause code used should correspond to the sequence of events regardless of which caused the most serious injury.

8) No external cause code needed in certain circumstances

No external cause code from Chapter 20 is needed if the external cause and intent are included in a code from another chapter (e.g. T36.0x1- Poisoning by penicillins, accidental (unintentional)).

b. Place of occurrence guideline

Codes from category Y92, Place of occurrence of the external cause, are secondary codes for use after other external cause codes to identify the location of the patient at the time of injury or other condition.

A place of occurrence code is used only once, at the initial encounter for treatment. No 7th characters are used for Y92. Only one code from Y92 should be recorded on a medical record. A place of occurrence code should be used in conjunction with an activity code, Y93.

Do not use place of occurrence code Y92.9 if the place is not stated or is not applicable.

c. Activity code

Assign a code from category Y93, Activity code, to describe the activity of the patient at the time the injury or other health condition occurred.

An activity code is used only once, at the initial encounter for treatment. Only one code from Y93 should be recorded on a medical record. An activity code should be used in conjunction with a place of occurrence code, Y92.

The activity codes are not applicable to poisonings, adverse effects, misadventures or sequela.

Do not assign Y93.9, Unspecified activity, if the activity is not stated.

A code from category Y93 is appropriate for use with external cause and intent codes if identifying the activity provides additional information about the event.

d. Place of occurrence, activity, and status codes used with other external cause code

When applicable, place of occurrence, activity, and external cause status codes are sequenced after the main external cause code(s). Regardless of the number of external cause codes assigned, there should be only one place of occurrence code, one activity code, and one external cause status code assigned to an encounter.

e. If the reporting format limits the number of external cause codes

If the reporting format limits the number of external cause codes that can be used in reporting clinical data, report the code for the cause/intent most related to the principal diagnosis. If the format

permits capture of additional external cause codes, the cause/intent, including medical misadventures, of the additional events should be reported rather than the codes for place, activity, or external status.

f. Multiple external cause coding guidelines

More than one external cause code is required to fully describe the external cause of an illness or injury. The assignment of external cause codes should be sequenced in the following priority:

If two or more events cause separate injuries, an external cause code should be assigned for each cause. The first-listed external cause code will be selected in the following order:

External codes for child and adult abuse take priority over all other external cause codes.

See Section I.C.19., Child and Adult abuse guidelines.

External cause codes for terrorism events take priority over all other external cause codes except child and adult abuse.

External cause codes for cataclysmic events take priority over all other external cause codes except child and adult abuse and terrorism.

External cause codes for transport accidents take priority over all other external cause codes except cataclysmic events, child and adult abuse and terrorism.

Activity and external cause status codes are assigned following all causal (intent) external cause codes.

The first-listed external cause code should correspond to the cause of the most serious diagnosis due to an assault, accident, or self-harm, following the order of hierarchy listed above.

g. Child and adult abuse guideline

Adult and child abuse, neglect and maltreatment are classified as assault. Any of the assault codes may be used to indicate the external cause of any injury resulting from the confirmed abuse.

For confirmed cases of abuse, neglect and maltreatment, when the perpetrator is known, a code from Y07, Perpetrator of maltreatment and neglect, should accompany any other assault codes.

See Section I.C.19. Adult and child abuse, neglect and other maltreatment

h. Unknown or undetermined intent guideline

If the intent (accident, self-harm, assault) of the cause of an injury or other condition is unknown or unspecified, code the intent as accidental intent. All transport accident categories assume accidental intent.

1) Use of undetermined intent

External cause codes for events of undetermined intent are only for use if the documentation in the record specifies that the intent cannot be determined.

i. Sequelae (Late Effects) of external cause guidelines

1) Sequelae external cause codes

Sequela are reported using the external cause code with the 7th character extension "S" for sequela. These codes should be used with any report of a late effect or sequela resulting from a previous injury.

2) Sequela external cause code with a related current injury

A sequela external cause code should never be used with a related current nature of injury code.

3) Use of sequela external cause codes for subsequent visits

Use a late effect external cause code for subsequent visits when a late effect of the initial injury is being treated. Do not use a late effect external cause code for subsequent visits for follow-up care (e.g., to assess healing, to receive rehabilitative therapy) of the injury when no late effect of the injury has been documented.

j. Terrorism guidelines

1) Cause of injury identified by the Federal Government (FBI) as terrorism

When the cause of an injury is identified by the Federal Government (FBI) as terrorism, the first-listed external cause code should be a code from category Y38, Terrorism. The definition of terrorism employed by the FBI is found at the inclusion note at the beginning of category Y38. Use additional code for place of occurrence (Y92.-). More than one Y38 code may be assigned if the injury is the result of more than one mechanism of terrorism.

2) Cause of an injury is suspected to be the result of terrorism

When the cause of an injury is suspected to be the result of terrorism a code from category Y38 should not be assigned. Suspected cases should be classified as assault.

3) Code Y38.9, terrorism, secondary effects

Assign code Y38.9, Terrorism, secondary effects, for conditions occurring subsequent to the terrorist event. This code should not be assigned for conditions that are due to the initial terrorist act.

It is acceptable to assign code Y38.9 with another code from Y38 if there is an injury due to the initial terrorist event and an injury that is a subsequent result of the terrorist event.

k. External cause status

A code from category Y99, External cause status, should be assigned whenever any other external cause code is assigned for an encounter, including an Activity code, except for the events noted below. Assign a code from category Y99, External cause status, to indicate the work status of the person at the time the event occurred. The status code indicates whether the event occurred during military activity, whether a non-military person was at work, whether an individual including a student or volunteer was involved in a non-work activity at the time of the causal event.

A code from Y99, External cause status, should be assigned, when applicable, with other external cause codes, such as transport accidents and falls. The external cause status codes are not applicable to poisonings, adverse effects, misadventures or late effects.

Do not assign a code from category Y99 if no other external cause codes (cause, activity) are applicable for the encounter.

An external cause status code is used only once, at the initial encounter for treatment. Only one code from Y99 should be recorded on a medical record.

Do not assign code Y99.9, Unspecified external cause status, if the status is not stated.

21. Chapter 21: Factors Influencing Health Status and Contact with Health Services (Z00-Z99)

Note: The chapter specific guidelines provide additional information about the use of Z codes for specified encounters.

a. Use of Z codes in any healthcare setting

Z codes are for use in any healthcare setting. Z codes may be used as either a first-listed (principal diagnosis code in the inpatient setting) or secondary code, depending on the circumstances of the encounter. Certain Z codes may only be used as first-listed or principal diagnosis.

b. Z Codes indicate a reason for an encounter

Z codes are not procedure codes. A corresponding procedure code must accompany a Z code to describe any procedure performed.

c. Categories of Z codes

1) Contact/exposure

Category Z20 indicates contact with, and suspected exposure to, communicable diseases. These codes are for patients who do not show any sign or symptom of a disease but are suspected to have been exposed to it by close personal contact with an infected individual or are in an area where a disease is epidemic.

Category Z77, indicates contact with and suspected exposures hazardous to health.

Contact/exposure codes may be used as a first-listed code to explain an encounter for testing, or, more commonly, as a secondary code to identify a potential risk.

2) Inoculations and vaccinations

Code Z23 is for encounters for inoculations and vaccinations. It indicates that a patient is being seen to receive a prophylactic inoculation against a disease. Procedure codes are required to identify the actual administration of the injection and the type(s) of immunizations given. Code Z23 may be used as a secondary code if the inoculation is given as a routine part of preventive health care, such as a well-baby visit.

3) Status

Status codes indicate that a patient is either a carrier of a disease or has the sequelae or residual of a past disease or condition. This includes such things as the presence of prosthetic or mechanical devices resulting from past treatment. A status code is informative, because the status may affect the course of treatment and its outcome. A status code is distinct from a history code. The history code indicates that the patient no longer has the condition.

A status code should not be used with a diagnosis code from one of the body system chapters, if the diagnosis code includes the information provided by the status code. For example, code Z94.1, Heart transplant status, should not be used with a code from subcategory T86.2, Complications of heart transplant. The status code does not provide additional information. The complication code indicates that the patient is a heart transplant patient.

For encounters for weaning from a mechanical ventilator, assign a code from subcategory J96.1, Chronic respiratory failure, followed by code Z99.11, Dependence on respirator [ventilator] status.

The status Z codes/categories are:

Z14   Genetic carrier

Genetic carrier status indicates that a person carries a gene, associated with a particular disease, which may be passed to offspring who may develop that disease. The person does not have the disease and is not at risk of developing the disease.

Z15   Genetic susceptibility to disease

Genetic susceptibility indicates that a person has a gene that increases the risk of that person developing the disease.

Codes from category Z15 should not be used as principal or first-listed codes. If the patient has the condition to which he/she is susceptible, and that condition is the reason for the encounter, the code for the current condition should be sequenced first. If the patient is being seen for follow-up after completed treatment for this condition, and the condition no longer exists, a follow-up code should be sequenced first, followed by the appropriate personal history and genetic susceptibility codes. If the purpose of the encounter is genetic counseling associated with procreative management, code Z31.5, Encounter for genetic counseling, should be assigned as the first-listed code, followed by a code from category Z15. Additional codes should be assigned for any applicable family or personal history.

Z16   Resistance to antimicrobial drugs

This code indicates that a patient has a condition that is resistant to antimicrobial drug treatment. Sequence the infection code first.

Z17   Estrogen receptor status

Z18   Retained foreign body fragments

Z21   Asymptomatic HIV infection status

This code indicates that a patient has tested positive for HIV but has manifested no signs or symptoms of the disease.

Z22   Carrier of infectious disease

Carrier status indicates that a person harbors the specific organisms of a disease without manifest symptoms and is capable of transmitting the infection.

Z28.3   Underimmunization status

Z33.1   Pregnant state, incidental

This code is a secondary code only for use when the pregnancy is in no way complicating the reason for visit. Otherwise, a code from the obstetric chapter is required.

Z66   Do not resuscitate

This code may be used when it is documented by the provider that a patient is on do not resuscitate status at any time during the stay.

Z67   Blood type

Z68   Body mass index (BMI)

Z74.01   Bed confinement status

Z76.82   Awaiting organ transplant status

Z78   Other specified health status

Code Z78.1, Physical restraint status, may be used when it is documented by the provider that a patient has been put in restraints during the current encounter. Please note that this code should not be reported when it is documented by the provider that a patient is temporarily restrained during a procedure.

Z79   Long-term (current) drug therapy

Codes from this category indicate a patient's continuous use of a prescribed drug (including such things as aspirin therapy) for the long-term treatment of a condition or for prophylactic use. It is not for use for patients who have addictions to drugs. This subcategory is not for use of medications for detoxification or maintenance programs to prevent withdrawal symptoms in patients with drug dependence (e.g., methadone maintenance for opiate dependence). Assign the appropriate code for the drug dependence instead.

Assign a code from Z79 if the patient is receiving a medication for an extended period as a prophylactic measure (such as for the prevention of deep vein thrombosis) or as treatment of a chronic condition (such as arthritis) or a disease requiring a lengthy course of treatment (such as cancer). Do not assign a code from category Z79 for medication being administered for a brief period of time to treat an acute illness or injury (such as a course of antibiotics to treat acute bronchitis).

Z88   Allergy status to drugs, medicaments and biological substances

Except: Z88.9, Allergy status to unspecified drugs, medicaments and biological substances status

Z89   Acquired absence of limb

Z90   Acquired absence of organs, not elsewhere classified

Z91.0-   Allergy status, other than to drugs and biological substances

Z92.82   Status post administration of tPA (rtPA) in a different facility within the last 24 hours prior to admission to a current facility

Assign code Z92.82, Status post administration of tPA (rtPA) in a different facility within the last 24 hours prior to admission to current facility, as a secondary diagnosis when a patient is received by transfer into a facility and documentation indicates they were administered tissue plasminogen activator (tPA) within the last 24 hours prior to admission to the current facility.

This guideline applies even if the patient is still receiving the tPA at the time they are received into the current facility.

The appropriate code for the condition for which the tPA was administered (such as cerebrovascular disease or myocardial infarction) should be assigned first.

Code Z92.82 is only applicable to the receiving facility record and not to the transferring facility record.

Z93   Artificial opening status

Z94   Transplanted organ and tissue status

Z95   Presence of cardiac and vascular implants and grafts

Z96   Presence of other functional implants

Z97   Presence of other devices

Z98   Other postprocedural states

Assign code Z98.85, Transplanted organ removal status, to indicate that a transplanted organ has been previously removed. This code should not be assigned for the encounter in which the transplanted organ is removed. The complication necessitating removal of the transplant organ should be assigned for that encounter.

See section I.C19.g.3. for information on the coding of organ transplant complications.

Z99   Dependence on enabling machines and devices, not elsewhere classified

Note: Categories Z89-Z90 and Z93-Z99 are for use only if there are no complications or malfunctions of the organ or tissue replaced, the amputation site or the equipment on which the patient is dependent.

4) **History (of)**

There are two types of history Z codes, personal and family. Personal history codes explain a patient's past medical condition that no longer exists and is not receiving any treatment, but that has the potential for recurrence, and therefore may require continued monitoring.

Family history codes are for use when a patient has a family member(s) who has had a particular disease that causes the patient to be at higher risk of also contracting the disease.

Personal history codes may be used in conjunction with follow-up codes and family history codes may be used in conjunction with screening codes to explain the need for a test or procedure. History codes are also acceptable on any medical record regardless of the reason for visit. A history of an illness, even if no longer present, is important information that may alter the type of treatment ordered.

The history Z code categories are:

Z80 Family history of primary malignant neoplasm

Z81 Family history of mental and behavioral disorders

Z82 Family history of certain disabilities and chronic diseases (leading to disablement)

Z83 Family history of other specific disorders

Z84 Family history of other conditions

Z85 Personal history of malignant neoplasm

Z86 Personal history of certain other diseases

Z87 Personal history of other diseases and conditions

Z91.4- Personal history of psychological trauma, not elsewhere classified

Z91.5 Personal history of self-harm

Z91.8- Other specified personal risk factors, not elsewhere classified

Exception: Z91.83, Wandering in diseases classified elsewhere

Z92 Personal history of medical treatment

Except: Z92.0, Personal history of contraception

Except: Z92.82, Status post administration of tPA (rtPA) in a different facility within the last 24 hours prior to admission to a current facility

5) Screening

Screening is the testing for disease or disease precursors in seemingly well individuals so that early detection and treatment can be provided for those who test positive for the disease (e.g., screening mammogram).

The testing of a person to rule out or confirm a suspected diagnosis because the patient has some sign or symptom is a diagnostic examination, not a screening. In these cases, the sign or symptom is used to explain the reason for the test.

A screening code may be a first-listed code if the reason for the visit is specifically the screening exam. It may also be used as an additional code if the screening is done during an office visit for other health problems. A screening code is not necessary if the screening is inherent to a routine examination, such as a pap smear done during a routine pelvic examination.

Should a condition be discovered during the screening then the code for the condition may be assigned as an additional diagnosis.

The Z code indicates that a screening exam is planned. A procedure code is required to confirm that the screening was performed.

The screening Z codes/categories:

Z11 Encounter for screening for infectious and parasitic diseases

Z12 Encounter for screening for malignant neoplasms

Z13 Encounter for screening for other diseases and disorders

Except: Z13.9, Encounter for screening, unspecified

Z36 Encounter for antenatal screening for mother

6) Observation

There are two observation Z code categories. They are for use in very limited circumstances when a person is being observed for a suspected condition that is ruled out. The observation codes are not for use if an injury or illness or any signs or symptoms related to the suspected condition are present. In such cases the diagnosis/symptom code is used with the corresponding external cause code.

The observation codes are to be used as principal diagnosis only. Additional codes may be used in addition to the observation code but only if they are unrelated to the suspected condition being observed.

Codes from subcategory Z03.7, Encounter for suspected maternal and fetal conditions ruled out, may either be used as a first-listed or as an additional code assignment depending on the case. They are for use in very limited circumstances on a maternal record when an encounter is for a suspected maternal or fetal condition that is ruled out during that encounter (for example, a maternal or fetal condition may be suspected due to an abnormal test result). These codes should not be used when the condition is confirmed. In those cases, the confirmed condition should be coded. In addition, these codes are not for use if an illness or any signs or symptoms related to the suspected condition or problem are present. In such cases the diagnosis/symptom code is used.

Additional codes may be used in addition to the code from subcategory Z03.7, but only if they are unrelated to the suspected condition being evaluated.

Codes from subcategory Z03.7 may not be used for encounters for antenatal screening of mother. See Section I.C.21.c.5, Screening.

For encounters for suspected fetal condition that are inconclusive following testing and evaluation, assign the appropriate code from category O35, O36, O40 or O41.

The observation Z code categories:

Z03 Encounter for medical observation for suspected diseases and conditions ruled out

Z04 Encounter for examination and observation for other reasons

Except: Z04.9, Encounter for examination and observation for unspecified reason

7) Aftercare

Aftercare visit codes cover situations when the initial treatment of a disease has been performed and the patient requires continued care during the healing or recovery phase, or for the long-term consequences of the disease. The aftercare Z code should not be used if treatment is directed at a current, acute disease. The diagnosis code is to be used in these cases. Exceptions to this rule are codes Z51.0, Encounter for antineoplastic radiation therapy, and codes from subcategory Z51.1, Encounter for antineoplastic chemotherapy and immunotherapy. These codes are to be first-listed, followed by the diagnosis code when a patient's encounter is solely to receive radiation therapy, chemotherapy, or immunotherapy for the treatment of a neoplasm. If the reason for the encounter is more than one type of antineoplastic therapy, code Z51.0 and a code from subcategory Z51.1 may be assigned together, in which case one of these codes would be reported as a secondary diagnosis.

The aftercare Z codes should also not be used for aftercare for injuries. For aftercare of an injury, assign the acute injury code with the appropriate 7th character (for subsequent encounter).

The aftercare codes are generally first-listed to explain the specific reason for the encounter. An aftercare code may be used as an additional code when some type of aftercare is provided in addition to the reason for admission and no diagnosis code is applicable. An example of this would be the closure of a colostomy during an encounter for treatment of another condition.

Aftercare codes should be used in conjunction with other aftercare codes or diagnosis codes to provide better detail on the specifics of an aftercare encounter visit, unless otherwise directed by the classification. Should a patient receive multiple types of antineoplastic therapy during the same encounter, code Z51.0, Encounter for antineoplastic radiation therapy, and codes from subcategory Z51.1, Encounter for antineoplastic chemotherapy and immunotherapy, may be used together on a record. The sequencing of multiple aftercare codes depends on the circumstances of the encounter.

Certain aftercare Z code categories need a secondary diagnosis code to describe the resolving condition or sequelae. For others, the condition is included in the code title.

Additional Z code aftercare category terms include fitting and adjustment, and attention to artificial openings.

Status Z codes may be used with aftercare Z codes to indicate the nature of the aftercare. For example code Z95.1, Presence of aortocoronary bypass graft, may be used with code Z48.812, Encounter for surgical aftercare following surgery on the circulatory system, to indicate the surgery for which the aftercare is being performed. A status code should not be used when the aftercare code indicates the type of status, such as using Z43.0, Encounter for attention to tracheostomy, with Z93.0, Tracheostomy status.

The aftercare Z category/codes:

Z42   Encounter for plastic and reconstructive surgery following medical procedure or healed injury

Z43   Encounter for attention to artificial openings

Z44   Encounter for fitting and adjustment of external prosthetic device

Z45   Encounter for adjustment and management of implanted device

Z46   Encounter for fitting and adjustment of other devices

Z47   Orthopedic aftercare

Z48   Encounter for other postprocedural aftercare

Z49   Encounter for care involving renal dialysis

Z51   Encounter for other aftercare

8) Follow-up

The follow-up codes are used to explain continuing surveillance following completed treatment of a disease, condition, or injury. They imply that the condition has been fully treated and no longer exists. They should not be confused with aftercare codes, or injury codes with a 7th character for subsequent encounter, that explain ongoing care of a healing condition or its sequelae. Follow-up codes may be used in conjunction with history codes to provide the full picture of the healed condition and its treatment. The follow-up code is sequenced first, followed by the history code.

A follow-up code may be used to explain multiple visits. Should a condition be found to have recurred on the follow-up visit, then the diagnosis code for the

condition should be assigned in place of the follow-up code.

The follow-up Z code categories:

Z08   Encounter for follow-up examination after completed treatment for malignant neoplasm

Z09   Encounter for follow-up examination after completed treatment for conditions other than malignant neoplasm

Z39   Encounter for maternal postpartum care and examination

9) Donor

Codes in category Z52, Donors of organs and tissues, are used for living individuals who are donating blood or other body tissue. These codes are only for individuals donating for others, not for self-donations. They are not used to identify cadaveric donations.

10) Counseling

Counseling Z codes are used when a patient or family member receives assistance in the aftermath of an illness or injury, or when support is required in coping with family or social problems. They are not used in conjunction with a diagnosis code when the counseling component of care is considered integral to standard treatment.

The counseling Z codes/categories:

Z30.0-   Encounter for general counseling and advice on contraception

Z31.5   Encounter for genetic counseling

Z31.6-   Encounter for general counseling and advice on procreation

Z32.2   Encounter for childbirth instruction

Z32.3   Encounter for childcare instruction

Z69   Encounter for mental health services for victim and perpetrator of abuse

Z70   Counseling related to sexual attitude, behavior and orientation

Z71   Persons encountering health services for other counseling and medical advice, not elsewhere classified

Z76.81 Expectant mother prebirth pediatrician visit

11) Encounters for obstetrical and reproductive services

See Section I.C.15. Pregnancy, Childbirth, and the Puerperium, for further instruction on the use of these codes.

Z codes for pregnancy are for use in those circumstances when none of the problems or complications included in the codes from the Obstetrics chapter exist (a routine prenatal visit or postpartum care). Codes in category Z34, Encounter for supervision of normal pregnancy, are always first-listed and are not to be used with any other code from the OB chapter. Codes in category Z3A, Weeks of gestation, may be assigned to provide additional information about the pregnancy.

The outcome of delivery, category Z37, should be included on all maternal delivery records. It is always a secondary code. Codes in category Z37 should not be used on the newborn record.

Z codes for family planning (contraceptive) or procreative management and counseling should be included on an obstetric record either during the pregnancy or the postpartum stage, if applicable.

Z codes/categories for obstetrical and reproductive services:

Z30   Encounter for contraceptive management

Z31   Encounter for procreative management

Z32.2 Encounter for childbirth instruction

Z32.3 Encounter for childcare instruction

Z33   Pregnant state

Z34   Encounter for supervision of normal pregnancy

Z36   Encounter for antenatal screening of mother

Z3A   Weeks of gestation

Z37   Outcome of delivery

Z39   Encounter for maternal postpartum care and examination

Z76.81 Expectant mother prebirth pediatrician visit

12) Newborns and Infants

See Section I.C.16. Newborn (Perinatal) Guidelines, for further instruction on the use of these codes.

Newborn Z codes/categories:

Z76.1 Encounter for health supervision and care of foundling

Z00.1- Encounter for routine child health examination

Z38   Liveborn infants according to place of birth and type of delivery

13) Routine and administrative examinations

The Z codes allow for the description of encounters for routine examinations, such as, a general check-up, or, examinations for administrative purposes, such as, a pre-employment physical. The codes are not to be used if the examination is for diagnosis of a suspected condition or for treatment purposes. In such cases the diagnosis code is used. During a routine exam, should a diagnosis or condition be discovered, it should be coded as an additional code. Pre-existing and chronic conditions and history codes may also be included as additional codes as long as the examination is for administrative purposes and not focused on any particular condition.

Some of the codes for routine health examinations distinguish between "with" and "without" abnormal findings. Code assignment depends on the information that is known at the time the encounter is being coded. For example, if no abnormal findings were found during the examination, but the encounter is being coded before test results are back, it is acceptable to assign the code for "without abnormal findings." When assigning a code for "with abnormal findings," additional code(s) should be assigned to identify the specific abnormal finding(s).

Pre-operative examination and pre-procedural laboratory examination Z codes are for use only in those situations when a patient is being cleared for a procedure or surgery and no treatment is given.

The Z codes/categories for routine and administrative examinations:

Z00   Encounter for general examination without complaint, suspected or reported diagnosis

Z01   Encounter for other special examination without complaint, suspected or reported diagnosis

Z02   Encounter for administrative examination

Except: Z02.9, Encounter for administrative examinations, unspecified

Z32.0- Encounter for pregnancy test

14) Miscellaneous Z codes

The miscellaneous Z codes capture a number of other health care encounters that do not fall into one of the other categories. Certain of these codes identify the reason for the encounter; others are for use as additional codes that provide useful information on circumstances that may affect a patient's care and treatment.

Prophylactic Organ Removal

For encounters specifically for prophylactic removal of an organ (such as prophylactic removal of breasts due to a genetic susceptibility to cancer or a family history of cancer), the principal or first-listed code should be a code from category Z40, Encounter for prophylactic surgery, followed by the appropriate codes to identify the associated risk factor (such as genetic susceptibility or family history).

If the patient has a malignancy of one site and is having prophylactic removal at another site to prevent either a new primary malignancy or metastatic disease, a code for the malignancy should also be assigned in addition to a code from subcategory Z40.0, Encounter for prophylactic surgery for risk factors related to malignant neoplasms. A Z40.0 code should not be assigned if the patient is having organ removal for treatment of a malignancy, such as the removal of the testes for the treatment of prostate cancer.

Miscellaneous Z codes/categories:

Z28   Immunization not carried out

Except: Z28.3, Underimmunization status

Z40   Encounter for prophylactic surgery

Z41   Encounter for procedures for purposes other than remedying health state

Except: Z41.9, Encounter for procedure for purposes other than remedying health state, unspecified

Z53   Persons encountering health services for specific procedures and treatment, not carried out

Z55   Problems related to education and literacy

Z56   Problems related to employment and unemployment

Z57   Occupational exposure to risk factors

Z58   Problems related to physical environment

Z59   Problems related to housing and economic circumstances

Z60   Problems related to social environment

Z62   Problems related to upbringing

Z63   Other problems related to primary support group, including family circumstances

Z64   Problems related to certain psychosocial circumstances

Z65   Problems related to other psychosocial circumstances

Z72   Problems related to lifestyle

Z73   Problems related to life management difficulty

Z74   Problems related to care provider dependency

Except: Z74.01, Bed confinement status

Z75   Problems related to medical facilities and other health care

Z76.0 Encounter for issue of repeat prescription

Z76.3 Healthy person accompanying sick person

Z76.4 Other boarder to healthcare facility

Z76.5 Malingerer [conscious simulation]

Z91.1- Patient's noncompliance with medical treatment and regimen

Z91.83 Wandering in diseases classified elsewhere

Z91.89 Other specified personal risk factors, not elsewhere classified

15) Nonspecific Z codes

Certain Z codes are so non-specific, or potentially redundant with other codes in the classification, that there can be little justification for their use in the inpatient setting. Their use in the outpatient setting should be limited to those instances when there is no further documentation to permit more precise coding. Otherwise, any sign or symptom or any other reason for visit that is captured in another code should be used.

Nonspecific Z codes/categories:

Z02.9   Encounter for administrative examinations, unspecified

Z04.9   Encounter for examination and observation for unspecified reason

Z13.9   Encounter for screening, unspecified

Z41.9   Encounter for procedure for purposes other than remedying health state, unspecified

Z52.9   Donor of unspecified organ or tissue

Z86.59 Personal history of other mental and behavioral disorders

Z88.9   Allergy status to unspecified drugs, medicaments and biological substances status

Z92.0   Personal history of contraception

16) Z codes that may only be principal/first-listed diagnosis

The following Z codes/categories may only be reported as the principal/first-listed diagnosis, except when there are multiple encounters on the same day and the medical records for the encounters are combined:

Z00   Encounter for general examination without complaint, suspected or reported diagnosis

Z01   Encounter for other special examination without complaint, suspected or reported diagnosis

Z02   Encounter for administrative examination

Z03   Encounter for medical observation for suspected diseases and conditions ruled out

Z04   Encounter for examination and observation for other reasons

Z31.81 Encounter for male factor infertility in female patient

Z31.82 Encounter for Rh incompatibility status

Z31.83 Encounter for assisted reproductive fertility procedure cycle

Z31.84 Encounter for fertility preservation procedure

Z33.2 Encounter for elective termination of pregnancy

Z34   Encounter for supervision of normal pregnancy

Z38   Liveborn infants according to place of birth and type of delivery

Z39   Encounter for maternal postpartum care and examination

Z42   Encounter for plastic and reconstructive surgery following medical procedure or healed injury

Z51.0 Encounter for antineoplastic radiation therapy

Z51.1- Encounter for antineoplastic chemotherapy and immunotherapy

Z52   Donors of organs and tissues

    Except: Z52.9, Donor of unspecified organ or tissue

Z76.1 Encounter for health supervision and care of foundling

Z76.2 Encounter for health supervision and care of other healthy infant and child

Z99.12 Encounter for respirator [ventilator] dependence during power failure

Section II. Selection of Principal Diagnosis

The circumstances of inpatient admission always govern the selection of principal diagnosis. The principal diagnosis is defined in the Uniform Hospital Discharge Data Set (UHDDS) as "that condition established after study to be chiefly responsible for occasioning the admission of the patient to the hospital for care."

The UHDDS definitions are used by hospitals to report inpatient data elements in a standardized manner. These data elements and their definitions can be found in the July 31, 1985, Federal Register (Vol. 50, No, 147), pp. 31038-40.

Since that time the application of the UHDDS definitions has been expanded to include all non-outpatient settings (acute care, short term, long term care and psychiatric hospitals; home health agencies; rehab facilities; nursing homes, etc).

In determining principal diagnosis the coding conventions in the ICD-10-CM, the Tabular List and Alphabetic Index take precedence over these official coding guidelines.

(See Section I.A., Conventions for the ICD-10-CM)

The importance of consistent, complete documentation in the medical record cannot be overemphasized. Without such documentation the application of all coding guidelines is a difficult, if not impossible, task.

A. Codes for symptoms, signs, and ill-defined conditions

Codes for symptoms, signs, and ill-defined conditions from Chapter 18 are not to be used as principal diagnosis when a related definitive diagnosis has been established.

B. Two or more interrelated conditions, each potentially meeting the definition for principal diagnosis

When there are two or more interrelated conditions (such as diseases in the same ICD-10-CM chapter or manifestations characteristically associated with a certain disease) potentially meeting the definition of principal diagnosis, either condition may be sequenced first, unless the circumstances of the admission, the therapy provided, the Tabular List, or the Alphabetic Index indicate otherwise.

C. Two or more diagnoses that equally meet the definition for principal diagnosis

In the unusual instance when two or more diagnoses equally meet the criteria for principal diagnosis as determined by the circumstances of admission, diagnostic workup and/or therapy provided, and the Alphabetic Index, Tabular List, or another coding guidelines does not provide sequencing direction, any one of the diagnoses may be sequenced first.

D. Two or more comparative or contrasting conditions

In those rare instances when two or more contrasting or comparative diagnoses are documented as "either/or" (or similar terminology), they are coded as if the diagnoses were confirmed and the diagnoses are sequenced according to the circumstances of the admission. If no further determination can be made as to which diagnosis should be principal, either diagnosis may be sequenced first.

E. A symptom(s) followed by contrasting/comparative diagnoses

When a symptom(s) is followed by contrasting/comparative diagnoses, the symptom code is sequenced first. All the contrasting/comparative diagnoses should be coded as additional diagnoses.

F. Original treatment plan not carried out

Sequence as the principal diagnosis the condition, which after study occasioned the admission to the hospital, even though treatment may not have been carried out due to unforeseen circumstances.

G. Complications of surgery and other medical care

When the admission is for treatment of a complication resulting from surgery or other medical care, the complication code is sequenced as the principal diagnosis. If the complication is classified to the T80-T88 series and the code lacks the necessary specificity in describing the complication, an additional code for the specific complication should be assigned.

H. Uncertain diagnosis

If the diagnosis documented at the time of discharge is qualified as "probable", "suspected", "likely", "questionable", "possible", or "still to be ruled out", or other similar terms indicating uncertainty, code the condition as if it existed or was established. The bases for these guidelines are the diagnostic workup, arrangements for further workup or observation, and initial therapeutic approach that correspond most closely with the established diagnosis.

Note: This guideline is applicable only to inpatient admissions to short-term, acute, long-term care and psychiatric hospitals.

I. Admission from observation unit

1. **Admission Following Medical Observation**
   When a patient is admitted to an observation unit for a medical condition, which either worsens or does not improve, and is subsequently admitted as an inpatient of the same hospital for this same medical condition, the principal diagnosis would be the medical condition which led to the hospital admission.

2. **Admission Following Post-Operative Observation**
   When a patient is admitted to an observation unit to monitor a condition (or complication) that develops following outpatient surgery, and then is subsequently admitted as an inpatient of the same hospital, hospitals should apply the Uniform Hospital Discharge Data Set (UHDDS) definition of principal diagnosis as "that condition established after study to be chiefly responsible for occasioning the admission of the patient to the hospital for care."

J. Admission from outpatient surgery

When a patient receives surgery in the hospital's outpatient surgery department and is subsequently admitted for continuing inpatient care at the same hospital, the following guidelines should be followed in selecting the principal diagnosis for the inpatient admission:

- If the reason for the inpatient admission is a complication, assign the complication as the principal diagnosis.
- If no complication, or other condition, is documented as the reason for the inpatient admission, assign the reason for the outpatient surgery as the principal diagnosis.
- If the reason for the inpatient admission is another condition unrelated to the surgery, assign the unrelated condition as the principal diagnosis.

Section III. Reporting Additional Diagnoses

GENERAL RULES FOR OTHER (ADDITIONAL) DIAGNOSES

For reporting purposes the definition for "other diagnoses" is interpreted as additional conditions that affect patient care in terms of requiring:

> clinical evaluation; or
>
> therapeutic treatment; or
>
> diagnostic procedures; or
>
> extended length of hospital stay; or
>
> increased nursing care and/or monitoring.

The UHDDS item #11-b defines Other Diagnoses as "all conditions that coexist at the time of admission, that develop subsequently, or that affect the treatment received and/or the length of stay. Diagnoses that relate to an earlier episode which have no bearing on the current hospital stay are to be excluded." UHDDS definitions apply to inpatients in acute care, short-term, long term care and psychiatric hospital setting. The UHDDS definitions are used by acute care short-term hospitals to report inpatient data elements in a standardized manner. These data elements and their definitions can be found in the July 31, 1985, Federal Register (Vol. 50, No, 147), pp. 31038-40.

Since that time the application of the UHDDS definitions has been expanded to include all non-outpatient settings (acute care, short term, long term care and psychiatric hospitals; home health agencies; rehab facilities; nursing homes, etc).

The following guidelines are to be applied in designating "other diagnoses" when neither the Alphabetic Index nor the Tabular List in ICD-10-CM provide direction. The listing of the diagnoses in the patient record is the responsibility of the attending provider.

A. Previous conditions

If the provider has included a diagnosis in the final diagnostic statement, such as the discharge summary or the face sheet, it should ordinarily be coded. Some providers include in the diagnostic statement resolved conditions or diagnoses and status-post procedures from previous admission that have no bearing on the current stay. Such conditions are not to be reported and are coded only if required by hospital policy.

However, history codes (categories Z80-Z87) may be used as secondary codes if the historical condition or family history has an impact on current care or influences treatment.

B. Abnormal findings

Abnormal findings (laboratory, x-ray, pathologic, and other diagnostic results) are not coded and reported unless the provider indicates their clinical significance. If the findings are outside the normal range and the attending provider has ordered other tests to evaluate the condition or prescribed treatment, it is appropriate to ask the provider whether the abnormal finding should be added.

Please note: This differs from the coding practices in the outpatient setting for coding encounters for diagnostic tests that have been interpreted by a provider.

C. Uncertain Diagnosis

If the diagnosis documented at the time of discharge is qualified as "probable", "suspected", "likely", "questionable", "possible", or "still to be ruled out" or other similar terms indicating uncertainty, code the condition as if it existed or was established. The bases for these guidelines are the diagnostic workup, arrangements for further workup or observation, and initial therapeutic approach that correspond most closely with the established diagnosis.

Note: This guideline is applicable only to inpatient admissions to short-term, acute, long-term care and psychiatric hospitals.

Section IV. Diagnostic Coding and Reporting Guidelines for Outpatient Services

These coding guidelines for outpatient diagnoses have been approved for use by hospitals/ providers in coding and reporting hospital-based outpatient services and provider-based office visits.

Information about the use of certain abbreviations, punctuation, symbols, and other conventions used in the ICD-10-CM Tabular List (code numbers and titles), can be found in Section IA of these guidelines, under "Conventions Used in the Tabular List." Information about the correct sequence to use in finding a code is also described in Section I.

The terms encounter and visit are often used interchangeably in describing outpatient service contacts and, therefore, appear together in these guidelines without distinguishing one from the other.

Though the conventions and general guidelines apply to all settings, coding guidelines for outpatient and provider reporting of diagnoses will vary in a number of instances from those for inpatient diagnoses, recognizing that:

> The Uniform Hospital Discharge Data Set (UHDDS) definition of principal diagnosis applies only to inpatients in acute, short-term, long-term care and psychiatric hospitals.

> Coding guidelines for inconclusive diagnoses (probable, suspected, rule out, etc.) were developed for inpatient reporting and do not apply to outpatients.

A. **Selection of first-listed condition**

In the outpatient setting, the term first-listed diagnosis is used in lieu of principal diagnosis.

In determining the first-listed diagnosis the coding conventions of ICD-10-CM, as well as the general and disease specific guidelines take precedence over the outpatient guidelines.

Diagnoses often are not established at the time of the initial encounter/visit. It may take two or more visits before the diagnosis is confirmed.

The most critical rule involves beginning the search for the correct code assignment through the Alphabetic Index. Never begin searching initially in the Tabular List as this will lead to coding errors.

1. **Outpatient surgery**

When a patient presents for outpatient surgery (same day surgery), code the reason for the surgery as the first-listed diagnosis (reason for the encounter), even if the surgery is not performed due to a contraindication.

2. **Observation stay**

When a patient is admitted for observation for a medical condition, assign a code for the medical condition as the first-listed diagnosis.

When a patient presents for outpatient surgery and develops complications requiring admission to observation, code the reason for the surgery as the first reported diagnosis (reason for the encounter), followed by codes for the complications as secondary diagnoses.

B. **Codes from A00.0 through T88.9, Z00-Z99**

The appropriate code(s) from A00.0 through T88.9, Z00-Z99 must be used to identify diagnoses, symptoms, conditions, problems, complaints, or other reason(s) for the encounter/visit.

C. **Accurate reporting of ICD-10-CM diagnosis codes**

For accurate reporting of ICD-10-CM diagnosis codes, the documentation should describe the patient's condition, using terminology which includes specific diagnoses as well as symptoms, problems, or reasons for the encounter. There are ICD-10-CM codes to describe all of these.

D. **Codes that describe symptoms and signs**

Codes that describe symptoms and signs, as opposed to diagnoses, are acceptable for reporting purposes when a diagnosis has not been established (confirmed) by the provider. Chapter 18 of ICD-10-CM, Symptoms, Signs, and Abnormal Clinical and Laboratory Findings Not Elsewhere Classified (codes R00-R99) contain many, but not all codes for symptoms.

E. **Encounters for circumstances other than a disease or injury**

ICD-10-CM provides codes to deal with encounters for circumstances other than a disease or injury. The Factors Influencing Health Status and Contact with Health Services codes (Z00-Z99) are provided to deal with occasions when circumstances other than a disease or injury are recorded as diagnosis or problems.

See Section I.C.21. Factors influencing health status and contact with health services.

F. **Level of Detail in Coding**

1. **ICD-10-CM codes with *3, 4, 5, 6 or 7 characters***

ICD-10-CM is composed of codes with 3, 4, 5, 6 or 7 characters. Codes with three characters are included in ICD-10-CM as the heading of a category of codes that may be further subdivided by the use of fourth, fifth, sixth or seventh characters to provide greater specificity.

2. **Use of full number of *characters* required for a code**

A three-character code is to be used only if it is not further subdivided. A code is invalid if it has not been coded to the full number of characters required for that code, including the 7th character extension, if applicable.

G. **ICD-10-CM code for the diagnosis, condition, problem, or other reason for encounter/visit**

List first the ICD-10-CM code for the diagnosis, condition, problem, or other reason for encounter/visit shown in the medical record to be chiefly responsible for the services provided. List additional codes that describe any coexisting conditions. In some cases the first-listed diagnosis may be a symptom when a diagnosis has not been established (confirmed) by the physician.

H. **Uncertain diagnosis**

Do not code diagnoses documented as "probable", "suspected," "questionable," "rule out," or "working diagnosis" or other similar terms indicating uncertainty. Rather, code the condition(s) to the highest degree of certainty for that encounter/visit, such as symptoms, signs, abnormal test results, or other reason for the visit.

Please note: This differs from the coding practices used by short-term, acute care, long-term care and psychiatric hospitals.

I. **Chronic diseases**

Chronic diseases treated on an ongoing basis may be coded and reported as many times as the patient receives treatment and care for the condition(s)

J. **Code all documented conditions that coexist**

Code all documented conditions that coexist at the time of the encounter/visit, and require or affect patient care treatment or management. Do not code conditions that were previously treated and no longer exist. However, history codes (categories Z80-Z87) may be used as secondary codes if the historical condition or family history has an impact on current care or influences treatment.

K. **Patients receiving diagnostic services only**

For patients receiving diagnostic services only during an encounter/visit, sequence first the diagnosis, condition, problem, or other reason for encounter/visit shown in the medical record to be chiefly responsible for the outpatient services provided during the encounter/visit. Codes for other diagnoses (e.g., chronic conditions) may be sequenced as additional diagnoses.

For encounters for routine laboratory/radiology testing in the absence of any signs, symptoms, or associated diagnosis, assign Z01.89, Encounter for other specified special examinations. If routine testing is performed during the same encounter as a test to evaluate a sign, symptom, or diagnosis, it is appropriate to assign both the Z code and the code describing the reason for the non-routine test.

For outpatient encounters for diagnostic tests that have been interpreted by a physician, and the final report is available at the time of coding, code any confirmed or definitive diagnosis(es) documented in the interpretation. Do not code related signs and symptoms as additional diagnoses.

Please note: This differs from the coding practice in the hospital inpatient setting regarding abnormal findings on test results.

L.   Patients receiving therapeutic services only

For patients receiving therapeutic services only during an encounter/visit, sequence first the diagnosis, condition, problem, or other reason for encounter/visit shown in the medical record to be chiefly responsible for the outpatient services provided during the encounter/visit. Codes for other diagnoses (e.g., chronic conditions) may be sequenced as additional diagnoses.

The only exception to this rule is that when the primary reason for the admission/encounter is chemotherapy or radiation therapy, the appropriate Z code for the service is listed first, and the diagnosis or problem for which the service is being performed listed second.

M.   Patients receiving preoperative evaluations only

For patients receiving preoperative evaluations only, sequence first a code from subcategory Z01.81, Encounter for pre-procedural examinations, to describe the pre-op consultations. Assign a code for the condition to describe the reason for the surgery as an additional diagnosis. Code also any findings related to the pre-op evaluation.

N.   Ambulatory surgery

For ambulatory surgery, code the diagnosis for which the surgery was performed. If the postoperative diagnosis is known to be different from the preoperative diagnosis at the time the diagnosis is confirmed, select the postoperative diagnosis for coding, since it is the most definitive.

O.   Routine outpatient prenatal visits

See Section I.C.15. Routine outpatient prenatal visits.

P.   Encounters for general medical examinations with abnormal findings

The subcategories for encounters for general medical examinations, Z00.0-, provide codes for with and without abnormal findings. Should a general medical examination result in an abnormal finding, the code for general medical examination with abnormal finding should be assigned as the first-listed diagnosis. A secondary code for the abnormal finding should also be coded.

Q.   Encounters for routine health screenings

See Section I.C.21. Factors influencing health status and contact with health services, Screening

Appendix I. Present on Admission Reporting Guidelines

Introduction

These guidelines are to be used as a supplement to the *ICD-10-CM Official Guidelines for Coding and Reporting* to facilitate the assignment of the Present on Admission (POA) indicator for each diagnosis and

external cause of injury code reported on claim forms (UB-04 and 837 Institutional).

These guidelines are not intended to replace any guidelines in the main body of the *ICD-10-CM Official Guidelines for Coding and Reporting*. The POA guidelines are not intended to provide guidance on when a condition should be coded, but rather, how to apply the POA indicator to the final set of diagnosis codes that have been assigned in accordance with Sections I, II, and III of the official coding guidelines. Subsequent to the assignment of the ICD-10-CM codes, the POA indicator should then be assigned to those conditions that have been coded.

As stated in the Introduction to the *ICD-10-CM Official Guidelines for Coding and Reporting*, a joint effort between the healthcare provider and the coder is essential to achieve complete and accurate documentation, code assignment, and reporting of diagnoses and procedures. The importance of consistent, complete documentation in the medical record cannot be overemphasized. Medical record documentation from any provider involved in the care and treatment of the patient may be used to support the determination of whether a condition was present on admission or not. In the context of the official coding guidelines, the term "provider" means a physician or any qualified healthcare practitioner who is legally accountable for establishing the patient's diagnosis.

These guidelines are not a substitute for the provider's clinical judgment as to the determination of whether a condition was/was not present on admission. The provider should be queried regarding issues related to the linking of signs/symptoms, timing of test results, and the timing of findings.

General Reporting Requirements

All claims involving inpatient admissions to general acute care hospitals or other facilities that are subject to a law or regulation mandating collection of present on admission information.

Present on admission is defined as present at the time the order for inpatient admission occurs -- conditions that develop during an outpatient encounter, including emergency department, observation, or outpatient surgery, are considered as present on admission.

POA indicator is assigned to principal and secondary diagnoses (as defined in Section II of the Official Guidelines for Coding and Reporting) and the external cause of injury codes.

Issues related to inconsistent, missing, conflicting or unclear documentation must still be resolved by the provider.

If a condition would not be coded and reported based on UHDDS definitions and current official coding guidelines, then the POA indicator would not be reported.

Reporting Options

    Y – Yes

    N – No

    U – Unknown

    W – Clinically undetermined

    Unreported/Not used (or "1" for Medicare usage) – (Exempt from POA reporting)

Reporting Definitions

    Y – present at the time of inpatient admission

    N – not present at the time of inpatient admission

    U – documentation is insufficient to determine if condition is present on admission

    W – provider is unable to clinically determine whether condition was present on admission or not

Timeframe for POA Identification and Documentation

There is no required timeframe as to when a provider (per the definition of "provider" used in these guidelines) must identify or

---

document a condition to be present on admission. In some clinical situations, it may not be possible for a provider to make a definitive diagnosis (or a condition may not be recognized or reported by the patient) for a period of time after admission. In some cases it may be several days before the provider arrives at a definitive diagnosis. This does not mean that the condition was not present on admission. Determination of whether the condition was present on admission or not will be based on the applicable POA guideline as identified in this document, or on the provider's best clinical judgment.

If at the time of code assignment the documentation is unclear as to whether a condition was present on admission or not, it is appropriate to query the provider for clarification.

Assigning the POA Indicator

Condition is on the "Exempt from Reporting" list
Leave the "present on admission" field blank if the condition is on the list of ICD-10-CM codes for which this field is not applicable. This is the only circumstance in which the field may be left blank.

POA Explicitly Documented
Assign "Y" for any condition the provider explicitly documents as being present on admission.

Assign "N" for any condition the provider explicitly documents as not present at the time of admission.

Conditions diagnosed prior to inpatient admission
Assign "Y" for conditions that were diagnosed prior to admission (example: hypertension, diabetes mellitus, asthma).

Conditions diagnosed during the admission but clearly present before admission
Assign "Y" for conditions diagnosed during the admission that were clearly present but not diagnosed until after admission occurred.

Diagnoses subsequently confirmed after admission are considered present on admission if at the time of admission they are documented as suspected, possible, rule out, differential diagnosis, or constitute an underlying cause of a symptom that is present at the time of admission.

Condition develops during outpatient encounter prior to inpatient admission
Assign "Y" for any condition that develops during an outpatient encounter prior to a written order for inpatient admission.

Documentation does not indicate whether condition was present on admission
Assign "U" when the medical record documentation is unclear as to whether the condition was present on admission. "U" should not be routinely assigned and used only in very limited circumstances. Coders are encouraged to query the providers when the documentation is unclear.

Documentation states that it cannot be determined whether the condition was or was not present on admission
Assign "W" when the medical record documentation indicates that it cannot be clinically determined whether or not the condition was present on admission.

Chronic condition with acute exacerbation during the admission
If a single code identifies both the chronic condition and the acute exacerbation, see POA guidelines pertaining to combination codes.

If a single code only identifies the chronic condition and not the acute exacerbation (e.g., acute exacerbation of chronic leukemia), assign "Y."

Conditions documented as possible, probable, suspected, or rule out at the time of discharge
If the final diagnosis contains a possible, probable, suspected, or rule out diagnosis, and this diagnosis was based on signs, symptoms or clinical findings suspected at the time of inpatient admission, assign "Y."

If the final diagnosis contains a possible, probable, suspected, or rule out diagnosis, and this diagnosis was based on signs, symptoms or clinical findings that were not present on admission, assign "N".

Conditions documented as impending or threatened at the time of discharge
If the final diagnosis contains an impending or threatened diagnosis, and this diagnosis is based on symptoms or clinical findings that were present on admission, assign "Y".

If the final diagnosis contains an impending or threatened diagnosis, and this diagnosis is based on symptoms or clinical findings that were not present on admission, assign "N".

Acute and Chronic Conditions
Assign "Y" for acute conditions that are present at time of admission and N for acute conditions that are not present at time of admission.

Assign "Y" for chronic conditions, even though the condition may not be diagnosed until after admission.

If a single code identifies both an acute and chronic condition, see the POA guidelines for combination codes.

Combination Codes
Assign "N" if any part of the combination code was not present on admission (e.g., COPD with acute exacerbation and the exacerbation was not present on admission; gastric ulcer that does not start bleeding until after admission; asthma patient develops status asthmaticus after admission).

Assign "Y" if all parts of the combination code were present on admission (e.g., patient with acute prostatitis admitted with hematuria).

If the final diagnosis includes comparative or contrasting diagnoses, and both were present, or suspected, at the time of admission, assign "Y".

For infection codes that include the causal organism, assign "Y" if the infection (or signs of the infection) was present on admission, even though the culture results may not be known until after admission (e.g., patient is admitted with pneumonia and the provider documents pseudomonas as the causal organism a few days later).

Same Diagnosis Code for Two or More Conditions
When the same ICD-10-CM diagnosis code applies to two or more conditions during the same encounter (e.g. two separate conditions classified to the same ICD-10-CM diagnosis code):

Assign "Y" if all conditions represented by the single ICD-10-CM code were present on admission (e.g. bilateral unspecified age-related cataracts).

Assign "N" if any of the conditions represented by the single ICD-10-CM code was not present on admission (e.g. traumatic secondary and recurrent hemorrhage and seroma is assigned to a single code T79.2, but only one of the conditions was present on admission).

Obstetrical conditions

Whether or not the patient delivers during the current hospitalization does not affect assignment of the POA indicator. The determining factor for POA assignment is whether the pregnancy complication or obstetrical condition described by the code was present at the time of admission or not.

If the pregnancy complication or obstetrical condition was present on admission (e.g., patient admitted in preterm labor), assign "Y".

If the pregnancy complication or obstetrical condition was not present on admission (e.g., 2nd degree laceration during delivery, postpartum hemorrhage that occurred during current hospitalization, fetal distress develops after admission), assign "N".

If the obstetrical code includes more than one diagnosis and any of the diagnoses identified by the code were not present on admission assign "N". (e.g., Category O11, Pre-existing hypertension with pre-eclampsia).

Perinatal conditions

Newborns are not considered to be admitted until after birth. Therefore, any condition present at birth or that developed in utero is considered present at admission and should be assigned "Y". This includes conditions that occur during delivery (e.g., injury during delivery, meconium aspiration, exposure to streptococcus B in the vaginal canal).

Congenital conditions and anomalies

Assign "Y" for congenital conditions and anomalies except for categories Q00-Q99, Congenital anomalies, which are on the exempt list. Congenital conditions are always considered present on admission.

External cause of injury codes

Assign "Y" for any external cause code representing an external cause of morbidity that occurred prior to inpatient admission (e.g., patient fell out of bed at home, patient fell out of bed in emergency room prior to admission).

Assign "N" for any external cause code representing an external cause of morbidity that occurred during inpatient hospitalization (e.g., patient fell out of hospital bed during hospital stay, patient experienced an adverse reaction to a medication administered after inpatient admission).

Categories and Codes Exempt from Diagnosis Present on Admission Requirement

Note: "Diagnosis present on admission" for these code categories are exempt because they represent circumstances regarding the healthcare encounter or factors influencing health status that do not represent a current disease or injury or are always present on admission.

B90–B94	Sequelae of infectious and parasitic diseases
E64	Sequelae of malnutrition and other nutritional deficiencies
I25.2	Old myocardial infarction
I69	Sequelae of cerebrovascular disease
O09	Supervision of high risk pregnancy
O66.5	Attempted application of vacuum extractor and forceps
O80	Encounter for full-term uncomplicated delivery
O94	Sequelae of complication of pregnancy, childbirth, and the puerperium
P00	Newborn (suspected to be) affected by maternal conditions that may be unrelated to present pregnancy
Q00 – Q99	Congenital malformations, deformations and chromosomal abnormalities

S00-T88.9	Injury, poisoning and certain other consequences of external causes with 7th character representing subsequent encounter or sequela
V00- V09	**Pedestrian injured in transport accident**
	Except: V00.81-, Accident with wheelchair (powered) V00.83-, Accident with motorized mobility scooter
V10-V19	**Pedal cycle rider injured in transport accident**
V20-V29	**Motorcycle rider injured in transport accident**
V30-V39	**Occupant of three-wheeled motor vehicle injured in transport accident**
V40-V49	Car occupant injured in transport accident
V50-V59	**Occupant of pick-up truck or van injured in transport accident**
V60-V69	**Occupant of heavy transport vehicle injured in transport accident**
V70-V79	**Bus occupant injured in transport accident**
V80-V89	Other land transport accidents
V90-V94	Water transport accidents
V95-V97	Air and space transport accidents
V98-V99	**Other and unspecified transport accidents**
W03	Other fall on same level due to collision with another person
W09	Fall on and from playground equipment
W14	**Fall from tree**
W15	Fall from cliff
W17.0	Fall into well
W17.1	Fall into storm drain or manhole
W18.01	Striking against sports equipment with subsequent fall
W20.8	Other cause of strike by thrown, projected or falling object
W21	Striking against or struck by sports equipment
W30	Contact with agricultural machinery
W31	Contact with other and unspecified machinery
W32-W34	Accidental handgun discharge and malfunction
W35- W40	Exposure to inanimate mechanical forces
W52	Crushed, pushed or stepped on by crowd or human stampede
W56	**Contact with nonvenomous marine animal**
W58	**Contact with crocodile or alligator**
W61	**Contact with birds (domestic) (wild)**
W62	**Contact with nonvenomous amphibians**
W89	Exposure to man-made visible and ultraviolet light
X02	Exposure to controlled fire in building or structure
X03	Exposure to controlled fire, not in building or structure
X04	Exposure to ignition of highly flammable material
X52	Prolonged stay in weightless environment
X71	**Intentional self-harm by drowning and submersion**
	Except: X71.0-, Intentional self-harm by drowning and submersion while in bath tub
X72	**Intentional self-harm by handgun discharge**
X73	**Intentional self-harm by rifle, shotgun and larger firearm discharge**
X74	**Intentional self-harm by other and unspecified firearm and gun discharge**
X75	**Intentional self-harm by explosive material**
X76	**Intentional self-harm by smoke, fire and flames**
X77	**Intentional self-harm by steam, hot vapors and hot objects**
X81	**Intentional self-harm by jumping or lying in front of moving object**
X82	**Intentional self-harm by crashing of motor vehicle**
X83	**Intentional self-harm by other specified means**

X71-X83	Intentional self-harm	Z44	Encounter for fitting and adjustment of external prosthetic device
Y21	Drowning and submersion, undetermined intent	Z45	Encounter for adjustment and management of implanted device
Y22	Handgun discharge, undetermined intent	Z46	Encounter for fitting and adjustment of other devices
Y23	Rifle, shotgun and larger firearm discharge, undetermined intent	Z47.8	Encounter for other orthopedic aftercare
Y24	Other and unspecified firearm discharge, undetermined intent	Z49	Encounter for care involving renal dialysis
Y30	Falling, jumping or pushed from a high place, undetermined intent	Z51	Encounter for other aftercare
		Z51.5	Encounter for palliative care
Y35	Legal intervention	Z51.8	Encounter for other specified aftercare
Y36	Operations of war	Z52	Donors of organs and tissues
Y37	Military operations	Z59	Problems related to housing and economic circumstances
Y38	Terrorism	Z63	Other problems related to primary support group including family circumstances
Y92	Place of occurrence of the external cause	Z65	Problems related to other psychosocial circumstances
Y93	Activity code	Z65.8	Other specified problems related to psychosocial circumstances
Y99	External cause status	Z67.1-Z67.9	Blood type
Z00	Encounter for general examination without complaint, suspected or reported diagnosis	Z68	Body mass index (BMI)
Z01	Encounter for other special examination without complaint, suspected or reported diagnosis	Z72	Problems related to lifestyle
		Z74.01	Bed confinement status
Z02	Encounter for administrative examination	Z76	Persons encountering health services in other circumstances
Z03	Encounter for medical observation for suspected diseases and conditions ruled out	Z77.110-	Environmental pollution and hazards in the physical environment
Z08	Encounter for follow-up examination following completed treatment for malignant neoplasm	Z77.128	
		Z78	Other specified health status
Z09	Encounter for follow-up examination after completed treatment for conditions other than malignant neoplasm	Z79	Long term (current) drug therapy
		Z80	Family history of primary malignant neoplasm
Z11	Encounter for screening for infectious and parasitic diseases	Z81	Family history of mental and behavioral disorders
Z11.8	Encounter for screening for other infectious and parasitic diseases	Z82	Family history of certain disabilities and chronic diseases (leading to disablement)
Z12	Encounter for screening for malignant neoplasms	Z83	Family history of other specific disorders
Z13	Encounter for screening for other diseases and disorders	Z84	Family history of other conditions
Z13.4	Encounter for screening for certain developmental disorders in childhood	Z85	Personal history of primary malignant neoplasm
		Z86	Personal history of certain other diseases
Z13.5	Encounter for screening for eye and ear disorders	Z87	Personal history of other diseases and conditions
Z13.6	Encounter for screening for cardiovascular disorders	Z87.828	Personal history of other (healed) physical injury and trauma
Z13.83	Encounter for screening for respiratory disorder NEC	Z87.891	Personal history of nicotine dependence
Z13.89	Encounter for screening for other disorder	Z88	Allergy status to drugs, medicaments and biological substances
Z14	Genetic carrier	Z89	Acquired absence of limb
Z15	Genetic susceptibility to disease	Z90.710	Acquired absence of both cervix and uterus
Z17	Estrogen receptor status	Z91.0	Allergy status, other than to drugs and biological substances
Z18	Retained foreign body fragments	Z91.4	Personal history of psychological trauma, not elsewhere classified
Z22	Carrier of infectious disease	Z91.5	Personal history of self-harm
Z23	Encounter for immunization	Z91.8	Other specified risk factors, not elsewhere classified
Z28	Immunization not carried out and underimmunization status	Z92	Personal history of medical treatment
Z28.3	Underimmunization status	Z93	Artificial opening status
Z30	Encounter for contraceptive management	Z94	Transplanted organ and tissue status
Z31	Encounter for procreative management	Z95	Presence of cardiac and vascular implants and grafts
Z34	Encounter for supervision of normal pregnancy	Z97	Presence of other devices
Z36	Encounter for antenatal screening of mother	Z98	Other postprocedural states
Z37	Outcome of delivery	Z99	Dependence on enabling machines and devices, not elsewhere classified
Z38	Liveborn infants according to place of birth and type of delivery		
Z39	Encounter for maternal postpartum care and examination		
Z41	Encounter for procedures for purposes other than remedying health state		
Z42	Encounter for plastic and reconstructive surgery following medical procedure or healed injury		
Z43	Encounter for attention to artificial openings		

Glossary

abortion. Premature expulsion or extraction of the products of conception.

abrasion. Removal of layers of the skin occurring as a superficial injury, or a procedure for removal of problematic skin or skin lesions.

abscess. Circumscribed collection of pus resulting from bacteria, frequently associated with swelling and other signs of inflammation.

abuse. In medical reimbursement, an incident that is inconsistent with accepted medical, business, or fiscal practices and directly or indirectly results in unnecessary costs to the Medicare program, improper reimbursement, or reimbursement for services that do not meet professionally recognized standards of care or which are medically unnecessary.

achalasia. Failure of the smooth muscles within the gastrointestinal tract to relax at points of junction; most commonly referring to the esophagogastric sphincter's failure to relax when swallowing.

acne. Inflammatory skin disease affecting the sebaceous glands and hair follicles resulting in comedones, papular, and pustular skin eruptions.

acquired. Produced by outside influences and not by genetics or birth defect.

acquired immune deficiency syndrome. Contagious retroviral disease resulting from infection with human immunodeficiency virus (HIV) that can, in severe cases, suppress vital immunity. Several opportunistic infections, such as Kaposi's sarcoma and pneumocystitis pneumonia, are associated with this syndrome. Synonyms: AIDS, ARC, symptomatic HIV.

acronym. Word formed from the initial letters of a name or by combining initial letters or parts of a series of words.

acute. Sudden, severe.

acute alcohol intoxication. Psychic and physical state resulting from alcohol ingestion characterized by slurred speech, unsteady gait, poor coordination, flushed face, nystagmus, sluggish reflexes, strong smell of alcohol, loud speech, emotional instability (e.g., jollity followed by gloominess), excessive socializing, talkativeness, and poorly inhibited sexual and aggressive behavior.

acute alcoholism. Psychic and physical state resulting from alcohol ingestion characterized by slurred speech, unsteady gait, poor coordination, flushed face, nystagmus, sluggish reflexes, strong smell of alcohol, loud speech, emotional instability (e.g., jollity followed by gloominess), excessive socializing, talkativeness, and poorly inhibited sexual and aggressive behavior.

acute care facility. Health care institution primarily engaged in providing treatment to inpatients and diagnostic and therapeutic services for medical diagnosis, treatment, and care of injured, disabled, or sick persons who are in an acute phase of illness.

acute fractures. Complicated limb fracture with severe bony comminution, extensive soft tissue damage, or multiple trauma. External fixation may be required.

adenocarcinoma. Malignant tumor of a gland.

adjuvant therapy. Therapy intended to enhance the primary therapy.

administrative code sets. Code sets that characterize a general business situation, rather than a medical condition or service. Under HIPAA, these are sometimes referred to as nonclinical or nonmedical code sets.

administrative simplification. Title II, subtitle of HIPAA, that gives HHS the authority to mandate the use of standards for the electronic exchange of health care data; to specify what medical and administrative code sets should be used within those standards; to require the use of national identification systems for health care patients, providers, payers (or plans), and employers (or sponsors); and to specify the types of measures required to protect the security and privacy of personally identifiable health care information. This is also the name of Title II, subtitle F, part C of HIPAA.

admission. Formal acceptance of a patient by a health care facility.

alcohol dependence syndrome. Chronic, progressive state of dependence upon alcohol that is both psychological and physical with periodic or continuous episodes impairing health and the ability to function emotionally, socially, and occupationally.

analgesia. Absence of a normal sense of pain without loss of consciousness.

angina. Chest pain that occurs secondary to the inadequate delivery of oxygen to the heart muscle and may be described as a heavy or squeezing pain in the midsternal area of the chest.

anomaly. Irregularity in the structure or position of an organ or tissue.

anterior. Situated in the front area or toward the belly surface of the body.

anterior chamber. Space in the eye located between the cornea and the lens that contains aqueous humor. The anterior chamber is bounded by the sclera and cornea in front and the ciliary body, iris, and pupillary portion of the lens in the back.

anteroposterior. Front to back.

anticoagulant. Substance that reduces or eradicates the blood's ability to clot.

antineoplastic. Any agent with the ability to inhibit the growth of new tumors by keeping the proliferation of malignant cells in check.

apical. End portion of the tooth root.

artery. Vessel through which oxygenated blood passes away from the heart to any part of the body.

avulsion. Forcible tearing away of a part, by surgical means or traumatic injury.

bacteremia. Nonspecific laboratory finding of bacteria in the blood in the absence of signs of illness; not to be confused with septicemia, the more acute infectious illness progressing from bacteremia, or with urosepsis, the presence of pus or bacteria found in the urine.

benign. Mild or nonmalignant in nature.

benign lesion. Neoplasm or change in tissue that is not cancerous (nonmalignant).

benign prostatic hyperplasia. Benign enlargement of the prostate caused by proliferation of fibrostromal elements of the gland and commonly affecting men older than age 50. BPH is often characterized by urination difficulties such as slow start, weak stream, dribbling, nocturia (night-time urination), and urinary obstruction as the urethra is compressed as the gland enlarges. Synonym: BPH.

bifurcated. Having two branches or divisions, such as the left pulmonary veins that split off from the left atrium to carry oxygenated blood away from the heart.

bilateral. Consisting of or affecting two sides.

blind hypertensive eye. Vision loss due to painful, high intraocular pressure.

BMI. Body mass index. Tool for calculating weight appropriateness in adults. The Centers for Disease Control and Prevention places adult BMIs in the following categories: below 18.5, underweight; 18.5 to 24.9, normal; 25.0 to 29.9 overweight; 30.0 and above, obese. BMI may be a factor in determining medical necessity for bariatric procedures.

bypass graft. Surgically created alternative blood vessel used to reroute blood flow around an area of obstruction or disease.

carcinoid tumor. Benign or malignant tumor that arises from neuroendocrine cells located throughout the body. The most common sites are the appendix, bronchi, rectum, small intestine, and stomach.

carcinoma. Malignant growth of epithelial cells in the coverings and linings of organs and tissues. The cells tend to spread to other locations via the bloodstream or lymphatic channels.

carcinoma in situ. Malignancy that arises from the cells of the vessel, gland, or organ of origin that remains confined to that site or has not invaded neighboring tissue.

cartilage. Variety of fibrous connective tissue that is inherently nonvascular. Usually found in the joints, it aids in movement and provides a cushion to absorb jolts and shocks.

cataract. Clouding or opacities of the lens that stop clear images from forming on the retina, causing vision impairment or blindness.

catheter. Flexible tube inserted into an area of the body for introducing or withdrawing fluid.

catheterization. Use or insertion of a tubular device into a duct, blood vessel, hollow organ, or body cavity for injecting or withdrawing fluids for diagnostic or therapeutic purposes.

Centers for Medicare and Medicaid Services. Federal agency that oversees the administration of the public health programs such as Medicare, Medicaid, and State Children's Insurance Program.

cervical. Relation to the cervical spine or to the cervix.

cesarean section. Delivery of fetus by incision made in the upper part of the uterus, or corpus uteri, via an abdominal peritoneal approach when a vaginal delivery is not possible or advisable; often referred to as a classic c-section. Low cervical approach is a type of c-section by an incision in the lower segment of the uterus, either through a transperitoneal incision or extraperitoneally with the peritoneal fold being displaced upwards.

chemotherapy. Treatment of disease, especially cancerous conditions, using chemical agents.

chordee. Ventral (downward) curvature of the penis due to a fibrous band along the corpus spongiosum seen congenitally with hypospadias, or a downward curvature seen on erection in disease conditions, causing a lack of distensibility in the tissues.

choroid. Thin, nourishing vascular layer of the eye that supplies blood to the retina, arteries, and nerves to structures in the anterior part of the eye.

chronic. Persistent, continuing, or recurring.

chronic kidney disease. Decreased renal efficiencies resulting in reduced ability of the kidney to filter waste. The National Kidney Foundation's classification includes five clinical stages, based on the glomerular filtration rate (GFR). The stages of CKD are as follows: stage 1, some kidney damage with normal or slightly increased GFR (>90); stage 2, mild kidney damage with a GFR value of 60 to 89; stage 3, moderate kidney damage with a GFR value of 30 to 59; stage 4, severe kidney damage and a GFR value of 15 to 29; and stage 5, severe kidney damage that has progressed to a GFR value of less than 15. Dialysis or transplantation is required at stage 5. Synonym: CKD.

ciliary body. Structure of the eye that produces the aqueous humor within the anterior chamber.

circumcise. Circular cutting around the genitals to remove the prepuce or foreskin.

classification. The systematic arrangement, based on established criteria, of similar entities. ICD-10 is a disease classification. The particular criterion on which the arrangement is based is called the axis of classification. The primary axis of the disease classification as a whole is by anatomy. Other axes have been used, such as etiology and morphology.

cleft palate. Congenital fissure or defect of the roof of the mouth opening to the nasal cavity due to failure of embryonic cells to fuse completely. A cleft palate can be unilateral (left or right of the midline of the mouth) or bilateral (on both the left and right of the midline of the mouth) and complete (extending to nose) or incomplete (does not involve the nose).

closed dislocation. Simple displacement of a body part without an open wound.

closed fracture. Break in a bone without a concomitant opening in the skin.

code set. Under HIPAA, any set of codes used to encode data elements, such as tables of terms, medical concepts, medical diagnosis codes, or medical procedure codes. This includes both the codes and their descriptions.

coder. Professional who translates documented, written diagnoses and procedures into numeric and alphanumeric codes.

coding conventions. Each space, typeface, indentation, and punctuation mark determining how ICD-10-CM codes are interpreted. These conventions were developed to help match correct codes to the diagnoses documented.

coding guidelines. Criteria that specifies how procedure, diagnosis, or supply codes are to be translated and used in various situations. Coding guidelines are issued by the AHA, AMA, CMS, NCHVS, and various other groups. Guidelines may vary by payer, type of coding system, and intended use.

coding rules. Official rules and coding conventions used for diagnosis and procedure coding.

coding specificity. Selection of classification codes that provide the highest degree of accuracy and completeness based on clinical documentation. For example, a three-character ICD-10-CM code cannot be reported when the specific code requires a fourth-character. Similarly, a four-character code cannot be reported when the specific code requires a fifth-character.

colostomy. Artificial surgical opening anywhere along the length of the colon to the skin surface for the diversion of feces.

compliance. Satisfying official coding and/or billing requirements.

compliance date. Under HIPAA, date by which a covered entity must comply with a standard, implementation specification, or modification. This is usually 24 months after the effective date of the associated final rule for most entities but 36 months after the effective date for small health plans. For future changes in the standards, the compliance date would be at least 180 days after the effective date, but may be longer for small health plans and complex changes.

complicated fracture. Open or closed fracture in which a bone fragment has injured a neighboring organ or adjacent tissue.

complication. Condition arising after the beginning of observation and treatment that modifies the course of the patient's illness or the medical care required, or an undesired result or misadventure in medical care.

condyle. Rounded end of a bone that forms an articulation.

congenital. Present at birth, occurring through heredity or an influence during gestation up to the moment of birth.

congestive heart failure. Condition caused by the heart's inability to adequately pump and circulate blood, resulting in fluid accumulation in the lungs and other tissues.

conjunctiva. Mucous membrane lining of the eyelids and covering of the exposed, anterior sclera.

connective tissue. Body tissue made from fibroblasts, collagen, and elastic fibrils that connects, supports, and holds together other tissues and cells and includes cartilage, collagenous, fibrous, elastic, and osseous tissue.

contusion. Superficial injury (bruising) produced by impact without a break in the skin.

cornea. Five-layered, transparent structure that forms the anterior or front part of the sclera of the eye.

coronary atherosclerosis. Chronic condition marked by thickening and loss of elasticity of the coronary artery, caused by deposits of plaque containing cholesterol, lipoid material, and lipophages.

coxsackie virus. Heterogenous group of viruses associated with aseptic meningitis, myocarditis, pericarditis, and acute onset juvenile diabetes.

culture. Growth of microorganisms in a medium conducive to their development.

cyst. Elevated encapsulated mass containing fluid, semisolid, or solid material with a membranous lining.

decubitus ulcer. Progressively eroding skin lesion produced by inflamed necrotic tissue as it sloughs off. A decubitus ulcer is caused by continual pressure to a localized area, especially over bony areas, where blood circulation is cut off when a patient lies still for too long without changing position. Synonyms: bedsore, pressure ulcer.

delirium. Transient organic psychotic condition with a short course in which there is a rapidly developing onset of disorganization of higher mental processes manifested by some degree of impairment of information processing, impaired or abnormal attention, perception, memory, and thinking. Manifested by clouded consciousness, confusion, disorientation, delusions, illusions, and vivid hallucinations.

delivery. Expulsion or extraction of a child and the afterbirth.

dementia. Progressive decrease in intellectual functioning of sufficient severity to interfere with occupational or social performance, with impairment of memory and abstract thinking, the ability to learn new skills, problem solving, and judgment. May involve personality change or impairment in impulse control.

Department of Health and Human Services. Cabinet department that oversees the operating divisions of the federal government responsible for health and welfare. HHS oversees the Centers for Medicare and Medicaid Services, Food and Drug Administration, Public Health Service, and other such entities.

depression. Disproportionate depressive state with behavior disturbance that is usually the result of a distressing experience and may include preoccupation with the psychic trauma and anxiety.

dermis. Skin layer found under the epidermis that contains a papillary upper layer and the deep reticular layer of collagen, vascular bed, and nerves.

diabetes mellitus. Endocrine disease manifested by high blood glucose levels and resulting in the inability to successfully metabolize carbohydrates, proteins, and fats, due to defects in insulin production and secretion, insulin action, or both.

diagnosis. Determination or confirmation of a condition, disease, or syndrome and its implications.

diagnosis code. Alphanumeric code that describes the patient's medical condition, symptoms, or the reason for the encounter.

diagnostic coding. Claims submitted to Medicare require diagnostic codes from the International Classification of Diseases, Clinical Modification, Ninth Edition (ICD-9-CM), through September 30, 2014. Claims for certain services, especially when local policy has been established, may be denied based on diagnosis, so correct code selection is important. In the next several years, the current system will be replaced by ICD-10-CM, effective October 1, 2014. Information about ICD-10-CM is available from the National Center of Health Statistics (NCHS), which is a department under the Centers for Disease Control (CDC).

dialysis. Artificial filtering of the blood to remove contaminating waste elements and restore normal balance.

digestion. Mechanical, chemical, and enzymatic process whereby ingested food is converted into material suitable for assimilation for synthesis of tissues or release of energy.

dislocation. Displacement of a bone in relation to its neighboring tissue, especially a joint.

disseminated. Spread over an extensive area.

distal. Located farther away from a specified reference point.

diverticulosis. Saclike pouches of the mucous membrane lining the intestine, herniating through the muscular wall of the colon, and occurring without inflammation.

documentation. Physician's written or transcribed notations about a patient encounter, including a detailed operative report or written notes about a routine encounter. Source documentation must be the treating provider's own account of the encounter and may be transcribed from dictation, dictated by the physician into voice recognition software, or be hand- or typewritten. A signature or authentication accompanies each entry.

Down syndrome. Common birth defect due to an error in the formation of the 21st chromosome.

drug abuse. Individual, for whom no other diagnosis is possible, has come under medical care because of the maladaptive effect of a drug on which he is not dependent (see Drug dependence) and that he has taken on his own initiative to the detriment of his health or social functioning.

drug dependence. Psychic and physical dependence, resulting from taking a drug, characterized by behavioral and other responses that always include a compulsion to take a drug on a continuous or periodic basis to experience its psychic effects, and sometimes to avoid the discomfort of its absence.

duodenum. First portion of the small intestine connected to the stomach at the pylorus and extending to the jejunum.

dysphagia. Difficulty and pain upon swallowing.

E code. ICD-9-CM diagnosis code that describes the circumstance that caused an injury, not the nature of the injury. E codes are used to classify external causes of injury, poisoning, or other adverse effects. An E code should not be used as a principal diagnosis because the intermediary will reject the claim.

eclampsia. Tetany and toxemia producing seizure activity or coma in a pregnant patient who most often has presented with prior preeclampsia (i.e., hypertension, albuminuria, and edema). Eclampsia most commonly occurs during the third trimester or within the first 48 hours following birth.

ectopic pregnancy. Fertilized ovum that implants and develops outside the uterus. The ovum may implant itself in different sites, such as the fallopian tube, the ovary, the abdomen, or the cervix.

ectropion. Drooping of the lower eyelid away from the eye or outward turning or eversion of the edge of the eyelid, exposing the palpebral conjunctiva and causing irritation.

electronic data interchange. Transference of claims, certifications, quality assurance reviews, and utilization data via computer in X12 format. May refer to any electronic exchange of formatted data.

embolism. Obstruction of a blood vessel resulting from a clot or foreign substance.

embryo. Developing cells of a new organism that will become a fetus; the period defined from the fourth day after fertilization to the end of the eighth week.

encounter. Direct personal contact between a patient and a physician, or other person who is authorized by state licensure law and, if applicable, by hospital staff bylaws, to order or furnish hospital services for diagnosis or treatment of the patient.

end-stage renal disease. Chronic, advanced kidney disease requiring renal dialysis or a kidney transplant to prevent imminent death.

endometriosis. Aberrant uterine mucosal tissue appearing in areas of the pelvic cavity outside of its normal location, lining the uterus, and inflaming surrounding tissues often resulting in infertility and spontaneous abortion.

entropion. Inversion of the eyelid, turning the edge in toward the eyeball and causing irritation from contact of the lashes with the surface of the eye.

enucleation. Removal of a growth or organ cleanly so as to extract it in one piece.

epidermis. Outermost, nonvascular layer of skin that contains four to five differentiated layers depending on its body location: stratum corneum, lucidum, granulosum, spinosum, and basale.

epidermolysis bullosa. Group of uncommon, inherited skin disorders manifested by frequently occurring painful blisters and open sores. Epidermolysis bullosa often occurs as a result of minor trauma, due to the skin's abnormally fragile state.

epididymis. Coiled tube on the back of the testis that is the site of sperm maturation and storage and where spermatozoa are propelled into the vas deferens toward the ejaculatory duct by contraction of smooth muscle.

epispadias. Male anomaly in which the urethral opening is abnormally located on the dorsum of the penis, appearing as a groove with no upper urethral wall covering.

eponym. Name of a drug, structure, disease, or procedure based on or derived from the name of a person.

erythema multiforme. Complex of symptoms with a varied pattern of skin eruptions, such as macular, bullous, popular, nodose, or vesicular lesions on the neck, face, and legs. Gastritis and rheumatoid pain are also present as the first noticeable symptoms. This complex is secondary to a number of factors including infections, ingestants, physical agents, malignancy, and pregnancy.

Escherichia coli. Gram negative, anaerobic of the family Enterobacteriaceae found in the large intestine of warm-blooded animals, generally as a non-pathologic entity aiding in digestion. They become pathogenic when an opportunity to grow somewhere outside this relationship presents itself, such as ingestion of fecal contaminated food or water. The species coli is the principle organism found in the human intestine and has both pathogenic and nonpathogenic strains. The enterotoxigenic form causes cholera-like illness while the enteroinvasive form causes dysentery by invading the epithelial cells of the human colon. Bloody stools are seen with the enterohemorrhagic strain. A relatively new strain of E. coli has been identified as E. coli O157:H7, found in undercooked beef and unpasteurized apple juice.

esophagus. Muscular tube that carries swallowed liquids and foods from the pharynx to the stomach.

ESRD. End stage renal disease. Progression of chronic renal failure to lasting and irreparable kidney damage that requires dialysis or renal transplant for survival.

examination. Comprehensive visual and tactile screening and specific testing leading to diagnosis or, as appropriate, to a referral to another practitioner.

extraocular muscles. Six orbital muscles (extrinsic) that move the eyeball.

facet. Smooth surface area where the transverse and articular processes of certain vertebrae articulate with another vertebra.

facility. Place of patient care, including inpatient and outpatient, acute or long term.

failure. Inability to function.

fascia. Fibrous sheet or band of tissue that envelops organs, muscles, and groupings of muscles.

Federal Register. Government publication listing changes in regulations and federally mandated standards, including coding standards such as HCPCS Level II and ICD-9-CM.

first-degree burn. Superficial partial-thickness burn in which only the epidermis or a portion of the dermis is involved, displaying redness but no blister formation.

flexor. Muscle/tendon that bends or flexes a limb or part as opposed to extending it.

follow-up. Visits or treatment following a procedure.

foreign body. Any object or substance found in an organ and tissue that does not belong under normal circumstances.

fracture. Break in bone or cartilage.

fracture types. There are three basic degrees of fracture: type I: a small crack in the bone without displacement; type II: a fracture in which the bone is slightly displaced; type III: a fracture in which there are more than three broken pieces of bone that cannot fit together.

gastroesophageal reflux disease. Weakening of the lower esophageal sphincter allowing reflux of the stomach contents into the esophagus. One form is commonly defined as "heartburn." Synonym: GERD.

general equivalence mapping. Translation tool that maps codes from one system (e.g., ICD-9-CM) to another (e.g., ICD-10-CM). The mappings are generally described as forward (mapping from ICD-9-CM to ICD-10-CM or ICD-10-PCS) or backwards (mapping ICD-10-CM or ICD-10-PCS to ICD-9-CM). Size, structure, and scope of the two systems may be completely different, which may require some decision making on the part of the user. Synonym: GEM.

generalized convulsive epilepsy (tonic-clonic epilepsy). Abnormalities in the brain's electrical activity that cause convulsive seizures with tension of limbs (tonic) or rhythmic contractions (clonic).

gestational diabetes. Glucose intolerance that develops in pregnant women who do not have a history of diabetes, most commonly developing in mid-pregnancy and resolving at delivery. It is treated primarily with diet but insulin may be required in some cases. Certain risk factors may predispose a woman to gestational diabetes, including being older than 25 years of age, obesity, a family history of diabetes, previous stillbirth, birth of a large infant, or one with a birth defect.

glaucoma. Rise in intraocular pressure, restricting blood flow and decreasing vision.

graft. Tissue implant from another part of the body or another person.

graft-versus-host disease. Acute or chronic complication of blood transfusion, bone marrow transplant, or any organ transplant in which white blood cells are present in the transplanted organ. Acute cases may result in skin disruption, diarrhea, hyperbilirubinemia, and an increase in susceptibility to infection. Chronic cases typically begin more than three months post-transplant. In addition to the symptoms noted above, dry eyes and mouth, loss of hair, and lung disorders may be present.

granuloma. Abnormal, dense collections or cells forming a mass or nodule of chronically inflamed tissue with granulations that is usually associated with an infective process.

guidelines. Information appearing at the beginning of each of the six major sections of the CPT book. They also may appear at the beginning of subsections and code ranges. The information contained in the guidelines provides definitions, explanations of terms, and factors relevant to the section.

haemophilus influenzae. Gram negative, aerobic or facultatively anaerobic rod shaped or coccobacillus from the family Pasturellaceae causing pneumonia, meningitis, septicemia, and infections in other conditions coded elsewhere. Synonym: Pfeiffer's bacillus.

Health Insurance Portability and Accountability Act of 1996. Federal law that allows persons to qualify immediately for comparable health insurance coverage when they change their employment relationships. Title II, subtitle F, of HIPAA gives the Department of Health and Human Services the authority to mandate the use of standards for the electronic exchange of health care data; to specify what medical and administrative code sets should be used within those standards; to require the use of national identification systems for health care patients, providers, payers (or plans), and employers (or sponsors); and to specify the types of measures required to protect the security and privacy of personally identifiable health care information. Synonyms: HIPAA, K2, Kassenbaum-Kennedy Bill, Kennedy-Kassenbaum Bill, Public Law 104-191.

hemiplegia. Paralysis of one side of the body.

hemodialysis. Cleansing of wastes and contaminating elements from the blood by virtue of different diffusion rates through a semipermeable membrane, which separates blood from a filtration solution that diffuses other elements out of the blood.

hemorrhage. Internal or external bleeding with loss of significant amounts of blood.

hemorrhoid. Dilated, varicose vein in the anal region caused by continually increased venous pressure. Reversed blood flow and clotted blood within a vein that extends beyond the anus.

hernia. Protrusion of a body structure through tissue.

hiatal hernia. Protrusion of an abdominal organ, mainly the stomach, through the esophageal opening within the diaphragm.

hyperemesis gravidarum. Persistent and severe nausea and vomiting in early pregnancy (before 22 completed weeks of gestation) that affects the management of the pregnancy. Synonym: HG.

hypertension. Abnormally increased pressure, usually referring to arterial pressure, exceeding an acceptable range.

hypertrophy. Overgrowth or enlargement of normal cells in tissue.

hypospadias. Fairly common birth defect in males in which the meatus, or urinary opening, is abnormally positioned on the underside of the penile shaft or in the perineum, requiring early surgical correction.

iatrogenic. Adversely induced in the patient; caused by medical treatment.

ICD-10-CM. International Classification of Diseases, 10th Revision, Clinical Modification. It is a clinical modification of the alphanumeric classification of diseases used by the World Health Organization, already in use in much of the world, and used for mortality reporting in the United States. The implementation date for ICD-10-CM diagnostic coding system to replace ICD-9-CM in the United States is October 1, 2014.

ICD-10-PCS. International Classification of Diseases, 10th Revision, Procedure Coding System. Beginning October 1, 2014, inpatient hospital services and surgical procedures must be coded using ICD-10-PCS codes, replacing the current ICD-9-CM, Volume 3 for procedures.

ICD-9-CM. International Classification of Diseases, 9th Revision, Clinical Modification. Clinical modification of the international statistical coding system used to report, compile, and compare health care data, using numeric and alphanumeric (E codes and V codes) codes to help plan, deliver, reimburse, and quantify medical care in the United States.

indexing. Listing diseases and conditions according to classification system.

infarction. Area of necrosis in tissue, due to ischemia from lack of circulation, usually from a thrombus or an embolus.

infection. Presence of microorganisms in body tissues that may result in cellular damage.

infusion. Introduction of a therapeutic fluid, other than blood, into the bloodstream.

inhalation. Act of drawing in by breathing.

injury. Harm or damage sustained by the body.

insufficiency. Inadequate closure of the valve that allows abnormal backward blood flow.

integumentary. Skin system covering the body that includes the epidermis, dermis, hair, nails, and glands.

internal fixation. Wires, pins, screws, and plates placed through or within the fractured area to stabilize and immobilize the injury.

International Classification of Diseases, 10th Revision. Classification of diseases by alphanumeric code, used by the World Health Organization but not yet adopted in the United States.

International Classification of Diseases, 10th Revision, Clinical Modification. Clinical modification of ICD-10 developed for use in the United States. Scheduled to replace ICD-9-CM October 1, 2014.

International Classification of Diseases, 10th Revision, Procedure Coding System. Procedure coding system developed by 3M HIS under contract with the Centers for Medicare and Medicaid Services. Scheduled to replace ICD-9-CM Volume 3, October 1, 2014.

International Classification of Diseases, 9th Revision, Clinical Modification. Clinical modification of the international statistical coding system used to report, compile, and compare health care data, using numeric and alphanumeric codes to help plan, deliver, reimburse, and quantify medical care in the United States.

intraocular lens. Artificial lens implanted into the eye to replace a damaged natural lens or cataract.

IOP. Intra-ocular pressure. High IOP is glaucoma.

iris. Pigmented membrane behind the cornea and in front of the lens that contracts and expands to enlarge or shrink the size of the pupil to regulate the light entering the eye.

ischemia. Deficiency in blood supply causing tissues to be deprived of oxygen, resulting from trauma, mechanical or functional constriction of blood vessels, or a physical obstruction.

IUGR. Intrauterine growth restriction. Fetal size smaller than the gestational age would predict.

jejunum. Highly vascular upper two-fifths of the small intestine, extending from the duodenum to the ileum.

joint. Area of contact, or juncture, between two or more bones, often articulating with each other.

joint replacement. Insertion of new substitute material in place of damaged or diseased joint tissue to restore function and movement.

labor. Rhythmic, progressive contractions of the uterus that cause retraction and dilation of the cervix, resulting in the birth of a child.

laceration. Tearing injury; a torn, ragged-edged wound.

larynx. Musculocartilaginous structure between the trachea and the pharynx that functions as the valve preventing food and other particles from entering the respiratory tract, as well as the voice mechanism.

late effect. Abnormality, dysfunction, or other residual condition produced after the acute phase of an illness, injury, or disease is over. There is no time limit on when late effects can appear.

left heart. Area of the heart consisting of the left atrium and left ventricle.

left heart failure. Inability of the left ventricle to adequately pump blood, resulting in fluid accumulation in the lungs.

lens. Convex disc of the eye, behind the iris and in front of the vitreous body, that refracts light entering the globe.

lesion. Area of damaged tissue that has lost continuity or function, due to disease or trauma.

leukemia. Malignancy of the blood and blood-forming organs manifested by abnormal proliferation or development of leukocytes and their developmental precursors in the blood and bone marrow. Acute and chronic classifications in leukemia refer to the degree that the malignant cells have differentiated and not to the length of the disease itself. The predominant type of cell involved, whether myelogenous or lymphocytic, also determines classification.

leukopenia. Sudden and severe condition caused by a reduced number of white blood cells (WBC). The type of leukopenia is classified according to what kind of WBC is deficient (i.e., agranulocytosis for granulocytes or neutropenia for neutrophils). Synonyms: agranulocytosis, aleukia, aleukocytosis, leukocytopenia, neutropenia.

level of specificity. Diagnosis codes reported to their highest number of available characters. The final level of subdivision in a classification category is a subcategory. The final level of subdivision in a subcategory is a valid code.

LGA. Large for gestational age. Excessive growth of a fetus that is more developed than is considered normal for the gestational age, measured in weeks and calculated from the first day of the mother's last menstrual period to the current date. The most common cause for LGA is maternal diabetes.

ligament. Band or sheet of fibrous tissue that connects the articular surfaces of bones or supports visceral organs.

lymph nodes. Bean-shaped structures along the lymphatic vessels that intercept and destroy foreign materials in the tissue and bloodstream.

lymphoma. Tumors occurring in the lymphoid tissues that are most commonly malignant.

macrosomia. Abnormally large size, often in reference to a fetus or newborn.

major depressive disorder. Manic-depressive psychosis in which there is a widespread depressed mood of gloom and wretchedness with some degree of anxiety, reduced activity, or restlessness and agitation. There is a marked tendency to recurrence; in a few cases this may be at regular intervals.

malignant. Any condition tending to progress toward death, specifically an invasive tumor with a loss of cellular differentiation that has the ability to spread or metastasize to other areas in the body.

malignant neoplasm. Any cancerous tumor or lesion exhibiting uncontrolled tissue growth that can progressively invade other parts of the body with its disease-generating cells.

malposition. Congenital or acquired condition in which an organ or body part is in an abnormal or uncharacteristic position.

manic depression syndrome. Alternating major depressive and manic periods. Synonym: bipolar syndrome.

Marfan's syndrome. Unusually long extremities, subluxation of the lens, dilation of the aorta, and other symptoms.

maxilla. Pyramidally shaped bone forming the upper jaw, part of the eye orbit, nasal cavity, and palate and lodging the upper teeth.

maxillary. Located between the eyes and the upper teeth.

medical documentation. Patient care records, including operative notes; physical, occupational, and speech-language pathology notes; progress notes; physician certification and recertifications; and emergency room records; or the patient's medical record in its entirety.

medical necessity. Medically appropriate and necessary to meet basic health needs; consistent with the diagnosis or condition and national medical practice guidelines regarding type, frequency, and duration of treatment; rendered in a cost-effective manner.

Medicare code editor. Computer program used by Medicare contractors to identify coding inconsistencies in the information reported on an inpatient claim. In determining the appropriate DRG payment, the age, sex, discharge status, principal diagnosis, secondary diagnosis, and procedures performed are reviewed for accuracy and consistency with the other data reported on the claim. The MCE reviews codes, coverage, and clinical information.

Medicare Part A. Medicare coverage for hospital, nursing home, hospice, home health, and other inpatient care. Claims are submitted to intermediaries for reimbursement. Ten regional offices provide the Centers for Medicare and Medicaid Services (CMS) with decentralized administration and delivery of Medicare programs. Each regional office manages private insurance companies that contract with the government to process and make payment for Medicare services.

melanoma. Highly metastatic malignant neoplasm composed of melanocytes that occur most often on the skin from a preexisting mole or nevus but may also occur in the mouth, esophagus, anal canal, or vagina.

MEN syndrome. Multiple endocrine neoplasia syndromes. Men syndromes are a group of conditions in which several endocrine glands grow excessively (such as in adenomatous hyperplasia) and/or develop benign or malignant tumors. Tumors and hyperplasia associated with MEN often produce excess hormones, which impede normal physiology. There is no comprehensive cure known for MEN syndromes. Treatment is directed at the hyperplasia or tumors in each individual gland. Tumors are usually surgically removed and oral medications or hormonal injections are used to correct hormone imbalances.

meninges. Tough membranous protectors of the central nervous system that cover the brain and spinal cord comprising three layers: the dura mater, arachnoid mater, and pia mater.

meningitis. Inflammation of meningeal layers of the brain.

meniscus. Crescent-shaped fibrous cartilage found within the knee, temporomandibular, acromioclavicular, and sternoclavicular intraarticular joint.

Merkel cell carcinoma. Malignant cutaneous cancer predominantly found in immunocompromised and elderly patients with a history of sun exposure.

morbidity. Diseased condition or state.

mortality. Condition of being mortal (subject to death).

multigravida. Female who has had two or more pregnancies. Women in this category are considered to be at high risk during pregnancy.

multiparity. Condition of having had two or more pregnancies that resulted in viable fetuses; producing more than one fetus or offspring in the same gestation.

muscle graft. Muscle taken from a donor site or person and inserted into a new site or person.

muscle tissue. Network of specialized cells for performing contraction to produce voluntary or involuntary movement of body parts, and skeletal, cardiac, or visceral muscles.

myocardial infarction. Obstruction of circulation to the heart, resulting in necrosis.

myopathy. Any disease process within muscle tissue.

myopia. Defect in focusing in which the eye is overpowered and incoming distant light rays are focused in front of the retina because of a refractive or curvature defect in the lens. Malignant myopia is highly degenerative and complicated by serious disease of the choroid that leads to retinal detachment and blindness.

narrow angle glaucoma. Progressive optic nerve disease associated with high intraocular pressure that can lead to irreversible vision loss. The aqueous humor is the clear fluid filling the chambers of the eye that is continually drained and renewed, produced by the ciliary body and passing out through the pupil and trabecular meshwork. Narrow angle glaucoma causes an increase in intraocular pressure due to an impairment of aqueous outflow caused by a narrowing or closing of the anterior chamber angle as the iris comes into contact with the trabecular meshwork. This type of glaucoma is identified in four stages: latent, intermittent, acute, and chronic. In the latent and intermittent phases, minor or transient attacks of varying severity, duration, and frequency occur in which intraocular pressure (IOP) rises with accompanying pain and edema. Acute angle closure glaucoma is a grave medical emergency as IOP rises, the cornea swells, and excruciating pain radiates through the eye. Visual acuity falls rapidly as the eye swells and blindness may result if the IOP is not lowered. The chronic stage manifests as irreversible IOP increases from progressive damage and scar tissue closing the anterior angle. Synonyms: angle closure glaucoma, closed angle glaucoma, pupillary block glaucoma.

National Center for Health Statistics. Division of the Centers for Disease Control and Prevention that compiles statistical information used to guide actions and policies to improve the public health of U.S. citizens. The NCHS maintains the ICD-9-CM coding system.

National Committee for Vital Health Statistics. Federal advisory body within the Department of Health and Human Services that advises the secretary regarding potential changes to the HIPAA standards. Synonym: NCVHS.

necrosis. Death of cells or tissue within a living organ or structure.

necrotic. Pathological condition of death occurring in a group of cells or tissues within a living part or organism.

neonatal period. Period of an infant's life from birth to the age of 27 days, 23 hours, and 59 minutes.

neoplasm. New abnormal growth, tumor.

nephritis. Inflammation of the kidney, often due to infection, metabolic disorder, or an autoimmune process.

nephropathy. Disease or abnormality of the kidney.

nephrosis. Nephrotic syndrome characterized by proteinuria more than 3.5 g/100 ml, hypoalbuminemia less than 3.0 g/100 ml, hyperlipemia (cholesterol greater than 300 mg/100 ml), massive edema, and intercurrent infections. Nephrosis is usually due to some form of glomerulonephritis. It may progress to chronic renal failure.

nervous tissue. Highly specialized, organized cells for the function of the central peripheral nervous system, permitting information transfer between the brain and active tissue for both automatic and voluntary functions of skeletal, visceral, and cardiac muscle.

newborn intensive care unit. Special care unit for premature and seriously ill infants.

nodular prostate. Small mass of tissue that swells, knots, or is a protuberance in the prostate.

nonessential modifiers. Subterms listed to the right of the ICD-9-CM main term and enclosed in parentheses.

nonspecific code. Catch-all code that identifies the diagnosis as ill-defined, other, or unspecified. A nonspecific code may be a valid choice if no other code closely describes the diagnosis.

not elsewhere classified. Condition or diagnosis that is not provided with its own specified code in ICD-9-CM, but is included in a more broadly defined code for other specified conditions.

not otherwise specified. Condition or diagnosis that remains ill defined and lacks the necessary information for selecting a more specific code.

notice of proposed rule making. Document that describes and explains regulations the federal government proposes to adopt at some future date, and invites interested parties to submit comments related to them. These comments can then be used in developing a final regulation.

NPRM. Notice of proposed rule making. Document that describes and explains regulations the federal government proposes to adopt at some future date, and invites interested parties to submit comments related to them. These comments can then be used in developing a final regulation.

obstruction. Act or state of being clogged or blocked from allowing through passage.

open fracture. Exposed break in a bone, always considered compound due to its high risk of infection from the open wound leading to the fracture.

open wound. Opening or break of the skin.

ophthalmic. Relating to the eye.

optic nerve. Transmits visual information from the retina to the brain.

oral. Pertaining to the mouth.

orbit. Bony cavity that contains the eyeball, formed by seven bones of the skull: frontal, sphenoid, maxilla, zygomatic, palatine, lacrimal, and ethmoid.

osteo-. Having to do with bone.

osteoarthritis. Most common form of a noninflammatory degenerative joint disease with degenerating articular cartilage, bone enlargement, and synovial membrane changes.

osteogenesis imperfecta. Hereditary collagen disorder that produces brittle, osteoporotic bones that are easily fractured, with hypermobility of points, blue sclerae and a tendency to hemorrhage.

osteoporosis. Bone degeneration caused by the breakdown of the bony matrix without equivalent regeneration, resulting in a weak, porous, fragile bone structure.

other diagnosis. All conditions (secondary) that exist at the time of admission or that develop subsequently that affect the treatment received and/or the length of stay. Diagnoses that relate to an earlier episode and that have no bearing on the current hospital stay are not to be reported.

other specified. Term in ICD-9-CM referring to codes reported when a diagnosis has been made and there is

no code identifying it more specifically as with NEC, or not elsewhere classified.

outpatient. Person who has not been admitted as an inpatient but who is registered on the hospital or CAH records as an outpatient and receives services (rather than supplies alone) directly from the hospital or CAH. (Code of Federal Regulations, section 410.2)

outpatient services. Medical and other services, diagnostic or therapeutic, provided to a person who has not been admitted to the hospital as an inpatient but is registered on the hospital records as an outpatient. Outpatient services usually require a stay of less than 24 hours.

outpatient visit. Encounter in a recognized outpatient facility.

partial epilepsy. Transient brain function disturbance resulting in episodes of seizures caused by focal, localized brain lesions.

Parvovirus B19. Only known parvovirus to cause disease in humans. Manifestation is erythema infectiosum. This parvovirus is also associated with polyarthropathy, chronic anemia, red cell aplasia, and fetal hydrops.

pathologic fracture. Break in bone due to a disease process that weakens the bone structure, such as osteoporosis, osteomalacia, or neoplasia, and not traumatic injury.

pathological. Pertaining to, or relating to, disease.

pathological gambling. Disorder of impulse control characterized by a chronic and progressive preoccupation with gambling and urge to gamble, with subsequent gambling behavior that compromises, disrupts, or damages personal, family, and vocational pursuits.

patient. Individual who is receiving or who has received health care services. This could include a person who is deceased.

perineal. Pertaining to the pelvic floor area between the thighs; the diamond-shaped area bordered by the pubic symphysis in front, the ischial tuberosities on the sides, and the coccyx in back.

phalanx. Bones of the digits (fingers or toes).

pharmacological agent. Drug used to produce a chemical effect.

pharynx. Musculomembranous passage of the throat consisting of three regions: the nasopharynx is the passage at the back of the nostrils, above the level of the soft palate, and communicating with the eustachian tube.

physician. Legally authorized practitioners including a doctor of medicine or osteopathy, a doctor of dental surgery or of dental medicine, a doctor of podiatric medicine, a doctor of optometry, and a chiropractor only with respect to treatment by means of manual manipulation of the spine (to correct a subluxation).

polyp. Small growth on a stalk-like attachment projecting from a mucous membrane.

polypoid lesion. Lesion with a stalk, usually removed with a snare or loop forceps.

postpartum. Period of time following childbirth.

preeclampsia. Complication of pregnancy manifesting in the development of borderline hypertension, protein in the urine, and unresponsive swelling between the 20th week of pregnancy and the end of the first week following birth in mild to moderate cases. Severe preeclampsia presents with hypertension, associated with marked swelling, proteinuria, abdominal pain, and/or visual changes.

pregnancy. Conception until the birth of a child, usually 40 weeks.

premature infant. Neonate born before 37 weeks gestation or as documented by provider criteria. A premature infant is more susceptible to complications.

pressure ulcers. Progressively eroding skin lesion produced by inflamed necrotic tissue as it sloughs off, caused by continual pressure impeding blood circulation, especially over bony areas, when a patient lies still for too long without changing position.

principal diagnosis. Condition established after study to be chiefly responsible for occasioning the admission of the patient to the hospital for care.

prion. Abnormal infectious agent that can produce rare, progressive neurodegenerative disorders that can affect both humans and animals. Marked by long incubation periods and distinctive changes in the brain due to neuronal loss, prion diseases lead to brain damage and are typically rapidly progressive. Examples of prion diseases include Creutzfeldt-Jakob disease, fatal familial insomnia, Gerstmann-Straussler-Scheinker syndrome, and kuru.

prostate. Male gland surrounding the bladder neck and urethra that secretes a substance into the seminal fluid.

prostate hyperplasia. Enlargement of the prostate gland from an abnormal proliferation of fibrostromal tissue in the paraurethral glands. The outer prostate glands are pushed against the prostate capsule, resulting in a thick pseudocapsule and as enlargement continues and the intracapsular pressure increases, impingement of the urethra results in obstructed urinary flow.

prostatic hypertrophy. Overgrowth of the normal prostate tissue.

prosthesis. Man-made substitute for a missing body part.

prosthetic. Device that replaces all or part of an internal body organ or body part, or that replaces part of the function of a permanently inoperable or malfunctioning internal body organ or body part.

provider. All-inclusive, generic term for people or institutions that provide health care. The provider may be a physician, hospital, pharmacy, other facility, or other health care provider.

pseudomonas. Large genus of anaerobic, gram negative bacteria, with more than 100 species, some producing toxins, responsible for causing diseases such as glanders or melioidosis, septicemia, pyogenic arthritis, and bacterial meningitis.

pterygium. Benign, wedge-shaped, conjunctival thickening that advances from the inner corner of the eye toward the cornea.

puerperium. Postpartum period that begins immediately following delivery and continuing for six weeks.

pulp. Living connective tissue within the tooth's root canal space that supplies blood vessels and nerves to the tooth.

pyelonephritis. Infection of the renal pelvis and ureters that may be acute or chronic, often occurring as a result of a urinary tract infection, particularly in instances of vesicoureteric reflux, the backflow of urine from the bladder into the kidney pelvis or ureters.

radiotherapy. External source of high-energy rays (x-rays or gamma rays) or internally implanted radioactive substances used in destroying tissue and stopping the growth of malignant cells.

range of motion. Action of a body part throughout its extent of natural movement, measured in degrees of a circle.

reflux. Return or backward flow.

regurgitation. Abnormal backward flow.

renal failure. Inability of a kidney to eliminate metabolites and retain electrolytes at a normal level.

retina. Layer of tissue located at the back of the eye that is sensitive to light similar to that of film in a camera.

right heart. Areas of the right heart, including the right atrium and right ventricle.

Ritter's disease. Skin infection most commonly found in infants and children under the age of five. It is caused by certain strains of Staphylococcus bacteria, which damages the skin and results in shedding. Symptoms include fever, exfoliation of large areas of skin, pain, and redness over most of the body. Gentle pressure may cause the skin to slip off, leaving red, wet areas known as Nikolsky's sign. Synonyms: Staphylococcal scalded skin syndrome, SSS.

Romano-Ward syndrome. Potentially fatal condition precipitated by vigorous exertion, emotional upset, or startling moments due to an imbalance in the electrical timing mechanism that controls the pumping action of the heart's ventricles. This syndrome causes the patient to be susceptible to recurrent episodes of syncope, collapse, and possible ventricular fibrillation that can cause sudden death. Synonyms: long QT syndrome, prolonged QT interval syndrome.

rule of nines. Rapid measurement system used to calculate the total body surface area (TBSA) involved in burns, based upon dividing the total area into segments as multiples of 9 percent. The perineum or external genitals are 1 percent; each arm is 9 percent; the front and back of the trunk, and each leg are separately counted as 18 percent; and the head is another 9 percent in adults. For infants and children, the head is 18 percent involvement and the legs are 14 percent each, due to the larger surface area of a child's head in proportion to the body.

salmonella. Group of more than 1,500 serotypes of a genus of gram negative, facultative anaerobic bacteria of the family Enterobacteriacae. The major clinical symptom is food poisoning. Salmonella causes enteric fevers like typhoid and paratyphoid, acute gastroenteritis, and septicemias. Spread through contaminated food, infected turtles or lizards, infected dyes, or contaminated marijuana.

sclera. White, fibrous, outer coating of the eye continuous with the cornea anteriorly and the optic nerve sheath posteriorly that is covered with conjunctival tissue.

screening mammography. Radiologic images taken of the female breast for the early detection of breast cancer.

screening pap smear. Diagnostic laboratory test consisting of a routine exfoliative cytology test (Papanicolaou test) provided to a woman for the early detection of cervical or vaginal cancer. The exam includes a clinical breast examination and a physician's interpretation of the results.

screening test. Exam or study used by a physician to identify abnormalities, regardless of whether the patient exhibits symptoms.

scrotum. Skin pouch that holds the testes and supporting reproductive structures.

sebaceous cyst. Benign cyst of the skin or hair follicle filled with keratin and debris rich in lipids that may be treated by incision and drainage or puncture aspiration.

second-degree burn. Deep partial-thickness burn with destruction of the epidermis, the upper portion of the dermis, possibly some deeper dermal tissues, and blistering of the skin with fluid exudate.

seizure. Sudden, abnormal electrical activity in the brain due to any number of causes including medication, high fever, head injuries, epilepsy, and other diseases. Seizures fall into two main groups. Focal seizures, also called partial seizures, happen in just one section of the brain. Generalized seizures are the result of abnormal activity on both sides of the brain.

seminal vesicles. Paired glands located at the base of the bladder in males that release the majority of fluid into semen through ducts that join with the vas deferens forming the ejaculatory duct.

sepsis. Phase following septicemia in the infectious illness continuum, not to be used interchangeably with septicemia. Sepsis is defined for clinical coding purposes as septicemia that has advanced to involve the presence of two or more manifestations of systemic inflammatory response syndrome (SIRS), without organ dysfunction. This is a different clinical picture than septicemia, which has a different outcome.

septic shock. Progression from septicemic infection to severe sepsis with shock, which carries a greater than 50 percent mortality rate. Septic shock presents with severe sepsis with low blood pressure, decreased urine output, increased oxygen demands, followed by major organ failure, manifesting systemic inflammatory disease from bacterial toxins. Synonym: endotoxic shock.

septicemia. Systemic disease associated with the presence and persistence of pathogenic microorganisms and their toxins in the blood.

sequela. Abnormality, dysfunction, or other residual condition produced after the acute phase of an illness, injury, or disease is over. There is no time limit as to when sequelae can appear. It may be apparent early, as with a stroke, or it can occur years later, as in arthritis following an injury.

severity of illness. Relative levels of loss of function and mortality that may be experienced by patients with a particular disease.

sialolithiasis. Stone or concretion in the salivary duct.

sinus. Open space, cavity, or channel within the body or abnormal cavity, fistula, or channel created by a localized infection to allow the escape of pus.

skin. Outer protective covering of the body composed of the epidermis and dermis, situated above the subcutaneous tissues.

skin tag. Small skin-colored or brown appendage appearing on the neck and upper chest resembling a little epithelial polyp.

small intestine. First portion of intestine connecting to the pylorus at the proximal end and consisting of the duodenum, jejunum, and ileum.

SNOMED. Systemized nomenclature of medicine. Uniform lexicon of treatments and diseases added in 2004 into the National Library of Medicine's Unified Medical Language System. It contains more than 350,000 concepts in a hierarchal organization that reviews disease, clinical findings, therapies, and outcomes and is expected to play a role in the development of electronic health records.

soft tissue. Nonepithelial tissues outside of the skeleton.

spasm. Involuntary muscle contraction.

spasticity. Muscular rigidity, spasms, or passive stretch resistance, synonymous with being spastic.

specimen. Tissue cells or sample of fluid taken for analysis, pathologic examination, and diagnosis.

spermatic cord. Structure of the male reproductive organs that consists of the ductus deferens, testicular artery, nerves, and veins that drain the testes.

spondylosis. Degenerative changes of the spine, including those from osteoarthritis.

spontaneous abortion. Early expulsion of the products of conception from the uterus that occurs naturally, without chemical intervention or instrumentation, before completion of 22 weeks of gestation. Spontaneous abortion may be complete, in which all of the products of conception are expelled; or incomplete, in which parts of the placental material or fetus are retained.

sprain and strain. Injuries to a joint, in which the fibers of supporting ligaments or muscles are overstretched or slightly ruptured, with the ligaments and muscles maintaining continuity.

staging. Determination of the course of a disease, as in the case of a malignancy, to determine whether the malignancy is confined to the primary tumor, has spread to one or more lymph nodes, or has metastasized.

staphylococcus. Bacteria whose name originates from the Greek, meaning a bunch of grapes. These round clusters of gram-positive, motile, facultative anaerobes are of the family Micrococcaceae and can cause serious opportunistic infections.

status epilepticus. More than 30 minutes of continuous seizure or multiple sequential seizures without a return to consciousness in between. Treatment usually begins after five minutes of seizure activity.

status migrainosus. More than 72 hours of continuous migraine headache, often requiring hospitalization due to dehydration, indicative of an ongoing, active migraine.

stenosis. Narrowing or constriction of a passage.

stoma. Opening created in the abdominal wall from an internal organ or structure for diversion of waste elimination, drainage, and access.

strabismus. Misalignment of the eyes due to an imbalance in extraocular muscles. Synonym: heterotropia.

streptococcus group B colonization. Bacteria normally found in the vagina or lower intestine of many healthy adult women that may infect the fetus during childbirth, causing mental or physical handicaps or death. Women who test positive for streptococcus Group B during pregnancy are considered a "colonized" status and are treated with IV antibiotics at the time of delivery and may also be treated with oral antibiotics during the pregnancy. Synonyms: beta Strep, GBS, Group B Strep.

subcutaneous. Below the skin.

subungual. Under the nail.

syncope. Light-headedness or fainting caused by insufficient blood supply to the brain.

synonym. Word having the same or nearly the same meaning as another word or other words.

temporal lobe. Cerebral hemisphere.

tendon. Fibrous tissue that connects muscle to bone, consisting primarily of collagen and containing little vasculature.

testes. Male gonadal paired glands located in the scrotum that secrete testosterone and contain the seminiferous tubules where sperm is produced.

third-degree burn. Full-thickness burn with total destruction of the epidermis and dermis, while deeper underlying tissue may also be affected, including the loss of body parts (e.g., nose, ear, extremity).

TIA. Transient ischemic attack. Intermittent or brief cerebral dysfunction from lack of oxygenation with no persistent neurological deficits; associated with occlusive vascular disease.

tissue. Group of similar cells with a similar function that form definite structures and organs. Tissue types include epithelial tissue, muscle tissue, connective tissue, and nervous tissue.

tracheostomy. Formation of a tracheal opening on the neck surface with tube insertion to allow for respiration in cases of obstruction or decreased patency. A tracheostomy may be planned or performed on an emergency basis for temporary or long-term use.

tracheotomy. Formation of a tracheal opening on the neck surface with tube insertion to allow for respiration in cases of obstruction or decreased patency. A tracheotomy may be planned or performed on an emergency basis for temporary or long-term use.

transplant. Insertion of an organ or tissue from one person or site into another.

tympanic membrane. Thin, sensitive membrane across the entrance to the middle ear that vibrates in response to sound waves, allowing the waves to be transmitted via the ossicular chain to the internal ear.

tympanoplasty. Surgical repair of the structures of the middle ear, including the eardrum and the three small bones, or ossicles.

ulcer. Open sore or excavating lesion of skin or the tissue on the surface of an organ from the sloughing of chronically inflamed and necrosing tissue.

ulcerative colitis. Chronic recurrent inflammation of the large intestine (colon) causing mucosal and submucosal ulceration of unknown cause, and leading to symptoms of abdominal pain, diarrhea with passage of non-fecal discharges, and rectal bleeding.

unspecified. Codes for use when documentation is insufficient to assign a more specific code.

upper respiratory infection. Common cold. Mild viral infectious disease of the nose and throat, the upper respiratory system. Its symptoms include sneezing, sniffling, and running/blocked nose; scratchy, sore, or phlegmy throat; coughing; headache; and a general feeling of illness. It is the most common of all diseases. Synonym: URI.

ureter. Tube leading from the kidney to the urinary bladder made up of three layers of tissue: the mucous lining of the inner layer; the smooth, muscular middle layer that propels the urine from the kidney to the bladder by peristalsis; and the outer layer made of fibrous connective tissue. Each ureter leaves the kidney from the hilum, a concave notch on the middle surface, and enters the bladder through a narrow valve-like orifice that prevents the backflow of urine to the kidney.

urethra. Small tube lined with mucous membrane that leads from the bladder to the exterior of the body.

V code. Part of ICD-9-CM codes, V codes describe circumstances that influence a patient's health status and identify reasons for medical encounters resulting from circumstances other than a disease or injury already classified in the main part of ICD-9-CM.

vaccine. Preparation formed by microorganisms or viruses that have been altered to reduce their virulence but retain their ability to trigger the immune response.

variant. Nucleotide deviation from the normal sequence of a region. Variations are usually either substitutions or deletions. Substitution variations are the result of one nucleotide taking the place of another. A deletion occurs when one or more nucleotides are left out. In some cases, several in a reasonably close proximity on the same chromosome in a DNA strand. These variations result in amino acid changes in the protein made by the gene. However, the term variant does not itself imply a functional change. Intron variations are usually described in one of two ways: 1) the changed nucleotide is defined by a plus or a minus sign indicating the position relative to the first or last nucleotide to the intron, or 2) the second variant description is indicated relative to the last nucleotide of the preceding exon or first nucleotide of the following exon.

vas deferens. Duct that arises in the tail of the epididymis that stores and carries sperm from the epididymis toward the urethra.

vertebra. Any one of the 33 bones composing the spinal column, generally having a disc-shaped body, two transverse processes, and a spinal process centered posteriorly. Vertebrae are connected by the laminae between them and are attached to the body by pedicles, forming an enclosed, protective ring around the vertebral foramen through which the spinal cord runs.

vitreous. Clear gel filling the posterior segment of the eye and functioning as a refractive component in vision and as a method of maintaining pressure in the posterior segment.

WHO. World Health Organization. International agency comprising UN members to promote the physical, mental, and emotional health of the people of the world and to track morbidity and mortality statistics worldwide. WHO maintains the International Classification of Diseases (ICD) medical code set.

World Health Organization. International agency comprising UN members to promote the physical, mental, and emotional health of the people of the world and to track morbidity and mortality statistics worldwide. WHO maintains the International Classification of Diseases (ICD) medical code set.

NOTES

NOTES

NOTES

NOTES

NOTES

NOTES

NOTES

NOTES